DSM-IV-TR®
Casebook, Volume 2

Experts Tell How They Treated Their Own Patients

DSM-IV-TR® Casebook, Volume 2

Experts Tell How They Treated Their Own Patients

Edited by

Robert L. Spitzer, M.D.
Michael B. First, M.D.
Janet B.W. Williams, D.S.W.
Miriam Gibbon, M.S.W.

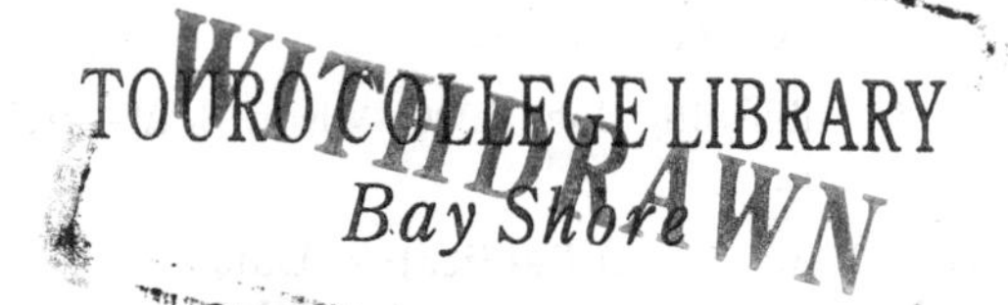

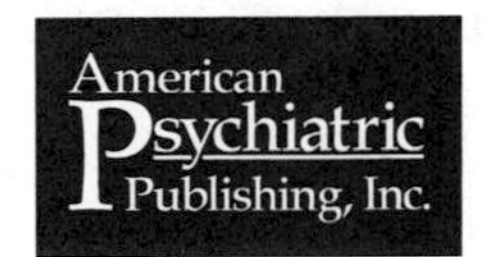
American Psychiatric Publishing, Inc.

Washington, DC
London, England

BS

Note: The authors have worked to ensure that all information in this book is accurate at the time of publication and consistent with general psychiatric and medical standards, and that information concerning drug dosages, schedules, and routes of administration is accurate at the time of publication and consistent with standards set by the U.S. Food and Drug Administration and the general medical community. As medical research and practice continue to advance, however, therapeutic standards may change. Moreover, specific situations may require a specific therapeutic response not included in this book. For these reasons and because human and mechanical errors sometimes occur, we recommend that readers follow the advice of physicians directly involved in their care or the care of a member of their family.

Books published by American Psychiatric Publishing, Inc., represent the views and opinions of the individual authors and do not necessarily represent the policies and opinions of APPI or the American Psychiatric Association.

To buy 25–99 copies of any APPI title at a 20% discount, please contact APPI Customer Service at appi@psych.org or 800-368-5777. To buy 100 or more copies of the same title, email bulksales@psych.org for a price quote.

Manufactured in the United States of America on acid-free paper
10 09 08 07 06 5 4 3 2 1
First Edition

Typeset in Adobe's Frutiger and Palatino.

American Psychiatric Publishing, Inc., 1000 Wilson Boulevard, Arlington, VA 22209-3901, www.appi.org

Library of Congress Cataloging-in-Publication Data
DSM-IV-TR casebook : experts tell how they treated their own patients / edited by Robert L. Spitzer ... [et al.].
p. ; cm.
"Volume 2."
Includes bibliographical references and index.
ISBN 1-58562-220-6 (pbk. : alk. paper) — ISBN 1-58562-219-2 (hardcover : alk. paper) 1. Mental illness—Treatment—Case studies. 2. Mental illness—Diagnosis—Case studies. 3. Mental illness—Classification. I. Spitzer, Robert L. II. American Psychiatric Publishing. III. Diagnostic and statistical manual of mental disorders. IV. Title: DSM-4-TR casebook. V. Title: DSM-four-TR casebook.
[DNLM: 1. Mental Disorders—diagnosis—Case Reports. 2. Mental Disorders—therapy—Case Reports. 3. Diagnosis, Differential—Case Reports. WM 40 D811 2006]
RC465.D76 2006
616.89'075—dc22 2006009424

British Library Cataloguing in Publication Data
A CIP record is available from the British Library.

3/13/08

Contents

PART III
Mental Disorders Due to a General Medical Condition

PART IV
Substance-Related Disorders

PART V
Schizophrenia and Other Psychotic Disorders

PART VI
Mood Disorders

PART IX
Factitious Disorders

PART X
Dissociative Disorders

PART XI
Sexual and Gender Identity Disorders

PART XII

Eating Disorders

PART XIII

Impulse-Control Disorders

PART XIV

Personality Disorders

About the Editors

Robert L. Spitzer, M.D.

Dr. Spitzer is Professor of Psychiatry at Columbia University and Chief of the Biometrics Research Department at the New York State Psychiatric Institute. He completed his psychiatric residency training at the Institute and has worked there since 1961. He has achieved national and international recognition as an authority in psychiatric assessment and the classification of mental disorders. He is the author of more than 250 articles on psychiatric assessment and diagnosis.

In 1974, the American Psychiatric Association (APA) appointed Dr. Spitzer to chair its Task Force on Nomenclature and Statistics. In this capacity, he assumed the leadership role in the development of the *Diagnostic and Statistical Manual of Mental Disorders, 3rd Edition* (DSM-III), published in 1980, which became the authoritative classification of mental disorders for the mental health professions, not only in the United States but also in the world.

In 1983, Dr. Spitzer was appointed to chair the APA's Work Group to Revise DSM-III. He coordinated the effort that resulted in the publication of the *Diagnostic and Statistical Manual of Mental Disorders, 3rd Edition, Revised* (DSM-III-R) in the spring of 1987. He was active in the development of the *Diagnostic and Statistical Manual of Mental Disorders, 4th Edition* (DSM-IV), as a special advisor to the APA's Task Force on DSM-IV.

In 1994, Dr. Spitzer received the APA's award for psychiatric research for his contributions to psychiatric assessment and diagnosis. In 2000, he received the Thomas William Salmon Medal from the New York Academy of Medicine. He has pioneered the development of several widely used diagnostic assessment procedures, including the Research Diagnostic Criteria, the Schedule for Affective Disorders and Schizophrenia, the Structured Clinical Interview for DSM-IV, and the PRIME-MD Patient Health Questionnaire.

Michael B. First, M.D.

Dr. First is a research psychiatrist in the Biometrics Department at the New York State Psychiatric Institute and is Professor of Clinical Psychiatry at Columbia University College of Physicians and Surgeons. He also maintains a schema-focused cognitive therapy and psychopharmacology practice in Manhattan. He is a nationally and internationally recognized expert on psychiatric diagnosis and assessment.

Dr. First is the editor and cochair of the *Diagnostic and Statistical Manual of Mental Disorders, 4th Edition, Text Revision* (DSM-IV-TR); editor of *Text and Criteria for DSM-IV*; editor of the *Diagnostic and Statistical Manual of Mental Disorders, 4th Edition: Primary Care Version*; and editor of the American Psychiatric Association's *Handbook of Psychiatric Measures*. He has coauthored and coedited a number of books, including *A Research Agenda for DSM-V; Advancing DSM: Dilemmas in Psychiatric Diagnosis; Am I OK? The Laymen's Guide to the Psychiatrist's Bible; DSM-IV-TR Guidebook; DSM-IV-TR Handbook of Differential Diagnosis*; the *Structured Clinical Interview for DSM-IV-TR;* and *DSM-IV-TR Casebook,* as well as various software packages for psychiatric diagnosis. Dr. First has trained thousands of clinicians and researchers in diagnostic assessment and differential diagnosis.

Janet B.W. Williams, D.S.W.

Dr. Williams is Professor of Clinical Psychiatric Social Work in the Departments of Psychiatry and Neurology at Columbia University College of Physicians and Surgeons and a research scientist and Deputy Chief of the Biometrics Research Department at the New York State Psychiatric Institute. Her career has focused on the development of psychiatric classifications and instruments to measure psychopathology, and she is well known for her interview guides for the Hamilton Rating Scales and the Montgomery-Åsberg Depression Rating Scale. She was heavily involved in the development of DSM-III, DSM-III-R, and DSM-IV and was made an American Psychiatric Association Honorary Fellow for her contributions. She collaborated on the development and testing of PRIME-MD, an interview guide designed to help primary care physicians make mental disorder diagnoses, and its self-report version, the PRIME-MD Patient Health Questionnaire. Dr. Williams is the author of many rating instruments and interview guides and more than 230 scholarly publications. She serves on the editorial boards of several psychiatric and social work journals and is an active consultant to clinical trials on depression and anxiety.

Dr. Williams holds a B.S. in biology from Tufts University, an M.S. in marine biology from the University of Massachusetts Dartmouth, and an M.S. and D.S.W. in social welfare from the Columbia University School of Social Work. In 1994, Dr. Williams founded the Society for Social Work and Research (now with more than 1,300 members) and served as its president for 2 years. She has been inducted into the Columbia University School of Social Work Alumni Association Hall of Fame. In 2000 she received a Lifetime Achievement Award from SSWR, and in 2005 she received the Knee/Wittman Outstanding Lifetime Achievement Award in Health and Mental Health Policy and Practice from the National Association of Social Workers Foundation.

Miriam Gibbon, M.S.W.

Ms. Gibbon is a research scientist in the Biometrics Department of the New York State Psychiatric Institute and is on the faculty of the Department of Psychiatry at Columbia University College of Physicians and Surgeons. She has been involved in the development of psychiatric evaluation and diagnostic instruments for 25 years and has served as a consultant to many research groups in the United States and in the world.

In the 1970s, Ms. Gibbon began working with the biometrics group to develop the Schedule for Affective Disorders and Schizophrenia (SADS). She is a coauthor of the Global Assessment Scale (GAS), which was part of the SADS, and of the Global Assessment of Functioning Scale, a revision of the GAS that became Axis V of DSM-III-R. Ms. Gibbon is also a coauthor of the *Structured Clinical Interview for DSM-IV-TR* (SCID) and the DSM casebooks and, with Dr. Michael First, produced the SCID 101 Videotape Training Program.

Ms. Gibbon has trained thousands of researchers and clinicians in the use of diagnostic and evaluation instruments, beginning with the SADS and continuing with the GAS, the Hamilton Depression and Anxiety Scales, and the SCID.

Foreword

WE KNOW, OF COURSE, that in all fields of medicine we deal with both the science and the art of diagnosis and treatment. Evidence-based medicine, the drumbeat of our time, relies on an important and burgeoning database testing the validity of specific diagnoses and studying treatment interventions, with randomized controlled trials whenever possible. In psychiatry, no system of classification has been as comprehensive and informative as that contained in the third edition of the *Diagnostic and Statistical Manual of Mental Disorders* (DSM-III), with the advent of its multi-axial, criteria-based framework. Subsequent editions of the DSM (DSM-III-R, DSM-IV, and DSM-IV-TR) have increasingly relied on published research findings to guide the revision process. Some have objected to the de-emphasis on theory in successive versions of the manual and to the reduced audibility of the clinician's voice; still others have contended that the manual is a product built by committees, with great unevenness in the degree to which diagnostic criteria and thresholds for various disorders have solid scientific foundations.

However, medicine is an inexact science, and it is a dynamic, changing science as new findings redirect our thinking. Furthermore, the very concerns expressed by some critics of our diagnostic system represent the most pertinent response to the concerns expressed by others. For example, those who lament the reduced voice of the seasoned, experienced clinician should note that it is precisely that voice that is called upon to guide diagnostic and treatment recommendations for patients with conditions for which research data are unavailable or insufficient, while patients with these diagnoses crowd our consulting rooms. Like it or not, we do not have sufficient evidence to guide us in all aspects of our work. There are at least two (and certainly many more) reasons for this: 1) some conditions and treatments are difficult to study, and 2) statistically significant results of carefully designed studies provide important information about classes or groups of patients but do not necessarily accurately predict the course or treatment response of any individual patient in that class. An example of the first reason is borderline personality disorder (BPD); at a 1992 conference jointly sponsored by the American Psychiatric Association (APA) and the National Institute of Mental Health to consider launching the APA Practice Guideline project, BPD was identified as a prevalent and challenging illness populating many inpatient beds and office practices, but about which there was insufficient research to guide treatment, and it was acknowledged that some system of clinical consensus would be needed. (As it turned out, almost 10 years later when a practice guideline for BPD was developed, new research studies had been accomplished to substantially inform the guideline process.) An example of the second reason is the well-known conundrum presented to clinicians in assessing suicide risk: risk factors that heighten concern about possible suicide are well known, yet accurately predicting the degree of risk in an individual patient is not possible.

A somewhat parallel dilemma is the now widely recognized difference between efficacy studies and effectiveness studies. Patients must be carefully selected for randomized controlled trials of a specific treatment, excluding many patients with comorbid conditions or with complications that would make it difficult to determine if the treatment itself is truly efficacious for the illness in question. Frequently, however, real-world patients do not conform to these highly selected efficacy study populations. There is now is growing support to fund effectiveness studies, utilizing large numbers of patients who resemble those in general clinical practice—for example, the CATIE study of patients with schizophrenia (Lieberman et al. 2005), and the STAR-D study of patients with depression (Trivedi et al. 2006) to guide our work of caring for more typical patients, those with complex multiple problems.

It is in the spirit of these concerns that this volume comes to us as a welcome compendium of invaluable real-world clinical cases. Here we have real patients in the hands of seasoned clinicians, and we have the wonderful opportunity to be the unseen observer, "listening" to diagnostic considerations (sometimes not so clear at first), the development of a treatment plan, and then the long-term implementation of that plan, with the inevitable need to individually adjust and revise the plan as needed.

No one is more widely associated with the challenging and changing landscape of diagnosis and assessment in psychiatric medicine than Robert Spitzer, whose energy and determination to guide the DSM-III to completion is by now legendary—it was a task that required the brain of a scientist, the arbitration skills of a lawyer, the perseverance of an obsessive person, and the patience of a saint! Fortunately for the field, not only did Spitzer shoulder that daunting task but he has remained a presence throughout all of the later versions of the DSM. He and a group of outstanding colleagues have provided us with a series of casebooks illustrating the diagnostic concepts in each successive edition of the DSM. The current volume is a welcome addition to this collection, but it is also unique by taking us into the offices of experienced psychiatric practitioners and allowing us to follow along, from intake to long-term treatment, on a case-by-case basis.

John M. Oldham, M.D., M.S.

REFERENCES

Lieberman JA, Stroup TS, McEvoy JP, et al: Effectiveness of antipsychotic drugs in patients with chronic schizophrenia. N Eng J Med 353:1209–1223, 2005

Trivedi MH, Rush AJ, Wisniewski SR, et al: Evaluation of outcomes with citalopram for depression using measurement-based care in STAR*D: implications for clinical practice. Am J Psychiatry 163:28–40, 2006

Preface

THIS CASEBOOK IS DIFFERENT from all existing casebooks, including our own, the *DSM-IV-TR Casebook* and the *Treatment Companion to the DSM-IV-TR Casebook.* All current casebooks include descriptions of cases from clinical practice, many include discussions of differential diagnosis, and some discuss suggested treatments; this book is different in that experts in a variety of treatment modalities describe their treatment of an interesting case from their own practice. In selecting the experts, we sought to ensure that they represented a wide range of psychiatric treatment approaches, including psychological, psychosocial, and pharmacological.

The experts were encouraged to go beyond just giving a standard case presentation. Our invitation to the experts asked them to send us a case write-up that included a summary of the patient's presenting symptoms, problems, and history of present and past illnesses; the expert's differential diagnosis, reasons for choosing the particular therapy applied, and initial treatment goals; how the expert explained the treatment to the patient and what the patient's reaction was; what actually occurred during the sessions (if treatment involved a talking therapy); the expert's thoughts and feelings during the treatment process; and how the patient changed over time.

The cases in this book—all new—are presented in the order in which the diagnoses appear in the DSM-IV-TR classification. To facilitate the reader's ability to quickly locate cases relevant to his or her practice, four separate indexesæone each by diagnosis, treatment modality, case name, and clinicianæhave been provided as appendixes.

We enjoyed working on this volume and have learned a great deal about treatment in the process. We hope you find it educational and stimulating as well.

PART I

Disorders Usually First Diagnosed in Infancy, Childhood, or Adolescence

CHAPTER 1

Bored At School

Multimodal Treatment of Tourette's Disorder

Glenn S. Hirsch, M.D.
Harold S. Koplewicz, M.D.

Glenn S. Hirsch, M.D., is Assistant Professor of Psychiatry and Medical Director of the New York University (NYU) Child Study Center at the NYU School of Medicine. In addition, Dr. Hirsch is Medical Director of the Division of Child and Adolescent Psychiatry at the NYU Medical Center and Bellevue Hospital Center. Dr. Hirsch has a clinical practice in child, adolescent, and adult psychiatry within the Child Study Center's Child and Family Associates. He specializes in diagnostic evaluation, psychopharmacology, pervasive developmental disorder, and anxiety and bipolar disorders. He is active in medical student education and the training and supervising of psychiatric residents. Dr. Hirsch is an associate editor of the *Journal of Child and Adolescent Psychopharmacology*.

Harold S. Koplewicz, M.D., was the founder and is currently the Director of the New York University Child Study Center. The center is dedicated to increasing the awareness of child mental health issues and expanding the scientific knowledge about and improving the treatment of child psychiatric illnesses. Dr. Koplewicz is the Arnold and Debbie Simon Professor of Child and Adolescent Psychiatry and serves as the Vice Chairman of the Department of Psychiatry and Professor of Pediatrics at the New York University School of Medicine. In addition, Dr. Koplewicz is the Director of the Division of Child and Adolescent Psychiatry at the Bellevue Hospital Center. Since 1997, Dr. Koplewicz is Editor-in-Chief of the *Journal of Child and Adolescent Psychopharmacology*.

HISTORY

Presenting Symptoms

Jesse was age 7 when I (G.S.H) first met him and his parents in the early spring of Jesse's second grade year. Jesse's parents brought him for an evaluation because of his increasing "boredom" at school and his irritability at home that resulted in frequent, daily verbal outbursts. During this period, he frequently stated that he wanted to run away from home, that nobody cared about him, and that he had no life. Jesse would make self-deprecating statements, such as saying that he was dumb, despite the fact that his teachers viewed him as gifted. His parents also remarked that he often sulked and was tearful. Jesse's parents demonstrated appropriate concern about these symptoms but were clearly exasperated with some of his other long-standing behavioral difficulties.

Jesse's teacher reported that Jesse's behavior had undergone a marked change early in his second-grade year, characterized by his lack of enthusiasm, severe oppositional behaviors, and a marked increase in disruptive behaviors as well as Jesse's saying that other children did not like him. Prior to the onset of this behavior, Jesse had always been seen as being markedly restless and fidgety, being easily distracted, having problems sustaining attention, and being impatient. These problematic symptoms first occurred during the preschool years. His behavior had always been intrusive in the classroom, but the new symptoms were a dramatic change. Although Jesse's teacher and teacher's assistant, who both knew him in first grade, reported that Jesse also displayed some tics, it was felt that those symptoms did not interfere with Jesse's functioning and tended to be ignored by his classmates.

Jesse's parents and teachers completed standardized questionnaires concerning Jesse, including the Achenbach Child Behavior Checklist, to examine a broad spectrum of his behavior, and the Conners Rating Scale, to obtain more detailed information on the symptoms of his disruptive behaviors.

Course of Illness

At age 4, Jesse developed a number of habits and tics. These included occasional eye blinking and a cough that was thought to be related to allergies. By the end of first grade, the symptoms progressed to include Jesse's licking the palm of his hand, clearing his throat, sniffing, and occasionally jerking his shoulder girdle. He was evaluated by a pediatric neurologist 6 months before coming to see me, diagnosed with a tic disorder, and treated with clonidine (0.1 mg tid). Clonidine is a medication that is generally used for hypertension but that has also been found to be helpful in reducing tics and the impulsive and hyperactive behaviors of attention-deficit/hyperactivity disorder (ADHD). The neurologist felt that the clonidine was only minimally helpful and agreed with Jesse's parents that it was causing Jesse to experience a fair amount of sedation. The partial efficacy of the clonidine and the onset of the current symptoms prompted the neurologist to refer Jesse for a psychiatric evaluation.

Jesse was the product of a full-term pregnancy. The pregnancy was unremarkable except for the mother's cigarette smoking. His delivery was by forceps, but there were no other birth-related complications. Jesse weighed 6 lb 6 oz at birth. He was breast-fed for 2 months but, after he developed severe colic, was weaned and tried on a number of formulas. He obtained language and motor milestones at a normal pace. His mother described him as always being very active and difficult.

Jesse began school at age 4. The teachers in his nursery and kindergarten programs noted that he was bright, had some social difficulties in that he seemed unaware of other children's personal space, was overly active, tended to "do his own thing," and had some fine motor difficulties. The latter included difficulties manipulating scissors and holding crayons and pencils. These difficulties resulted in an evaluation by his school that led to the implementation of occupational therapy for his motor deficits.

Jesse's medical history was unremarkable except for mild environmental allergies. His family history was positive for tics and obsessive-compulsive symptoms on the paternal side and depressive symptoms on the maternal side. Jesse had one younger sibling who was "fine."

Presenting Mental Status

At his initial presentation, Jesse was a neatly groomed, remarkably thin boy who was short for his age. He separated easily from his parents and initially sat in the waiting room while I met with his parents. His parents brought some play materials for him that supplemented the toys in the waiting area. During the first 30-minute meeting with his parents, Jesse barged into the office on several occasions—not to check on his parents but to complain about having to sit out in the waiting area. His parents asked him not to interrupt and to knock before entering, but their requests went unheeded. When Jesse was interviewed, he immediately complained of being bored despite the availability of a variety of play materials in the office. He frequently asked when we would be finished. He demonstrated some minor tics during the 30-minute meeting that included rapid eye blinking and an occasional cough. It was unclear if the latter was a tic because he also had a mild upper respiratory infection. Jesse made minimal eye contact with me and appeared angry and unhappy throughout the initial session. He complained that his parents "do not give me the things they have promised me" and stated that he hates school, saying, "It is boring; everything is boring." He acknowledged feeling unhappy, saying that nobody wanted to play with him. He did report that at times he wished he were dead, but he displayed no evidence of active suicidal ideation and was unable to indicate what events triggered those feelings. He also described himself as unhappier than anyone else he knew. His distress was palpable and painful.

DIAGNOSIS

At the time of my initial evaluation, I noted that by history and family report Jesse's tic symptoms met criteria for Tourette's disorder. Two main criteria are required to meet the DSM-IV-TR diagnosis for this disorder: 1) the patient must have had multiple motor tics and at least one vocal tic during the course of the illness, although it is not necessary for both kinds of tics to be present at the same time; and 2) the tics must be frequent, be present nearly every day, and occur several times a day for at least 1 year with no period of more than 3 months when tics were not present. In addition, the onset must be before age 18 and not be due to the effects of substances or another medical condition. Jesse's tics had been present for several years, and, although there had been periods of waxing and waning in their presence, he was never completely free of his tics. In addition to his motor tics, he had a variety of vocal tics including sniffing, throat clearing, and coughing. In addition, his behavior problems met full criteria for ADHD, combined type and his other symptoms fulfilled criteria for a diagnosis of major depressive disorder. Because 30%–60% of individuals with Tourette's disorder also have obsessive-compulsive disorder (OCD) (Cohen and Leckman 1994), I carefully examined him for OCD symptoms; both Jesse and his parents denied the existence of any of those symptoms. Because one of the possible side effects of clonidine is depression, a remaining question was whether the depression was in fact triggered by the clonidine and would therefore qualify for a diagnosis of clonidine-induced mood disorder (Hunt et al. 1991).

TREATMENT

Recommendations

I suggested to Jesse's parents that Jesse undergo a neuropsychological evaluation to assess the nature of his learning strengths and weaknesses, determine the degree of his "giftedness," and help develop an educational plan for him. However, this evaluation was deferred pending improvement of Jesse's ADHD symptoms. Although Jesse might have benefited from stimulant medication for the treatment of his ADHD, his parents were hesitant to permit the use of stimulants because they feared they could increase his tics. A behavioral therapy approach was then initiated. Treatment for Jesse's depressive symptoms was discussed and placed on hold while other treatments and evaluations were completed.

Finally, given the apparent lack of clear-cut efficacy of the clonidine in ameliorating his tics and decreasing his impulsive behaviors and the possibility that the drug had precipitated Jesse's depression, the clonidine was tapered and eventually discontinued while Jesse's blood pressure was carefully monitored for any signs of rebound hypertension.

Although my initial roles in Jesse's case were as therapist and psychopharmacologist, my role as a case coordinator of his treatment in the broadest sense—working in the context of Jesse's school system and with his parents, pediatrician, neurologist, and behavioral therapist—was equally important.

Treatment Course

Follow-up questionnaires administered after the clonidine was discontinued and a subsequent examination during an office visit revealed Jesse had multiple tics, including eye blinking, occasional head jerks, sniffing, and throat clearing. Although the symptoms did not appear to interfere with his daily functioning, reports about some of Jesse's behaviors, such as his calling out in class, displaying marked inattentiveness, and being unable to sit in his seat, demonstrated that his ADHD symptoms were quite disabling. After 2 weeks of being completely weaned from the clonidine, Jesse's symptoms of depression were no longer present, his tics were slightly more frequent but still did not impair his functioning, and his core ADHD symptoms remained unchanged. In the office, Jesse was much more engaged, looked happier, and had improved eye contact. The tics present at the first session were slightly more frequent and his cough was clearly tic-like.

After discussing the benefits and risks of stimulant treatment for a person with a tic disorder, a trial of the stimulant dextroamphetamine, 2.5 mg taken in the morning before school, was started. Adjustments to the dextroamphetamine dosage were made by evaluating Jesse's impulsive behavior and the frequency of his tics using parent and teacher reports.

Once Jesse's ADHD symptoms were under fair control, he underwent neuropsychological testing. The testing revealed that Jesse had a full-scale IQ in the very superior range with minimal difference between his performance and verbal IQ. (A difference of ≥15 points or more between the performance and verbal IQ would indicate the presence of a significant learning disorder.) The results of the testing demonstrated that Jesse had some fine motor difficulties that resulted in his having difficulty with handwriting and more importantly confirmed the absence of any learning disability.

Behavioral treatment that was initiated before the stimulants were prescribed was only minimally effective as Jesse's father was unable to attend the sessions regularly and had difficulty following through on behavioral assignments. This placed an extra burden on Jesse's mother. The father's resistance stemmed from his own symptoms that were suggestive of ADHD as well as his OCD. It was recommended that the father have his own evaluation, but he refused. My inability to engage the father at any level was frustrating and worrisome because I knew it would likely affect the success of Jesse's treatment.

A series of rewards and consequences for home and school using a behavioral program outlined by Barkley (1997) was developed for Jesse and his mother. Jesse's teacher was given a daily report card to fill out that inquired about homework completion, appropriate class participation, and following rules in school. We targeted Jesse's getting up and being ready in the morning as initial behaviors to improve at home. Many of his behaviors improved dramatically and quickly, but his social interaction with peers remained difficult. He continued to be seen as intrusive, silly, and immature. The behavioral therapy did appear to reduce the conflict within the family, and the parents became more united in their approach toward him.

Jesse continued to do fairly well for almost a year. Based on feedback from the school, I adjusted the dextroamphetamine dosage to 10 mg bid. Although Jesse complained of decreased appetite and initial insomnia, these side effects did not require a tapering of the dosage and Jesse continued to maintain his expected gains in weight and height.

Approximately 1 year after he began dextroamphetamine, Jesse's tic symptoms and behavioral symptoms worsened dramatically. His symptoms included sudden flinging movements of his arms; mouth movements, including expanding his cheeks and pursing his lips; eyelid squeezing; frequent coughing; and making a smacking sound with his lips. Increases in Jesse's impulsive behaviors that were unrelated to the tics were also noted, including his fighting and hitting peers. In addition, Jesse began having a variety of compulsive symptoms, including his needing to touch people when he walked by them, hoarding paper at home and in his knapsack, and needing to stare briefly at the four corners of a room when he came through a door. He displayed no evidence of obsessive thoughts or depressive symptoms. Jesse appeared unbothered by his tics and compulsions despite their occurring with a frequency that was painful to observe, and he initially denied having any behavioral problems in school. Despite the level of his difficulties, his teachers liked Jesse. During his visits to my office he was cooperative, and he was willing to superficially examine some of his apparently compulsive behaviors that were bothersome—especially the touching of others, which he felt got him into further difficulty with his peers.

I discussed with Jesse's parents the strategy of adjusting the dextroamphetamine dosage to examine the medication's potential role in Jesse's tic exacerbation. All options were explored: increasing the current dosage to decrease the impulsivity stemming from his ADHD, adding a second medication to control his tics, or discontinuing the dextroamphetamine. Although it is not uncommon to see marked periods of exacerbation of tic symptoms without a specific trigger, I did explore with Jesse and his parents any stressors that may have been influencing the exacerbations. None were found.

We agreed to discontinue the dextroamphetamine—although there was only a low level of suspicion that it was related to the exacerbation of his tics—and reevaluate Jesse's response after 2–4 weeks. We discussed this plan with Jesse's school, as any reemergence of symptoms as a result of stopping the medication would be problematic in the classroom and we wanted to ensure that the school remained an integral part of Jesse's treatment.

Immediately after he was withdrawn from the dextroamphetamine, Jesse's impulsivity in all areas of his life worsened, and after 3 weeks there was no evidence of any reduction in his tic or obsessive-compulsive symptoms. We decided to try the second strategy—adding a second medication to the stimulant to help control the tics. We briefly considered the use of habit reversal, a behavioral treatment for tics (Woods and Himle 2004), but felt that Jesse's lack of motivation would be a major impediment to the success of this approach. The dextroamphetamine was restarted and a trial of pimozide was initiated for the treatment of the tics. Pimozide is a conventional antipsychotic that has been well studied as an effective treatment of tics and Tourette's disorder, and for many years it was considered the first choice of medication for this disorder. Over the course of a month, Jesse's pimozide dosage was titrated to 6 mg qhs. Because this is a medication that has the potential to cause heart rhythm disturbances by slowing down the conduction of electrical impulses in the heart muscle, an electrocardiogram was performed at baseline and on several subsequent occasions as the pimozide dosage was increased.

Despite the addition of pimozide, Jesse's compulsive behaviors and tics continued to interfere with his schooling, and a conference was set up with his parents, teachers, and school guidance counselors to plan for his educational needs and educate the school personnel about the symptoms of Tourette's disorder. Our recommendations to the school included developing or finding a self-contained program that would challenge Jesse's intellect and include a behavioral intervention program. Although this program would be able to directly address Jesse's ADHD and OCD symptoms, it would only indirectly address his tics. To help the school better tolerate Jesse's tics, we decided to implement a process of psychoeducation to help school personnel and other students understand the symptoms of Tourette's disorder and the involuntary nature of the tics. The school agreed to these recommendations, and for fourth grade Jesse was placed in a new class with seven other children, one teacher, and two assistant teachers, one of whom had been trained in behavioral techniques.

After Jesse's dose of pimozide was eventually increased to 10 mg, there was still no reduction in Jesse's tics and he complained of severe tiredness; the pimozide was therefore discontinued. In the new classroom environment, Jesse's teachers reported that they were better able to manage his impulsiveness—including his calling out and interrupting class lessons—with a behavioral management plan that included frequent praise, tangible rewards, and daily feedback to home. However, Jesse's increasing compulsiveness included the need to ask multiple questions about every topic discussed in class, an urge to touch the heads of each classmate each day, and the need to pick at the skin of his lips until they bled. These symptoms were problematic at school and home and were resistant to school-based interventions. Jesse's insight into his compulsive behavior was poor. We decided to hold off on further direct treatment of the tics and instead attempted to treat the compulsive behaviors with the thought that a reduction in these symptoms might reduce the tics indirectly through an overall reduction in stress.

To treat his compulsive behavior, a trial of fluoxetine, a selective serotonin reuptake inhibitor, was begun at 5 mg, but Jesse became markedly disinhibited on the medication. His behaviors included his calling out more frequently in class, making silly faces at other children, and throwing paper balls. Therefore, the fluoxetine was discontinued and Jesse was started on clomipramine 25 mg/day, a tricyclic antidepressant with serotonin reuptake inhibition that has been shown to be especially effective in the treatment of OCD. This medication has a potential adverse effect that can cause heart irregularities through the same mechanism as pimozide. Therefore Jesse received serial electrocardiograms, which confirmed that Jesse's heart function remained healthy throughout the course of his taking this medication. Jesse's final dose was 225 mg, to which he had a fair response, with marked diminution of compulsive symptoms and some reduction in tics.

In the office, we used response prevention, as described by March et al. (1994), to further reduce Jesse's compulsive symptoms. This treatment is a form of cognitive-behavioral therapy that first teaches and provides patients with strategies to resist rituals and then exposes them to stimuli that will trigger a compulsive response. The therapist then works with the patient to resist the compulsion. This approach was met with limited success due to Jesse's poor insight and his parents' satisfaction with the level of improvement achieved by medication. As a result and because Jesse was demoralized by his lack of friends, we spent more time on Jesse's social difficulties. The ability and willingness of all professionals in Jesse's life to work as a team kept the treatment on track.

Improvements in Jesse's overall impulsivity and obsessive-compulsive symptoms were maintained through his elementary school years. Jesse continued receiving special educational services as he entered middle school. At that stage, he refused to continue with any psychotherapy and his parents reluctantly accepted his decision. Jesse continued to have impaired social skills and only rarely was involved in social activities. He continued to be maintained on dextroamphetamine and clomipramine. Jesse experienced side effects with these medications, including tiredness, decreased appetite, and dry mouth. I saw him every 3 months while his symptoms remained stable. Although he enjoyed his interactions with me and discussed some of his concerns about his illness, it was not possible to engage him in a more therapeutic dialogue. I also met with Jesse's mother every 6 weeks without Jesse to help her better deal with his continuing difficulties.

In the spring of eighth grade, Jesse's tics, which were still present but had slowly waned in intensity during the sixth and seventh grades, worsened and expanded to include lip licking, nose twitching, head jerking, arm swinging, abdominal jerks, barking sounds, and coprolalia. Coprolalia, a relatively rare symptom, is a complex vocal tic of uttering curses and obscenities. In addition to these worsened tics, Jesse's attention and interest in academic performance diminished.

Because Jesse had failed trials of clonidine and pimozide, the two most commonly used medications to treat tics, we decided on a trial of haloperidol, an antipsychotic medication that is usually used to treat schizophrenia but that has also been shown to be useful in the treatment of Tourette's disorder. Jesse's haloperidol dosage was slowly titrated to 1.5 mg/day, which resulted in a moderate degree of relief in his tics and cessation of his coprolalia. However, his attention and interest in academic matters continued to be poor.

During his high school years, Jesse remained in a special education program but put very little effort into his schoolwork despite the involvement of school personnel in developing a behavioral program to address his needs. Given that earlier testing revealed a youngster with superior intellect, Jesse's lack of effort and poor performance in school were disappointing to his mother and upsetting to me. I reexamined Jesse to see if there was perhaps an underlying depression or other issue that would help explain his lack of interest in school, but nothing was evident.

A group intervention in school was added to his educational plan to address his poor social skills. However, his social skills continued to be markedly deficient. In part this seemed to be secondary to his compulsive need to comment on everything and talk nonstop even when his comments were tangential to a group discussion. Although we wondered if the hypertalkativeness might be a manifestation of partially treated ADHD, Jesse felt strongly and we agreed that this symptom more closely resembled a compulsion rather than an impulsive behavior. He did not want to try increasing his dextroamphetamine, a strategy that might have helped answer this clinical question. His nonstop talking was evident in the office as well, and it was easy to see how others would find him annoying. Although he had some awareness of this problem, he seemed to be unable to address it in the group therapeutic setting. Attempts to work with him individually were met with marked resistance. We discussed making adjustments to the medication by increasing the clomipramine, but Jesse and his family were reluctant to do this.

Toward the end of his junior year of high school, Jesse's haloperidol dosage was tapered without any worsening of his tics. After graduating from high school, Jesse attended a community college for one semester, but the lack of structure at college was too difficult for him to handle. Afterward, he requested a trial off all medications. A 1-year drug-free trial resulted in a mild increase in his compulsive behaviors and marked worsening of his attentional problems.

Jesse is now working as an assistant at a pet store. He continues to talk too much, but his employer tolerates it. Jesse struggles with other social relationships, has minimal interest in romantic relationships, and has recently agreed to return to therapy, but has decided not to restart any medication.

DISCUSSION

Treating children is always complex. It involves much more than just giving a pill or talking to a child. It includes parents; teachers; at times, siblings; and others. In addition, the rapid pace of normal child development always presents new challenges and opportunities. At times, we shared the same hope as Jesse's family that we would be able to magically resolve all of his difficulties. It was disappointing that Jesse's psychopathology prevented him from reaching his academic potential. Although Jesse is content with some aspects of his functioning, it is still hard to accept the current scientific limitations in our field in treating children with complex disorders like Tourette's.

REFERENCES

Barkley RA: Defiant Children: A Clinician's Manual for Assessment and Parent Training, 2nd Edition. New York, Guilford, 1997

Cohen DJ, Leckman JF: Developmental psychopathology and neurobiology of Tourette's syndrome. J Am Acad Child Adolesc Psychiatry 33:2–15, 1994

Hunt RD, Lau S, Ryu J: Alternative therapies for ADHD, in Ritalin: Theory and Patient Management. Edited by Greenhill LL, Osman BB. New York, Mary Ann Liebert, 1991, pp 75–95

March J, Mulle K, Herbel B: Behavioral psychotherapy for children and adolescents with obsessive-compulsive disorder: an open trial of a new protocol driven treatment package. J Am Acad Child Adolesc Psychiatry 33:333–341, 1994

Woods DW, Himle MB: Creating tic suppression: comparing the effects of verbal instruction to differential reinforcement. J Appl Behav Anal 37:417–420, 2004

CHAPTER 2

A Ball of String

Comprehensive Treatment of Autistic Disorder

Fred R. Volkmar, M.D.

Fred R. Volkmar, M.D., is the Irving B. Harris Professor of Child Psychiatry, Pediatrics, and Psychology at the Child Study Center, Yale University. He is a graduate of the University of Illinois (Urbana) and Stanford University. Dr. Volkmar completed his child psychiatry training at Yale before joining the faculty in 1982. The author of over 100 research papers and several hundred chapters, he has served as an Associate Editor of the *Journal of Autism*, the *Journal of Child Psychiatry and Psychology*, and the *American Journal of Psychiatry*. He was an editor of the *Handbook of Autism and Pervasive Developmental Disorders*, 3rd Edition, and has served as Co-Chairperson of the Autism-Intellectual Disabilities Committee for the American Academy of Child and Adolescent Psychiatry. He coordinated the DSM-IV field trial for autistic disorder and served on the National Research Council panel, which authored *Educating Children with Autism*

HISTORY

Quentin was initially referred to us at age 30 months because of his parents' concern about his lack of speech and poor social skills. The younger of two children, he was born after an uncomplicated pregnancy; his labor and delivery were also unremarkable. Although he engaged in breast-feeding with no problems, Quentin had difficulties tolerating solid foods. His parents described him as a good baby who was relatively undemanding.

By the time Quentin was about age 1 year, his parents noted that he made limited eye contact with people and that he was delayed in achieving age-appropriate motor and communication milestones. He played with materials by lining them up and then using an adult's hand to reach a desired object; throughout this process he made no eye contact. Although the family physician initially told Quentin's parents to "watch and wait," the parents sought an evaluation from the state's early intervention program when Quentin reached age 2 years and still was not speaking. At that time he was noted to have marked delays in communication, socialization, and adaptive skills. He also exhibited attachments to unusual objects (e.g., he often carried around [and slept with] a soda bottle).

Nonintensive early intervention services were begun, consisting of 1 hour per week with a speech pathologist and another hour per week with an occupational therapist, with both treatments occurring in the home. Because of continued concerns about multiple aspects of his development, Quentin was referred to our center for comprehensive assessment. We noted at that time that Quentin's maternal cousin had autism.

DIAGNOSIS

Quentin's medical history at age 30 months was generally unremarkable apart from his recurrent ear infections. He was noted to have a small number of words that he used indiscriminately and noncontingently (e.g., saying "wow" or "hi" repeatedly but not in context). His eye contact was fleeting, and he was largely oblivious to bids for social interaction. He did have several stereotyped mannerisms that his parents reported had increased in frequency and complexity over time. For example, Quentin engaged in body rocking and complicated hand/finger mannerisms; he would also spend considerable time exploring nonfunctional aspects of materials (e.g., he repeatedly stroked toys rather than playing with them in typical ways). The stereotyped mannerisms often interfered with his learning and were more likely to occur when he was having difficulties (e.g., with a change in the environment), but he would also engage in them preferentially.

Quentin was preoccupied with aspects of the nonsocial environment (e.g., he spent long periods of time rubbing the carpet on the floor) and could be disrupted by a change in materials or extraneous environmental stimuli (e.g., even the sound of someone walking by in the hall). He exhibited occasional staring spells not associated with unusual movement or apparent loss of consciousness. His physical examination was unremarkable, and an electroencephalogram was within normal limits. His test results for fragile X syndrome, the most common form of inherited intellectual impairment, were also negative.

It was difficult to engage Quentin in assessment due to his lack of a "learning to learn" set; that is, it was hard to engage him in such basic activities as sitting still and paying attention unless he was held in his father's lap, and considerable time had to be spent to help him feel comfortable with the room and test materials. The language assessment showed that Quentin's expressive language was more delayed than his receptive language. He had a vocabulary consisting of a few words—mostly echoed and sometimes used idiosyncratically. His prosody (the musical aspects of speech) was unusual with somewhat nasal, loud, and monotonic word pronunciation. He did respond to some very simple requests involving a verb and a noun but not to more complex requests. His expressive language abilities were slightly above the 1-year level, and his receptive skills were close to the 15-month level. Quentin's nonverbal cognitive abilities, assessed using an instrument originally developed for deaf children, were close to his age level. He could match objects and size. On the Vineland Adaptive Behavior Scales, his scores for interpersonal and expressive language were at the 11-month level; his motor skills were shown to be an area of relative strength.

In considering a diagnosis for Quentin, our impression was that he had autistic disorder with significantly delayed language/communication and social abilities associated with unusual responses to the environment (American Psychiatric Association 1994). Although Quentin exhibited significant developmental delays and behavioral difficulties, we saw some positive prognostic signs, including the presence of limited language and his relatively preserved nonverbal cognitive abilities. We recommended a highly structured, comprehensive intervention program that could build on these areas of strength and address his multiple areas of vulnerability (National Research Council 2001). His parents were understandably upset with the news of this diagnosis. After a period of initial denial, they moved to a more active phase of positive coping.

TREATMENT

Quentin's parents were faced with the choice of several different programs and asked for our input on the choice of program. The programs available to them included a child-centered, but less-structured, approach in which the focus of treatment would follow Quentin's lead; a much more structured applied behavior analytic program; and a public school (eclectic) program in which he would be exposed to typically developing peers. Our recommendation was for the more highly structured, applied behavior analytic program; this program would use a more intrusive and intensive intervention approach in fostering Quentin's acquisition of skills and decreasing the frequency of his undesirable behaviors, with the goal of increasing his capacity to tolerate adult proximity and intrusion. The recommended program included considerable individual instruction and the use of reinforcement techniques and learning principles throughout the day. We recommended that the teaching environment be very simple and free of distractions to maximize Quentin's capacity to learn. Initial goals of the program would include establishing Quentin's ability to consistently engage in work routines, developing a list of effective reinforcers, explicitly teaching functional use of behaviors, and generalizing skills across settings. In developing his individual educational plan, we recommended that explicit goals be factored out from each objective (e.g., tolerating adult intrusion and leads, increasing social awareness, fostering cognitive skills). We emphasized that social engagement should be fostered to enhance Quentin's communication with others, and that occupational and physical therapy focus on developing his increased task engagement and self-awareness. His communication goals should include his increasing the frequency and consistency with which he communicated; to this end, we recommended use of both an augmentative approach (picture exchange in which a picture is used instead of a word) as well as spoken language and use of visual supports (an area of cognitive strength for Quentin) to help him organize himself. We also advocated for extensive family engagement to ensure Quentin's new skills could be generalized outside of the program setting and used to help his parents cope with his problem behaviors at home (National Research Council 2001; Volkmar et al. 1999).

Quentin was enrolled in the behavioral program and made significant gains over the next 2 years. He was seen for reassessment at age 5. At that point he continued to exhibit problems in social interaction, communication, and behavior consistent with a diagnosis of autism, but he had made significant gains in terms of his language and cognitive abilities. Although his language continued to be monotonic with a rather mechanical vocal tone, he was speaking in full sentences, could engage in simple conversations, and was generally more socially engaged, although his social approaches to others remained somewhat eccentric and one-sided. He had developed an interest in hoarding string and often carried a large ball of string around with him that he would sleep with at night. At times of distress or excitement, he would engage in some stereotyped mannerisms such as hand flapping and body rocking. His parents were pleased with his progress and, with the agreement of his special school and school district, they planned a transition back to the public school for kindergarten. He subsequently repeated kindergarten then was mainstreamed into the first grade, where he did well with support, including some pull-out special classes, speech/language services, and social skills training. He generally did well until the third grade when he experienced an exacerbation of some of his early behavioral difficulties (difficulties with change and a substantial increase in stereotyped mannerisms that interfered with his engagement in the educational program). Use of an atypical neuroleptic, risperidone, at a relatively low dose resulted in dramatic improvement in his behavior but was accompanied by significant weight gain. After 1 year he was gradually withdrawn from the medication (McCracken et al. 2002; Volkmar et al. 1999)

Presently Quentin is a high school student who continues to receive special services but who has made many gains. He is self-sufficient in daily activities, and job planning for his post–secondary school years has begun. At the time of his most recent assessment, he was functioning overall in the borderline range of intellectual functioning with his nonverbal skills rating significantly higher than his verbal ones. He continues to have difficulties with social interaction and communication. He has some acquaintances in the community and is actively involved in a supportive church youth program. Although he wants a girlfriend, his one-sided and rather eccentric social approaches to girls have posed an obstacle to his achieving this goal. He spends considerable time engaged in volunteer clerical work at a community center, which he and his family hope will facilitate his obtaining employment when he graduates from high school.

Quentin and his family have continued to use our services periodically. During adolescence Quentin had continued difficulties with behavioral rigidity and repetitive behaviors. A trial of sertraline, a selective serotonin reuptake inhibitor, led to behavioral activation; he has otherwise not received any behavior-modifying medications.

Despite the infrequent contact, Quentin and his family have developed a strong relationship with us and Quentin talks quite positively about coming for visits. Sometimes months or even a few years go by without our seeing him; at other times, he is seen on a weekly or more frequent basis. Focused psychotherapy has been helpful for Quentin as he has worked diligently to "learn the rules" for social interaction. His parents have been pleased with his progress and are working with Quentin and his support group to develop plans for supporting his independent living as an adult (Howlin and Goode 1998).

DISCUSSION

Several features of this case deserve discussion, including the issues of diagnosis, intervention, and longitudinal course. Autism is diagnosed based on characteristic problems in the areas of social development, communication, and play and on unusual patterns of environmental interest/responsivity (Volkmar and Klin 2005). In most cases, parents of children with autism become concerned about their child's development early in life; common presenting complaints include language delay, social isolation, and unusual responses to the environment, all with onset before age 3. As was true in this case, stereotyped mannerisms and difficulties with environmental change sometimes become more prominent around age 3. Such behaviors can pose a significant obstacle to educational and behavioral interventions (McCracken et al. 2002).

With growing public awareness of and research advances in autism, earlier diagnosis of the disorder is now more frequent. Pediatricians and health care providers are more aware of the diagnosis and are less likely to adopt a wait-and-see attitude; this is important given the substantial body of work on the effects of early intervention (National Research Council 2001). Several lines of emerging research will likely make it possible to screen for autism at progressively younger ages over the next decade. This will offer increased opportunities for early intervention, although it will also demand increased levels of service for this age group. It is clear that autism can be diagnosed in many cases before age 3, although for some children it is only around this time that all the features required for the diagnosis are observable.

The importance of early intervention is emphasized in this case. A comprehensive review of evidence-based interventions has shown that substantial gains can be made for children with autism through early intervention (Howlin and Good 1998). Although programs differ in some respects, such as with regard to theory, they share many practical similarities, including the importance of structured, intensive teaching and a focus on fostering communication and adaptive skills. Many children do make substantial gains in these programs; however, other children do not, despite their participation in good programs. Positive prognostic factors include the presence of communicative speech by age 5 and higher IQ (Howlin and Goode 1998). In this case, Quentin's language abilities substantially increased with early intervention and his relatively preserved nonverbal cognitive abilities consistently remained an important strength for him.

This case also illustrates the changes that children with autism exhibit over time. There are several points at which children with autism often have difficulties, such as with the transition to primary school programs and on entering adolescence. School-age children may make significant developmental gains, but progress with behavioral difficulties may be more problematic. For some children, substantial gains can be made in adolescence whereas for others losses are observed.

Although there is no consensus on the issue of understanding comorbid disorders in autism and related conditions, there is a growing body of work on the effectiveness of carefully selected pharmacological treatments; for example, placebo-controlled, double-blind studies of risperidone have shown significant benefit for certain target symptoms (McCracken et al. 2002). Higher rates of epilepsy are observed in children with autism; an electroencephalogram is indicated whenever symptoms or features suggestive of seizure disorder are observed (Volkmar et al. 1999).

It appears that with better and earlier case detection and more effective behavioral and educational interventions, the long-term outcome in autism has improved, with many autistic individuals being able to achieve self-sufficiency and independence in adulthood. Thus increased awareness of autism on the part of medical and educational professionals as well as of parents is particularly important. Because autism is a chronic, developmental disorder, it is not uncommon for individuals and their families to make extensive but episodic use of the services of mental health providers over time. A flexible approach in treating the child and supporting family members is needed.

REFERENCES

American Psychiatric Association: Diagnostic and Statistical Manual of Mental Disorders, 4th Edition. Washington, DC, American Psychiatric Association, 1994

Howlin P, Goode S: Outcome in adult life for people with autism and Asperger's syndrome, in Autism and Pervasive Developmental Disorders. Edited by Volkmar FR. New York, Cambridge University Press, 1998, pp 209–241

McCracken JT, McGough J, Shah B, et al: Risperidone in children with autism and serious behavioral problems. N Engl J Med 347:314–321, 2002

National Research Council: Educating Young Children With Autism. Washington, DC, National Academy Press, 2001

Volkmar FR, Klin A: Issues in the diagnosis and classification of autism and related conditions, in Handbook of Autism and Pervasive Developmental Disorders, 3rd Edition. Edited by Volkmar F, Klin A, Paul R, et al. New York, Wiley, 2005, pp 5–41

Volkmar F, Cook EH Jr, Pomeroy J, et al: Practice parameters for the assessment and treatment of children, adolescents, and adults with autism and other pervasive developmental disorders. American Academy of Child and Adolescent Psychiatry Working Group on Quality Issues. J Am Acad Child Adolesc Psychiatry 38 (suppl 12):32S–54S, 1999

PART II

Delirium, Dementia, and Amnestic and Other Cognitive Disorders

CHAPTER 3

Paranoid Retiree

Evaluation and Management of Delirium

Steven Fischel, M.D., Ph.D.
Benjamin Liptzin, M.D.

Steven Fischel, M.D., Ph.D., is the Medical Director of the Psychiatry Consultation Service at Baystate Medical Center, a 600-bed academic medical center in Springfield, Massachusetts, and Assistant Professor of Psychiatry at Tufts University School of Medicine. He is the Psychiatry Clerkship Director for third-year medical students from Tufts who have their psychiatric rotation at Baystate, the western campus of Tufts. He is also Vice-Chair of the Undergraduate Medical Education Committee at Baystate. Dr. Fischel has been recognized for excellence in teaching by Tufts medical students. He is a member of the Association of Directors of Medical Student Education in Psychiatry and a Fellow of the Academy of Psychosomatic Medicine.

Benjamin Liptzin, M.D., is Chairman of the Department of Psychiatry at Baystate Medical Center and is Professor and Deputy Chair of Psychiatry at Tufts University School of Medicine. He is an internationally recognized expert on delirium and a leader in geriatric psychiatry. His prior position was as Director of Geriatric Psychiatry at McLean Hospital where he also served as Associate Professor of Psychiatry and Director of the Geriatric Education Center at Harvard Medical School. He was the recipient of a Geriatric Mental Health Academic Award from the National Institute of Mental Health (NIMH) and was the Director of the NIMH-funded Geriatric Psychiatry Fellowship at McLean. He chaired the American Psychiatric Association Task Force on Nursing Homes and the Mentally Ill Elderly. He was a member of the DSM-IV Cognitive Impairment Disorders Work Group and helped conduct a literature review and data analysis that informed the development of the diagnostic criteria and text for delirium in DSM-IV. He is Secretary-Treasurer–elect of the American Association for Geriatric Psychiatry, a Board member of the Massachusetts chapter of the Alzheimer's Association, and Chair of the Committee on Aging of the Group for the Advancement of Psychiatry.

WILLIAM WAS A 75-YEAR-OLD married man with a history of bipolar I disorder, hypertension, and type 2 diabetes. He was brought to the emergency room by his wife because he was increasingly isolative, was not eating, was sleeping more than usual, and was fearful that people wanted to break into the house. In the emergency room, he was noted to have a fever and urinary tract infection, resulting in his admission to the medical unit. We were asked to consult regarding treatment of his depression and paranoia and to arrange an inpatient psychiatric admission once he was medically cleared.

HISTORY

William was a retired teacher. He had a long history of bipolar disorder and first presented with depression and suicidal ideation at age 30. He was hospitalized at that time and treated with the antidepressant imipramine. Several years later, he presented with his first manic episode for which lithium carbonate was prescribed; his mood disorder remained stabilized with the lithium for many years. His most recent psychiatric hospitalization occurred 1 year prior to the admission described herein, when he was hospitalized for depression.

At the time of William's admission, his medication regimen included lithium carbonate 450 mg qhs, which resulted in a lithium level of 1.0 mEq/L and which had previously stabilized his bipolar mood disorder; olanzapine, 2.5 mg qhs, an atypical neuroleptic for the psychotic symptoms of his bipolar disorder; fluoxetine, 20 mg/day, for treatment of his bipolar depression; donepezil, 10 mg qhs, for treatment of his Alzheimer's type dementia; and lisinopril, 10 mg/day, for his hypertension. His mood had stabilized on these medications, but over the previous year he had begun to pull back from socializing. He had also turned over management of the finances and checkbook to his spouse. His family noticed that he was more forgetful. They had him evaluated for his forgetfulness, and he was thought to have mild dementia most likely due to Alzheimer's type dementia. He had been started on the acetylcholinesterase inhibitor donepezil 6 months prior to his admission; the medication had been titrated up to his current dose with no significant side effects. One week prior to his admission, he abruptly became very isolative and was fearful that someone was trying to break into the house. At times he became angry with his wife because she did not see the people lurking outside the house. She hesitated to bring him to the hospital because his paranoia episodes were intermittent with periods of relative lucidity between them. However, when he stopped eating, refused to get out of bed, and seemed confused, his wife felt she could no longer handle him and brought him to the emergency room.

DIAGNOSIS

Given William's history, I (S.F.) was a little concerned about the state in which I would find him. I wondered whether his bipolar illness would be out of control, with a recurrence of his depression or manic state, either of which might require psychiatric hospitalization. Alternatively, his decompensation might be due to an as yet undiagnosed medical problem. His symptoms could also be due to a combination of medical and psychiatric factors. In person, William was quiet and withdrawn; he was unable to give a coherent history of his illness. He denied feeling depressed and displayed no evidence of suicidal ideation. His affect was blunted and his manner was withdrawn; he had a vacant look about him and appeared confused rather than depressed. His speech was sparse but fluent, except for anomia (difficulty naming familiar objects). Although he could not name simple objects, he could describe their function. His cognition was impaired, and he was oriented to person only. He could register three words but remembered none of them 5 minutes later. When asked to spell "world" backward, his halting response was "d-o." He did not appear to be hallucinating, as had been reported prior to his hospitalization. His insight and judgment were impaired by his confusion.

A medical workup included a physical exam conducted by the admitting physician, which showed a fever with temperature of 101°F. Chest and lungs were clear, making pneumonia unlikely; his abdomen was soft and nontender. There were no focal neurologic abnormalities to suggest a stroke. His white blood cell count was 8,800 with a high proportion of polys. Although this white cell count was within normal limits, the high percentage of polys suggested the possibility of an infectious process. The urinalysis was positive for leukocytes or white blood cells, nitrites, and moderate bacteria, suggesting a urinary tract infection. His electrolytes, including his serum levels of sodium, potassium, chloride, and calcium, were within normal limits. He had a serum urea nitrogen of 17 mg/dL and creatinine of 1.2 mg/dL, both indicators of normal kidney function. His blood glucose was 200 mg/dL, which was elevated but not enough to explain his symptoms. His lithium level was 0.9 mEq/L, which was within the normal therapeutic range for lithium of 0.6–1.2 mEq/L. The findings on his thyroid function tests were within normal limits. The results of a computed tomography scan of his head were unremarkable except for age-appropriate atrophy.

At this point in the evaluation, I was relieved to recognize a familiar scenario. William's presentation was not uncommon for a medically ill, hospitalized, older patient. An older patient, particularly one with an underlying dementia, is at high risk for developing delirium while experiencing an acute medical illness that requires hospitalization (Levkoff et al. 1992). The acute change in his mental status that led to his being brought to the hospital was characteristic of delirium, with impaired attention, disorientation, abrupt onset, and a waxing/waning course (American Psychiatric Association 2000). The challenge for me and the medical team was to identify the underlying cause or causes of his delirium. The urinary tract infection identified in the emergency department with its accompanying fever was a prime suspect, but some of William's symptoms concerned me and I did not want to come to premature closure on his diagnosis and risk missing something. Delirium is often multifactorial in its causation. William's anomia was unusual, and I was worried that he might have had an acute stroke. It was reassuring when his neurological examination did not identify any other neurological signs of a stroke and his computed tomograpy (CT) head scan did not reveal any features that were indicative of a stroke. Medications can also often be responsible for causing delirium, especially anticholinergic medications, but there had been no recent change in William's prescriptions or actual intake. Lithium toxicity can cause delirium, but William's lithium level was within normal limits and was not different from what it had been for several years. It is possible that with the onset of dementia, he was no longer able to tolerate his usual lithium level, but we were concerned about destabilizing his bipolar disorder and so left his lithium dose unchanged. The use of an angiotensin-converting enzyme inhibitor, such as lisinopril. can result in an increased lithium level, but William's outpatient psychiatrist had previously decreased the lithium dose to manage this interaction. Hypo- or hyperglycemia can also result in delirium, and atypical antipsychotics may precipitate hyperglycemia and diabetic ketoacidosis, but these potential problems did not seem to be present in this case.

What made this case more complicated and challenging was the patient's long history of bipolar disorder as well as his more recent history of dementia. Could his symptoms of isolation, decreased appetite, hypersomnia, and paranoia have been attributable to a recurrent major depressive episode with psychotic features? Certainly. But when he was seen, William did not appear to be depressed and his wife clearly felt his behavior was different from that during previous depressive episodes and was accompanied by more confusion than was usual for his depressive episodes.

I considered whether his symptoms could have been due to a slow progression of the Alzheimer's type dementia, causing a gradual decline in his abilities. Certainly there had been a slow decline in his memory and his ability to pay bills and manage his checkbook, despite his being started on donepezil. Alzheimer's patients on acetylcholinesterase inhibitors such as donepezil have been shown to score statistically better on cognitive tests than a comparative group of patients on placebo; however, over time they continue to decline cognitively and functionally (Kawas 2003). In unusual cases, some patients become more confused and agitated when first starting a cholinesterase inhibitor, but William had been stable on donepezil for 6 months.

The medical treatment team was initially impressed by the psychiatric symptoms and, given William's behavior problems and history of psychiatric hospitalizations, requested that he be transferred to the inpatient psychiatric unit. However, as consultants, we felt that his medical conditions would be better monitored and treated on a medical floor and that his psychiatric symptoms would likely clear as his medical condition improved. Consultation psychiatrists often have to negotiate between a medical team that is pushing for early transfer and a psychiatric unit that feels the patient is not medically stable. In this case, the acuteness of the patient's mental status changes, the alterations in his consciousness, and the fluctuating nature of his symptoms pointed toward a diagnosis of delirium rather than simply a worsening dementia.

TREATMENT

The key to managing a delirious patient is to try to identify the underlying medical problem and treat it. In this case, a careful history, physical examination, and screening laboratory studies by his medical attending physician identified a urinary tract infection, and an antibiotic was subsequently started. William had no known history of excessive alcohol use, but it is not unusual for hospitalized patients—even if they deny such use—to show signs of alcohol withdrawal several days into their hospitalization. For that reason, we have helped train nurses on our medical and surgical floors in the use of the Clinical Institute Withdrawal Assessment for Alcoholism, Revised, and the associated treatment protocol (Mayo-Smith 1997). Fortunately, William did not demonstrate any signs or symptoms of alcohol withdrawal during his hospitalization. It was important for the medical team to keep William well hydrated, ensure he took his medications, and keep him safe. His wife was encouraged to stay by his bedside as much as possible to provide reassurance to him when he was in a more confused and agitated state. The management of patients with delirium has been described as a marker for quality of care on a medical unit because of the possibility that patients will sustain falls or other injuries or develop bed sores (Inouye et al. 1999).

The request for psychiatric consultation for William was largely based on his symptoms of paranoia and agitation. I knew that I would need to convince the medical team that these behavioral symptoms were likely due to his medical condition. Once I explained my reasoning, the medical team was willing to continue treating William on the medical floor. I was also able to reassure them that I would continue to monitor him, make suggestions about the management of his illness, and arrange appropriate follow-up care for him, including inpatient psychiatric hospitalization, if the symptoms did not resolve with the treatment of the delirium.

Rather than just waiting for the antibiotic to successfully treat the infection, it was felt that some psychotropic medication was also required to treat his paranoia and hallucinations in order to keep William safe and comfortable. Clinical practice has favored the use of neuroleptic medication for this purpose despite the paucity of controlled clinical trials on such usage (Breitbart et al. 1996). For William, olanzapine (as needed) was ordered to treat any agitation because he had responded positively to a low dose of this antipsychotic in the past when he was manic. Given the possibility that olanzapine would aggravate his diabetes, his blood glucose levels were monitored carefully and ultimately remained unchanged. On occasion, lorazepam may be used to simply sedate a patient, especially if the behavior disturbance occurs at night when the patient should be sleeping and there are fewer staff members to manage the patient's agitation. Anecdotal reports (Gleason 2003) have also raised the possibility of using cholinesterase inhibitors to treat delirium, but William was already on donepezil so that was not an option.

It was also important to educate and reassure William's wife that William's acute symptoms were due to delirium and that it was likely they would resolve with medical treatment. This information was very helpful in allaying her fear that her husband would never get better and would have to be placed in a nursing home.

Over the next several days, I was relieved to see that William became more alert and less confused. He still had a poor recall of the week prior to his hospitalization, but his paranoia had resolved—he was no longer seeing figures lurking about. He was oriented to the date and place. He still had evidence of short-term memory impairment, as indicated by the fact that he was able to repeat to me the names of three objects but was unable to recall any of them 5 minutes later. I was especially pleased to see that William's initial difficulty naming objects shown to him had resolved. However, William continued to show some perseveration in his responses and could spontaneously generate the names of only three animals in 5 minutes. These symptoms suggested frontal lobe deficits that could be due to his resolving delirium or underlying dementia. He displayed a full range of affect and described his mood as "pretty good."

At this point, William wanted to go home, and his wife was comfortable with this plan. The medical team felt assured that his paranoia and agitation had resolved sufficiently so that he did not require a transfer to an inpatient psychiatric unit. He was discharged home with his usual psychiatric medications and was instructed to attend outpatient psychiatric follow-up. It was also suggested that his cognitive function be carefully followed. Most patients return to baseline upon resolution of their delirium; however, some patients with pre-existing dementia have residual symptoms and never return to their prior baseline (Levkoff et al. 1992). His spouse was also advised that William would be at risk for developing delirium in the future in response to acute medical illnesses, significant changes in medication, or surgical procedures requiring anesthesia. She was told that any changes in mental status should be reported to William's primary care physician, because delirium can be the first or only symptom of a serious underlying illness that requires treatment.

DISCUSSION

Delirium is a syndrome of generalized brain dysfunction which causes disturbances of attention and concentration and is common in hospitalized elderly patients. However, patients often present with psychiatric symptoms such as hallucinations, suspiciousness, and delusions, leading to a referral to a psychiatrist. It is essential to recognize the possibility of delirium and to examine the patient so as to identify the underlying medical cause or causes. Frequently, the delirium is due to the adverse effects of medications added to treat some medical condition or interactions with the patient's previously prescribed medications. Often an infection (e.g., urinary tract infection, pneumonia, etc.) is discovered. Withdrawal from alcohol or benzodiazepines can precipitate delirium in a patient with physical dependence and may not be suspected from the patient's history. Many other medical conditions (e.g., dehydration, congestive heart failure, hyperglycemia, etc.) can cause delirium. The key to treating delirium is to treat the underlying medical condition—until that resolves, it is essential to keep the patient safe and well hydrated. Psychotropic medications are sometimes used to treat agitation, hallucinations, and to provide some nighttime sedation. Generally, patients with delirium are best treated on a general medical inpatient, rather than a general psychiatric inpatient unit, where their medical needs can be addressed.

REFERENCES

American Psychiatric Association: Diagnostic and Statistical Manual of Mental Disorders, 4th Edition, Text Revision. Washington, DC, American Psychiatric Association, 2000

Breitbart W, Marotta R, Platt MM, et al: A double-blind trial of haloperidol, chlorpromazine, and lorazepam in the treatment of delirium in hospitalized AIDS patients. Am J Psychiatry 153:231–237, 1996

Gleason OC: Donepezil for postoperative delirium. Psychosomatics 44:437–438, 2003

Inouye SK, Schlesinger MJ, Lydon TJ: Delirium: a symptom of how hospital care is failing older persons and a window to improve quality of hospital care. Am J Med 106:565–573, 1999

Kawas CH: Early Alzheimer's disease. N Engl J Med 349:1056–1063, 2003

Levkoff SE, Evans DA, Liptzin B, et al: Delirium: the occurrence and persistence of symptoms among elderly hospitalized patients. Arch Intern Med 152:334–340, 1992

Mayo-Smith MF: Pharmacological management of alcohol withdrawal: a meta-analysis and evidence-based practice guideline. JAMA 278:144–151, 1997

SUGGESTED READINGS

Liptzin B, Jacobson SA: Delirium, in Kaplan and Sadock's Comprehensive Textbook of Psychiatry, 8th Edition. Edited by Sadock BJ, Sadock VA. Philadelphia, Lippincott Williams & Wilkins, 2005, pp 3693–3700

PART III

Mental Disorders Due to a General Medical Condition

CHAPTER 4

Mystery Diagnosis

Treatment of Neuropsychiatric Lyme Disease

Brian A. Fallon, M.D.

Brian A. Fallon, M.D., is Associate Professor of Clinical Psychiatry at the Columbia University College of Physicians and Surgeons, Director of Neuropsychiatry at Columbia University Medical Center, and Director of the Lyme Disease Research Program at the New York State Psychiatric Institute. In addition to his work on neuropsychiatric Lyme disease, Dr. Fallon's research interests include hypochondriasis and obsessive-compulsive disorder. Dr. Fallon recently completed a National Institutes of Health–funded study of chronic Lyme encephalopathy using both neurocognitive testing and brain imaging (PET and MRI) to determine the efficacy of a repeated course of intravenous antibiotic therapy. Currently, in addition to ongoing work on Lyme disease, Dr. Fallon is principal investigator on a multi-site study comparing pharmacologic and psychotherapeutic treatments for hypochondriasis. For more information about Lyme disease, see http://www.columbia-lyme.org.

DANIEL WAS A 66-YEAR-OLD man who was referred to me for the evaluation and treatment of hypochondriasis.

HISTORY

At age 65 and in good physical and mental health as he approached retirement, Daniel felt ready to leave work at his brokerage firm. However, during the spring of the following year, about 9 months after he had retired, Daniel began to worry that he might have a serious illness because he was experiencing weight loss, an increased need for sleep, frequent awakenings, marked fatigue during the day, memory problems, and tingling feelings in his hands. He consulted his primary care physician, who examined him and conducted a battery of tests (complete blood count to check for signs of infection or anemia; chemistry screen to look for abnormalities in electrolytes such as glucose, sodium, or potassium; thyroid studies, because thyroid abnormalities can cause a mood disorder; Lyme enzyme-linked immunosorbent assay [ELISA], a commonly used screening test for antibodies against the agent of Lyme disease; and tests for antinuclear antibodies to screen for autoimmune diseases and vitamin B_{12} because a B_{12} deficiency can cause neuropsychiatric disorders) to determine whether or not Daniel might have an underlying cause for his symptoms. The results of the evaluation and blood tests were unremarkable, except for indications of a mildly elevated serum glucose level. The physician assured Daniel that he was medically fine and that the primary cause of his symptoms was most likely psychological. Daniel was therefore referred to a psychiatrist.

The psychiatrist took a careful history and diagnosed Daniel with DSM-IV-TR hypochondriasis based on the patient's marked concern about having a serious illness despite his primary care doctor's reassurance to the contrary. Daniel's history, partly already known by the psychiatrist, revealed that 12 years earlier he had had a hypochondriacal episode accompanied by agitation during which he worried he might have cancer; that episode was quite severe, did not respond to treatment with a tricyclic antidepressant or a selective serotonin reuptake inhibitor (SSRI), and required electroconvulsive therapy (ECT), after which Daniel's agitated hypochondriacal state completely resolved. Daniel had been well over the subsequent years (a fact confirmed by his wife). The psychiatrist who had treated Daniel previously felt that the current hypochondriacal preoccupation was most likely precipitated by the stress associated with the change from a full-time job to retirement. Although Daniel denied being anxious about his retirement, the presence of unconscious conflicts over this life change seemed likely.

Given reports that patients with hypochondriasis may respond well to SSRIs (Fallon 2004; Fallon et al. 1993a), Daniel was initially treated with medications for obsessional disorders and generalized anxiety. Sertraline (Zoloft), up to 200 mg/day, was given for 10 weeks without benefit. This was followed by venlafaxine (Effexor) at dosages up to 300 mg/day with adjunctive risperidone (Risperdal), an atypical antipsychotic; however, this new medication regimen also was of no benefit and Daniel's agitation increased. The psychiatrist then recommended ECT because this had worked well previously. However, 10 ECT treatments were not beneficial. At this point, the psychiatrist felt a second opinion was needed and referred Daniel to me because I was conducting a clinical trial using fluvoxamine, another SSRI, for patients with hypochondriasis (Fallon et al. 2003).

DIAGNOSIS

On first meeting Daniel, I was struck by his high degree of anxiety. In a manner similar to that of the most severely ill obsessive-compulsive patient, he repeated his symptoms and his questions for reassurance over and over again. Spending 60 minutes with this man was difficult because of his profound distress, repetitive statements, and inability to be reassured for more than a short period of time. His wife sat quietly by his side and was supportive of him but was clearly very tired. Daniel told me that he was concerned that he might have a serious disease (e.g., cancer) because of his 25-lb weight loss the prior spring; the throbbing, pulsing feelings in his body; the tingling in his hands and feet; the episodic sharp stabbing pains in his right side; his severe daytime fatigue; and his concentration and memory problems. His wife added that he was easily startled by sounds and confirmed that he spent much of his day worrying about his illness. I reviewed the medical evaluation conducted thus far, which confirmed that there was no identifiable cause for Daniel's physical symptoms. I agreed to enter him into our study of hypochondriasis. My initial diagnosis for Daniel was hypochondriasis with poor insight. The term "poor insight" was applied because most of the time Daniel did not recognize that his concern about having an illness was excessive or unreasonable.

Initial Treatment Plan and Course

The treatment of Daniel's hypochondriasis with fluvoxamine entailed starting at 50 mg/day and increasing the daily dosage by 50 mg each week to a total final dosage of 300 mg/day. The dosage was started low because patients with marked anxiety and somatoform disorders are often hypersensitive to their bodily sensations and might react adversely to early side effects of the medication. I saw him in weekly sessions, alone for the first half of the session and accompanied by his wife for the second half. His anxiety was so dramatic and all consuming that I was not confident I could obtain a good history from him alone.

Over the course of the first several weeks of my work with Daniel, he continued to focus on the thought that he must have a serious disease as he was not getting better with the medication I was giving him. His feelings of tingling, throbbing, and numbness were extending to other parts of his body, and he had developed new-onset shooting pains down his arms and a couple of episodes of stabbing shoulder pains in his right side. He had consulted again with his primary care doctor who did another cursory set of laboratory tests and stated that this man might have an early "mild" diabetic condition that could be contributing to the tingling but that no intervention was indicated at this point.

I had three reactions to this patient. First, I was struck by the severity of his hypochondriasis and the intensity of his self-absorption. Given that he was not capable of putting his thoughts about his illness out of his mind, his waking moments were consumed by dread and repeated efforts to gain reassurance from his wife. Second, I admired the tenacity and endurance of his wife; given that I found spending 45 minutes with this man extremely trying, I wondered how she was able to handle him all day long. Third, as it became clear by the fifth week of treatment that he was not improving (by then he was taking 250 mg/day of fluvoxamine), I wondered if underneath it all Daniel might be right and that perhaps he did have a medical illness that had not yet been detected. However, I did not want to raise these doubts as I imagined that my questioning his medical diagnosis would raise his anxiety level even further.

Reevaluation of Diagnosis and Treatment Plan

In the midst of my doubts, I reconsidered the possibility of Daniel's having Lyme disease. Early in my work with patients with hypochondriasis, I had seen a few patients with multiple unexplained somatic symptoms who had been told that they had a somatization disorder or hypochondriasis but whom I felt might have undiagnosed and untreated Lyme disease. Those patients, however, were different from Daniel. They had the classic chronic fatigue–like symptom cluster of myalgias, arthralgias, marked fatigue, a need for 10–14 hours of sleep at night, memory problems, and headaches; the results of their blood tests also supported the diagnosis and so I referred them to internists who treated them with good results.

Because he lived in a Lyme endemic area and was an avid gardener, the probability of Daniel having been bitten by a tick was high. However, he did not recall finding a tick bite, nor did he recall having had the classic red circular expanding rash (*erythema migrans*) that is the diagnostic hallmark of Lyme disease. Some of his symptoms, however, were suggestive of neurological Lyme disease. These included his paresthesias (numbness and tingling) and radicular (shooting or stabbing) pains, which are signs of possible peripheral nerve and nerve root involvement, respectively; his memory and attention problems could be suggestive of encephalopathy. However, certainly the paresthesias might be explained by anxiety, as people who hyperventilate, for example, can easily self-induce sensations of numbness and tingling in their extremities. Furthermore, Daniel's memory and attention problems might reflect his poor attention secondary to severe anxiety, resulting in poor encoding and storage of memory.

As a researcher who specializes in neuropsychiatric manifestations of Lyme disease, I did not want to deprive this man of the additional testing that might help to clarify the diagnosis. However, as a clinician faced with a severely anxious man who clearly had a history of classic hypochondriasis, I did not want to raise questions that might worsen his anxiety.

At week 6, Daniel came to my office with his usual plethora of multiple somatic symptoms and severe, unimproved anxiety. Midway during the evaluation session, he asked if I would take a look at a rash on his chest. I agreed to do so. The rash was 5 inches in diameter with a crisp margin, not itchy, and red in color with faint discoloration in the center. The rash was a textbook Lyme rash. I looked at him and wondered, "Now what do I do? This sure looks like a Lyme rash. Do I tell this hypochondriacal patient that I think he has Lyme disease?"

Tentative Diagnosis: Lyme Disease

I decided to tell Daniel about my tentative diagnosis of the rash; in response he asked with dread in his voice, "Is it serious, Doc?" By that point in my academic career, I had written a number of papers documenting the serious neuropsychiatric effects of Lyme disease (Fallon and Nields 1994; Fallon et al. 1993b), a disease caused by a spirochete that, like the spirochete that causes syphilis, travels within days of the tick bite through the blood to the brain and can cause a variety of severe neuropsychiatric disorders, such as mania, psychosis, depression, memory loss, and prolonged unrelenting anxiety attacks. These patients can be ill for many months or years. I felt it reasonable that an undetected tick bite with spirochetal transmission the prior spring could account for many of Daniel's symptoms that had started 7 months earlier (spring is peak nymphal tick biting time), including Daniel's severe anxiety.

My response to his question was, "The good news about Lyme disease is that if you catch it early, people can do very well with treatment. I feel confident that you will do well." Given that I suspected he had contracted Lyme disease about 7 months earlier, his time frame of identification was not exactly early, but neither was it considered late (i.e., 2 or 3 years after infection). I indicated that we needed to do additional blood tests and discuss this situation with his primary care doctor.

The reader only superficially familiar with Lyme disease might wonder how Daniel could have Lyme disease when it was already indicated that the screening blood test was negative, or reason with himself or herself, "I thought the rash was a sign of early Lyme disease and that it occurs right after the tick bite. If that is true, then how could this man have Lyme disease as the explanation for the symptoms over the prior 7 months?" or, "This man didn't have joint swelling; how could he have Lyme disease?"

In answer to the first question, the blood tests, while helpful, are not always positive. One can test negative and have Lyme disease due to a poor antibody response to the invading organism or the poor sensitivity of the screening test for Lyme disease (sensitivity is about 70%). Because of the problems with the screening test (the ELISA), I usually order the more highly specific and informative follow-up Lyme Western blot test as my first line of testing. This test is more informative because the laboratory will tell you which bands, markers of the immune system's antibody response, are present. A healthy immune response against infection with the spirochete that causes Lyme disease (*Borrelia burgdorferi*) would be the development of five or more bands on the IgG Western blot, which would also count as a positive test by Centers for Disease Control and Prevention (CDC) standards. An immune response that has three or four of the CDC-specified bands would be considered suggestive of Lyme disease but would not meet the CDC criteria. Physicians ordering the Western blot test should add "please report all bands" to the script, as most laboratories will report only the 10 bands identified by the CDC as being specific to Lyme disease unless asked to do otherwise; other bands, such as the ones identified by the 31- or 34-kDa markers, are highly specific for Lyme disease as well and their presence would provide additional valuable information. The CDC does not include these in the list of the top 10 specific bands because in frequency of occurrence they are numbers 11 and 12, respectively; in other words, although highly specific (e.g., the 31-kDa marker was used to create early Lyme vaccines), these antibodies are not among the 10 most frequently seen. In ordering tests for Lyme disease, I avoid commercial laboratories, which tend to use tests with low sensitivity, and instead send the blood to two different Lyme reference laboratories that have different techniques but excellent quality control.

The second question is also a good one. The Lyme rash is the hallmark sign of early Lyme disease, but rashes can also appear later in the course of the illness. These late-appearing rashes, known as satellite rashes, are thought to be due to intermittent travel of the spirochete through the blood stream and seeding of the skin, resulting in the erythema migrans rash. I assumed that Daniel probably had had a rash last spring after the presumed tick bite but that it was not seen most likely because it occurred on a part of the body not easily visible (e.g., at the back of his knees, in his hair).

The third question is a common one. It is frequently assumed that Lyme disease is characterized only by a rash or swollen joints. In fact, in cases of neuropsychiatric Lyme disease, although many patients have joint pain, most do not have joint swelling and some do not have any joint involvement at all.

What happened with Daniel? I called his primary care doctor while Daniel was in the office with me and informed him of my suspicions. There was silence on the other end of the line. I imagined him thinking, "Who is this psychiatrist and why is he telling me that my patient who is an obvious hypochondriac actually has Lyme disease?" I immediately relieved him of the need to act by stating that I would order the blood work and forward the results to him. The primary care doctor expressed skepticism that Lyme disease was the correct diagnosis, but he was willing to provide the antibiotic treatment should the tests come back positive. He also agreed to see Daniel's rash, and he subsequently concurred with me that it looked like an erythema migrans rash.

The results of the blood tests were remarkable. The first laboratory reported a positive screening (ELISA) test but a negative confirmatory test (Western blot). The second laboratory reported a negative ELISA but a positive IgG Western blot that met full CDC criteria. I then told Daniel that his rash and these test results together supported our hypothesis that he had been exposed to an agent of Lyme disease and that one more set of tests should be considered: a lumbar puncture (spinal tap) and a brain single-photon emission computed tomography (SPECT) scan. Daniel had no interest in having the lumbar puncture, particularly when I informed him it had been well established in the literature (Coyle et al. 1995) that some patients with neurologic Lyme disease may have a misleadingly normal-appearing cerebrospinal fluid (negative Lyme ELISA, normal protein and white blood cell count); the lumbar puncture could help confirm the diagnosis only if the spinal fluid showed typical markers, but it could not exclude neurological Lyme disease.

Daniel was willing to go as an outpatient to the hospital's nuclear medicine division to obtain a brain SPECT scan. Most insurance policies cover the cost of a brain SPECT scan to evaluate a patient for possible Lyme disease. The scan procedure itself is relatively comfortable for patients. A peripheral intravenous catheter is placed in the arm and a small amount of a radioactive tracer that allows the SPECT cameras that circle around the head to assess the blood flow of the brain is injected. Daniel's SPECT scan showed a pattern of blood flow that is typically seen among patients with a vasculitis or encephalitis, as in Lyme disease. This pattern is one of moderately or severely decreased blood flow throughout the brain in a patchy pattern so that some areas have better flow than others. The official term for this pattern is *heterogeneous hypoperfusion*.

Revised and Final Diagnosis: Anxiety Disorder Due to Lyme Disease

Daniel's history of multiple somatic symptoms, residence in a Lyme endemic area, satellite erythema migrans rash, and positive blood tests confirmed the diagnosis of Lyme disease. His severe, unrelenting anxiety despite excellent prior psychiatric therapy was a critical clue to an underlying medical cause, and the abnormal results on the brain SPECT scan confirmed central nervous system involvement in his disorder.

TREATMENT

By the time all of this testing was completed, Daniel had had 9 weeks of fluvoxamine and his anxiety continued to be quite intense. Although he experienced some measure of relief in just knowing that he had a medical cause for his symptoms, he was still extremely agitated and compulsively sought reassurance that his symptoms would improve. I opted not to give him further psychiatric medication but rather to provide supportive psychotherapy as he entered the antibiotic phase of his treatment.

Although treatment with intravenous antibiotics is the usual recommendation for neurological Lyme disease, oral antibiotics may be sufficient if the blood-brain barrier is inflamed enough to allow antibiotics to cross. Certain antibiotics are better at crossing the blood-brain barrier than others, including the oral antibiotics doxycycline and minocycline and the intravenous antibiotics ceftriaxone and cefotaxime. Daniel's primary care doctor agreed to initially treat Daniel with doxcycline, a standard first-line treatment. I warned Daniel and his wife that it is not uncommon for patients to initially feel worse after beginning antibiotics. The emergence of transient arthritic or new neuropsychiatric symptoms in patients after treatment is usually interpreted as a positive sign that the treatment is resulting in bactericidal activity, leading to inflammation and hence new symptoms. Indeed, during the first week of treatment, Daniel experienced a few episodes of new sharp pains to his knees, a brief episode of transient paranoia (he suspected his neighbor of peering through his window), and more restless sleep. Therefore we knew that the treatment was working.

Within 6 weeks of beginning antibiotic treatment, Daniel began feeling markedly better. His paresthesias and radicular pains had remitted, his psychic anxiety had diminished, and his restlessness was improved. The paranoia did not return. By week 12, Daniel was nearly free of symptoms. Whereas previously he had been completely self-absorbed with his fear of illness, by the end of treatment he had independently chosen to volunteer his time working with the homeless population in his local town. The amelioration of his anxiety and the resolution of his physical symptoms were accompanied by a marked improvement in his personality as well. This man who had been so difficult to live with when ill became a generous, other-minded individual. His wife was grateful to have her husband back.

Although the optimal duration of antibiotic therapy for patients with neuropsychiatric Lyme disease is not known, in this case the recommendation was for 1 month beyond the point when the patient felt well. Daniel therefore received 4 months of doxycycline and, on follow-up 12 months later, was continuing to do well without the antibiotics. The every-other-week supportive therapy ended during his last month of antibiotic therapy. He was advised to contact me should any questions about neuropsychiatric Lyme disease arise in the future.

DISCUSSION

A Lyme disease patient's response to antibiotics is not always as rapid and complete as in this case. A patient's symptoms may partially improve with antibiotics, but the patient may be left with marked fatigue, symptoms of depression and hyperarousal syndromes, and/or cognitive problems. Further, the patient's marriage, family, or work life may be severely effected by the patient's Lyme symptoms. If a patient develops chronic symptoms that improve only gradually, then a reappraisal of the patient's life goals in light of the new limitations may be warranted. In these situations, mental health providers can be enormously helpful by working with these patients and using the full armamentarium of treatments, including supportive psychotherapy; pharmacotherapy of the attention, mood, fatigue, or hyperarousal syndromes; and/or marital and family therapy. After the initial course of antibiotics, psychotropic medications are much more likely to be beneficial. Because it is never entirely clear when the patient with chronic symptoms after contracting Lyme disease is cleared of all active infection, many patients are treated with repeated and/or longer courses of antibiotics accompanied by psychotropic medications. The goal of treatment by a mental health practitioner is to educate and support the patient while relieving his or her symptoms in an adjunctive fashion as the primary care doctor treats the underlying infection. The practitioner would also be wise to ensure that the primary care physician has ruled out other medical causes for the patient's marked fatigue and muscle pain, such as coinfection with the tick-borne agent *babesia microti*, which causes an illness called "babesiosis" that is commonly characterized by severe fatigue, muscle pains, and night sweats. Finally, the mental health provider should make use of the excellent cognitive-behavioral strategies for chronic fatigue (Prins et al. 2001). Teaching the patient that remaining in bed for long periods of time leads to muscle weakness from deconditioning and further fatigue during exertion can help motivate the individual to start a gradual and progressive exercise regimen.

This case demonstrates several important points. First, when a patient's psychiatric disorder does not respond to treatments that should work or have worked in the past, then the psychiatrist should reevaluate the diagnosis and search for an underlying medical disorder. This case underlines the point that hypochondriacal patients can become medically sick also. Second, knowledge about Lyme disease and the finer points of its diagnosis is essential for mental health providers who work in Lyme endemic areas; as in this case, being aware of the poor sensitivity of Lyme screening tests and increased sensitivity of the Western blot test, the variability in results across laboratories, and the utility of functional brain imaging can help to make a correct diagnosis. Third, not all cases of neuropsychiatric Lyme disease follow the typical pattern. Although most patients present with severe fatigue, depression, headaches, paresthesias, cognitive problems, and joint pain, some present, as did Daniel, with heightened anxiety and arousal with multisystemic complaints but few joint symptoms. Furthermore, although treatment for 4 months in Daniel's case led to a complete and sustained resolution of symptoms, relapse occurs in some patients several months to a year after the course of antibiotics has been completed. In these cases, retreatment with antibiotics can be helpful. Finally, as physicians, psychiatrists are in a unique position to work collaboratively with primary care doctors and internists. Psychiatrists order additional tests in cases of suspected Lyme disease, the results of which can supply helpful information for the primary care doctor who may be less familiar with the disease. In addition, a psychiatrist can support a primary care doctor's efforts by providing him or her with a consultation letter that summarizes the psychiatrist's impressions and findings, thereby bolstering the primary care doctor's confidence as he or she conducts the antibiotic treatment for a patient with neuropsychiatric Lyme disease.

REFERENCES

Coyle PK, Schutzer SE, Deng Z, et al: Detection of Borrelia burgdorferi–specific antigen in antibody-negative cerebrospinal fluid in neurologic Lyme disease. Neurology 45:2010–2015, 1995

Fallon BA: Pharmacotherapy of somatoform disorders. J Psychosom Res 56:455–460, 2004

Fallon BA, Nields JA: Lyme disease: a neuropsychiatric illness. Am J Psychiatry 151:1571–1583, 1994

Fallon BA, Liebowitz MR, Salmon E, et al: Fluoxetine for hypochondriacal patients without major depression. J Clin Psychopharmacol 13:438–441, 1993a

Fallon BA, Nields JA, Parsons B, et al: Psychiatric manifestations of Lyme borreliosis. J Clin Psychiatry 54:263–268, 1993b

Fallon BA, Qureshi AI, Schneier FR, et al: An open trial of fluvoxamine for hypochondriasis. Psychosomatics 44:298–303, 2003

Prins JB, Lleijenberg G, Bazelmans E, et al: Cognitive behavior therapy for chronic fatigue syndrome: a multicenter randomized controlled trial. Lancet 357:841–847, 2001

PART IV

Substance-Related Disorders

CHAPTER 5

Refinishing Without Rebuilding

Dual-Focus Schema Therapy for Personality Disorder and Addiction

Samuel A. Ball, Ph.D.
Bruce J. Rounsaville, M.D.

Samuel A. Ball, Ph.D., is an Associate Professor of Psychiatry at the Yale University School of Medicine and Director of Research for The APT Foundation, a private nonprofit agency providing treatment and research programs for substance abuse in the Greater New Haven area. After completing his Ph.D. in 1990, Dr. Ball joined the Yale faculty and has held several clinical and training leadership roles. He has directed both outpatient and residential programs and consulted to methadone maintenance and dual diagnosis programs. For the past 15 years, he has coordinated psychology training in the Division of Substance Abuse, supervised psychotherapy, taught a psychotherapy seminar, and now directs a research education program for psychology interns and psychiatry residents. Dr. Ball has been principal investigator or coinvestigator on numerous National Institute on Drug Abuse (NIDA)–funded diagnostic and treatment studies, including serving as the Director of Training for the New England Node of the NIDA Clinical Trials Network and Chairperson for its national training subcommittee. His research has focused on the assessment and treatment implications of personality dimensions, personality disorders, and multidimensional subtypes in substance abuse. Dr. Ball is the developer of dual-focus schema therapy for personality disorders and drug abuse (in collaboration with Jeffrey Young, Ph.D.), which has shown promising results in several clinical trials. Ongoing research is focused on intervention strategies for refractory drug abusers and diagnostic studies focused on the prevalence and correlates of personality disorders (particularly Cluster A) in homeless clients.

Bruce J. Rounsaville, M.D., is Professor of Psychiatry at the Yale University School of Medicine and Director of the U.S. Veterans Administration New England Mental Illness Research Education and Clinical Center. Since he joined the Yale faculty in 1977, Dr. Rounsaville has focused his clinical research career on the diagnosis and treatment of patients with alcohol and drug dependence. Using modern methods for psychiatric diagnosis, he was among the first to call attention to the high rates of dual diagnosis in drug abusers. As a member of the Work Group to Revise DSM-III, Dr. Rounsaville was a leader in adopting the drug dependence syndrome concept into the DSM-III-R and DSM-IV Substance Use Disorders criteria. He has been a strong advocate for adopting psychotherapies shown to be effective in rigorous clinical trials. Dr. Rounsaville has also played a key role in clinical trials on the efficacy of a number of important treatments, including outpatient clonidine/naltrexone for opioid detoxification, naltrexone for treatment of alcohol dependence, cognitive-behavioral treatment for cocaine dependence, and disulfiram treatment for cocaine abusers. He has contributed extensively to the psychiatric treatment research literature with over 300 articles and six books.

HISTORY

Frank was a 24-year-old, single, European-American, male, self-employed furniture refinisher who was referred by his substance abuse counselor to me (S.A.B.) for a psychotherapy research protocol for patients with a personality disorder. His counselor had referred him out of frustration over Frank's extreme inconsistency in an aftercare recovery group in which he was struggling to maintain abstinence and contribute productively to the group process.

Frank lived with his parents and grandparents in a two-family home in a small, urban, working class neighborhood. His grandparents were Holocaust survivors who had immigrated to the United States 50 years earlier. Frank's parents and grandparents wanted a better life for Frank and his younger sister and expressed this by imposing extremely rigid standards for behavior and expectations for achievement on them. Frank's grandparents communicated the beliefs that carelessness had deadly consequences and that people were either totally good or bad. The family atmosphere was one of intolerance for ambiguity and imperfection, and anxious preoccupation with the risk of sudden, traumatic death if mistakes in behavior or judgment were made. This environment apparently interacted powerfully with Frank's childhood temperament of negative emotionality, behavioral constraint, and preference for order and predictability. In contrast, his sister seemed to be easygoing, flexible, and better able to adapt to the family's anxious rigidity. Frank's mother was obsessed with the dead-end nature of her husband's factory job, and her achievement expectations for her two children became increasingly intense as her husband's work performance deteriorated due to his alcoholism. Frank's father judged careless mistakes and poor performance very harshly, and he could be physically abusive. During his early adolescence, Frank became attracted to a peer group that appeared to lack any sense of rigid standards, and he recalled experiencing a great relief from these friendships, referring to them as "my liberation from Auschwitz." With these friends, he used various drugs and engaged in drug-related delinquent behaviors (property destruction, theft and deceit, rule violation) consistent with a diagnosis of conduct disorder (adolescent onset, mild type). While at home and in school, he was a model son and student; on the weekends with friends, he developed a reputation for being out of control.

Frank began drinking alcohol at age 12 years and using marijuana at age 14; by his sophomore year in high school, he was a regular weekend user. A varsity athlete in football and baseball, Frank graduated high school near the top of his class and received an athletic and academic scholarship for college. During his freshman year, he began using cocaine and in his sophomore year began selling drugs on campus. After being arrested, he lost his scholarship and was cut from the baseball team. His drug use escalated, he failed classes for the first time in his life, and he dropped out of college subsequent to his being rearrested for selling cocaine and being sent to a long-term residential therapeutic community in lieu of incarceration. After an initial struggle with this demanding treatment environment, he became a model resident and thrived within a program emphasizing a strong hierarchy, unambiguous rules, and caring confrontation. He rose to the highest status level in the program and, through his assigned work position in the program's maintenance department, resumed an old hobby of refinishing furniture, for which he showed significant talent. After completing the program, he moved into a room in his parent's home and rapidly developed a successful small business refinishing antiques and other furniture. His family required that he attend outpatient aftercare as a condition of being allowed to live in the house. Shortly after beginning his outpatient group counseling, his refinishing work exposed him to a high potency solvent/stripper that he began to inhale more than was necessary. He reported enjoying "losing my mind while I worked" without recognizing that he had relapsed. His inhalation of this chemical increased and his behavior in group counseling at the outpatient program became increasingly erratic. He was then referred to the on-site psychotherapy research study.

DIAGNOSIS

As a patient in this research study, Frank underwent an extensive battery of tests to establish his baseline functioning and symptoms before beginning individual therapy. The findings from the Structured Clinical Interview for DSM-IV (First et al. 1997) indicated Axis I diagnoses of recent-onset inhalant abuse and longer-term cocaine, cannabis, and alcohol dependence. On Axis II, Frank's symptoms met structured diagnostic criteria for obsessive-compulsive personality disorder (OCPD) and antisocial personality disorder (ASPD). ASPD is a highly heterogeneous diagnosis in substance abusers (i.e., almost innumerable symptom combinations are possible) (Cecero et al. 1999), with most patients not having a classic psychopathic personality. Frank did not exhibit symptoms of aggression, disregard for others' safety, or lack of remorse. Careful interview probing (Rounsaville et al. 1998) indicated that his symptoms of unlawful behavior, deceitfulness, and impulsive and irresponsible behavior were best understood as secondary to his early-onset substance abuse.

Frank endorsed lifelong symptoms of overpreoccupation with details, perfectionism, rigidity, and overconscientiousness that were consistent with OCPD. These symptoms and OCPD are fairly uncommon in substance abusers, particularly those with ASPD (Rounsaville et al. 1998). However, this apparent contradiction characterized Frank quite well and seemed consistent with the split lifestyle he had developed. High perfectionism, achievement, and responsibility at home preceded the onset of substance abuse and continued in parallel with irresponsible, deceitful, and antisocial behavior with his drug-using peer group. Furthermore, on the NEO Five-Factor Inventory (Costa and McCrae 1992), Frank scored low on agreeableness and high on neuroticism and conscientiousness.

TREATMENT

Dual-Focus Schema Therapy

Dual-focus schema therapy (DFST) (Ball 1998, 2003) does not regard the Axis II diagnoses as being reliable or valid constructs for the purpose of treatment planning. Instead, DFST hypothesizes that personality disorders reflect combinations of extreme personality traits, Axis I symptoms, and maladaptive schemas and coping styles that provide better targets for psychoeducational and change strategies. Beck et al. (1990) and Young et al. (2003) have defined maladaptive schemas as enduring, unconditional, negative themes about oneself, others, and the environment that develop early in life and then become reinforced, elaborated on, and perpetuated in adulthood. They are triggered by everyday events and mood states and generate high levels of affect, self-defeating consequences, and harm to others and are deeply entrenched and difficult to change. According to Young et al.'s (2003) model, 18 early maladaptive schemas are grouped into five broad domains: 1) disconnection and rejection, 2) impaired autonomy and performance, 3) impaired limits, 4) other-directedness, and 5) overvigilance and inhibition. Frank's primary early maladaptive schema was unrelenting standards (one of the overvigilance/inhibition schemas), characterized by perfectionism, rigid rules, and preoccupation with time and efficiency. This core theme appeared to originate from the toxic interaction of his temperament and the intense family environment of anxious expectations. He also had a secondary schema of mistrust/abuse related to the physical and emotional abuse he experienced for careless mistakes and acting out with a delinquent peer group.

Maladaptive coping styles are long-standing responses to the distressing thoughts, feelings, memories, or impulses associated with schema activation. Individuals are often unaware of the various internal states and external situations that can activate their schemas and coping styles. Avoidant and compensatory coping strategies temporarily reduce the affect associated with schemas but have the unintended effect over time of perpetuating the schemas (Young et al. 2003). Frank had a long-standing pattern of putting enormous pressure on himself and others. Any minor deviation from perfectionistic goals or expectations imposed by authority figures (e.g., parents, teachers, coaches, addiction professionals) triggered in him an equally powerful desire to use drugs, be irresponsible, give up on himself, and act out antisocially to nullify these expectations. Whenever he anticipated that he could not master something, he became distressed and would avoid commitments, withdraw from the source of expectations, procrastinate, or "forget" to complete tasks. Drug use provided a ready-made excuse for why he could not meet the imposed expectations. These avoidance strategies inadvertently reinforced his unrelenting standards schema as he would then have to redouble his efforts to obtain desired outcomes or "make good" with the people he had disappointed. In some ways, his addictive behavior and associated duplicity became a kind of compensatory coping style, with antisocial acting out providing some mastery over his unrelenting standards. As mentioned, Frank's ASPD symptoms were conceptualized as secondary manifestations and expected to fully remit with complete abstinence from substance use, whereas his OCPD symptoms could conceivably worsen with abstinence.

Course and Components of Treatment

Frank was treated with DFST (Ball 1998, 2003) by me (S.A.B.) within the context of a 24-week individual psychotherapy research protocol. This manual-guided, cognitive-behavioral therapy integrates a schema-focused approach (Young et al. 2003) with symptom-focused relapse-prevention coping skills interventions (Kadden et al. 1992) to treat the interrelated symptoms of substance abuse and a personality disorder. It consists of a set of individualized core and elective topics. The first stage of DFST involves the integration of relapse-prevention work with an identification and education about early maladaptive schemas and coping styles and their association with substance use and other presenting life problems. A technically eclectic but theoretically integrated series of cognitive, behavioral, experiential, and therapy relationship change strategies for the schemas and coping styles defines the second stage of DFST.

Relapse Prevention and Problem Identification and Solving

At the beginning of DFST, Frank was abusing cocaine and the refinishing solvent once weekly and alcohol and marijuana every other day. During the first 2 months of therapy, I (S.A.B.) remained highly focused on helping him reestablish abstinence and prevent relapse. This work included the identification of intrapersonal and interpersonal precipitants for Frank's substance use and teaching him specific coping skills for these high-risk situations. For Frank, this involved assertiveness training to resist pressure from his friends to hang out, stopping his usual pattern of bar hopping on Fridays and Saturdays, refraining from purchasing volatile furniture strippers, and redeveloping leisure and athletic activities to cope with boredom and drug cravings. Our therapeutic alliance was strengthened by our focusing on these skills and addressing some of the issues arising in his concurrent group counseling sessions. Before he was referred to me, he had been a model group member and had maintained abstinence. He demanded much of himself and others in the group and was rigid about everyone making the correct decisions to support recovery. He rapidly lost his credibility in the group when he started missing appointments. His relapses were addressed in the group, and he found flaws in any suggestions made by fellow patients. In subsequent group sessions, Frank adopted a defensive stance whenever other patients noted the discrepancy between his high recovery standards and his actual behavior.

Psychoeducation and Case Conceptualization

After 1 month of DFST, Frank had reduced his substance use to weekends. Therapy shifted toward psychoeducation about the schema model through completion and review of four questionnaires developed by Young to measure 1) schemas, 2) parental origins, 3) avoidant coping, and 4) compensatory coping (Young 1994, 1995; Young and Brown 1994; Young and Rygh 1994). Frank also read all of the handouts on personality traits, schemas, and disorders given to him as homework and was eager to discuss in detail the similarities and differences of what he had read with his own unique situation.

Over this second month, I explained the interaction of his personality traits (especially his high neuroticism and conscientiousness on the NEO Five-Factor Inventory) (Costa and McCrae 1992) with his parents' and grandparents' behaviors and how these combined to foster the development of an "unrelenting standards" schema. I described how it appeared that during very early adolescence he began alternating between avoidant and overcompensating styles of coping aided by his substance abuse and peer group. Several sessions were devoted to revisiting this case formulation based on his very critical feedback. I found the minute level of detailed corrections he provided quite stifling and felt the collaborative spirit of our discussions had been lost. This became my first opportunity to introduce the different kinds of change strategies (described below) used to modify the schemas and coping styles. Specifically, I shared with Frank my frustration with our attempts to make the conceptualization 100% accurate, and he responded with disapproval of my characterization of him and indicated he felt trapped by the interpretations. I pointed out how our struggle around the conceptualization was an example of his schema in action. After becoming initially argumentative, Frank had a sudden moment of clarity for the value of such here-and-now work within the session. The push for significant changes in Frank's thinking, feeling, relating, and behaving began after he felt I understood the rationality for his self-defeating behavioral cycle and resistance to change.

Cognitive Change Strategies

The goal of cognitive change strategies is to identify dysfunctional thinking associated with schemas and coping ("When I can't do something exactly right, I should give up and get high"), disputing this schema-based thinking, and then learning the validity and value of alternative explanations ("Being human means being imperfect, and using drugs makes minor problems bigger"). Frank's high intelligence and tendency to argue over details served him well during these exercises. He appeared quite comfortable with rational disputes and role-play dialogues aimed at questioning the validity of his "unrelenting standards" schema or the usefulness of his maladaptive coping styles. His achievement of complete abstinence in the third month further suppressed his avoidant and compensatory coping, and the perfectionistic and achievement side of his identity became stronger. As his unrelenting standards schema intensified, he began trying to become a model therapy patient. A cost-benefit analysis of his "unrelenting standards" schema was conducted, and he took the risk of talking about some of his imperfections with group members and his father. Cognitive techniques aimed at changing his dichotomous view of his own and others' recovery as either all good/sober or all bad/relapsed were less successful.

Behavior Change Strategies

Behavior change strategies are not limited to any specific phase of DFST. Early in treatment, Frank and I (S.A.B) focused on changing his drug use and negative behavior in his counseling group. Later work focused on his developing adaptive coping skills specifically aimed at decreasing maladaptive avoidance and overcompensation. An important component of this work was his recognition (through our open discussion) of the self-defeating nature of his various all-or-nothing splits (good versus bad patient, avoiding versus overcompensating, OCPD versus ASPD symptoms, perfectionistic versus careless, recovering versus relapsed). We identified a new goal of not trying to suppress or dismiss his negative sides but rather to moderate the extreme nature of his behavioral choices so that he might express himself less intensely and rediscover some areas of fun in his life. Through graded-task assignments and in-session rehearsal, skills training focused particularly on communicating assertively rather than aggressively. Another important skill was learning to accept the smaller, incremental steps of good-enough work from himself and others, accepting directions from people he did not respect, and no longer procrastinating in his plan to resume athletic activity (e.g., join a softball league or gym).

Experiential and Affect Reprocessing Strategies

Although Frank seemed cognitively persuaded by many of our dispute exercises and through behavioral work gained some acceptance of his different sides, he did not experience much affective change with regard to his schemas. DFST uses experiential techniques to heighten emotional and cognitive awareness of schemas and their origins through allowing visualization of past upsetting events (typically from childhood), emotional ventilation, and the substitution of more adaptive (adult) explanations for what happened and why. Frank was quite adept at these guided mental imagery exercises, and he was able to develop an intellectual understanding for the early origins of his schemas and possible motivations of his parents and grandparents. In addition, he was able to see the ways that he had adopted or inherited his father's perfectionism, demands, expectations, and alcoholism, and he became convinced of the need to establish a different approach to his own adult life. However, he was mostly unwilling or unable to access emotions related to these past events and was unwilling to express anger toward or blame his family for his difficulties. Over the last months of therapy, Frank refused to do some experiential tasks such as writing exercises (e.g., expressing honest, painful feelings to his parents in a letter that was not sent) or role-play enactments.

Therapy Relationship Strategies

As with behavior change, therapy relationship strategies are not limited to a specific phase of DFST. An empathically nurturing and limit-setting approach is the overall therapeutic style. Young et al. (2003) also recommends providing schema-specific adjustments to this style (e.g., nonjudgmental flexibility for an unrelenting standards schema) for the purpose of "limited re-parenting" to provide what was not available during the patient's earlier development. Other relational strategies focused on the schema and coping styles that were activated in the therapy session. For example, through processing his "perfectionistic" versus his "acting out" identity split in his individual versus his group therapy work, Frank gradually reported feeling less pressure to behave in specific ways. As evidence of his growing acceptance of himself as an imperfect patient, I supportively pointed to Frank's willingness to challenge my conceptualization of his problems, episodic substance use, occasional homework noncompliance, and resistance to some of the emotion-focused work. I shared with him my view that he was doing very well and told him that I very much respected and liked him as a person. Other strategies included my modeling an acceptance of my own mistakes, processing the reasons for his homework noncompliance, and empathically confronting his dichotomous views of me and significant others in his life. Over time he became increasingly able to express anger or frustration with me and respect for his group counseling peers whose productivity and recovery he could not control.

Because of the time constraints of therapy and Frank's preference not to delve too deeply into emotional issues, I used an occupationally relevant, furniture restoration metaphor to frame our therapeutic relationship and goals. Specifically, we talked about how the goal of restoring a fine piece of furniture is not to completely rebuild it but to make necessary repairs and refinishing so that its basic character is displayed in a way that can be better appreciated. The elimination of all natural (e.g., biologically based traits) or acquired imperfections (e.g., early maladaptive experiences, schemas, coping behaviors, addictions) in the "wood" is neither a realistic nor a necessarily appropriate therapy or work goal. Rather, successful completion of a complex task involving work on something created in the past depends on targeted applications or interventions designed to bring out the inherent value of the "piece." Through this therapy relationship metaphor, I think Frank was able to experience some limited reparenting through my acceptance of both his virtues and his flaws as a human being.

DISCUSSION

DFST (Ball 1998, 2003) does not have the unrealistic goal of curing a chronic, life-defining personality disorder, and Frank's OCPD certainly did not go into full remission through a 24-week, manual-guided treatment focused on underlying schemas and coping styles. Instead, realistic treatment goals were achieved, including reduced Axis I symptoms (substance abuse) and improved self-esteem, relationships, and work functioning. Despite a course of treatment with several ups and downs, Frank appeared genuinely interested in improving himself, made some significant changes, and completed DFST. In addition to his reduced substance abuse, he also experienced significant reductions in psychiatric symptoms and interpersonal problems. After completing the individual therapy protocol, Frank continued in group therapy for another 3 months and terminated treatment when he began taking evening courses to finish his college degree. He became very active in Alcoholics Anonymous meetings, and he seemed to make excellent use of the structure, rules, steps, and commitments that came with these meetings. He also became involved in a romantic relationship with a woman he met at the 12-step meetings despite strong disapproval by his recovering peer group related to the potential relapse risk. In a follow-up phone call with me, he told me that he felt uncomfortable with people knowing about his relationship and guilty that he was not "following the program." Nonetheless, he was maintaining his sobriety, and I praised him for doing very well with the overall task even though he was not following a guideline and might be making a mistake.

During Frank's treatment, I experienced some reactions that were potentially countertherapeutic but that were adjusted through consultation. For example, I initially experienced some pride when Frank was doing well with me in individual therapy but was struggling with the group counseling; I attributed his progress in individual therapy to my skillful application of a psychotherapy model that was of high relevance for him and high interest for me. This briefly prevented me from recognizing that the more important issue was Frank's repetition of his maladaptive coping with perceived adult expectations by rapidly fluctuating between his perfectionistic and acting-out identity. My initial acceptance of this split pointed to another area of potential collusion. I initially did not see the integration of his perfectionistic and acting-out identity as a treatment goal, preferring to only suppress the acting-out side. This blind spot seemed rooted in my own maintenance of a similar split in identity during my earlier development. By monitoring my countertherapeutic reactions, I tried to avoid pushing Frank too little or too much to integrate these separate sides.

Frank's expectations of therapy evolved over our 6 months working together. He initially demanded that I "start at the beginning and rebuild" him. His anxiety and personality style, however, made him unwilling to delve into his emotions and the past in a way that might have made that kind of reconstructive work possible. This, in addition to the time constraints of this research treatment, precluded any attempt to "rebuild" him. At several points, the metaphor of furniture restoration helped keep the time-limited, focused therapy goals and relationship on track. By the end of therapy, Frank had come to understand and accept that, like an antique, the building of himself as a person had occurred in the past and could not be changed other than through destruction. However, targeted repairs and periodic refinishing could significantly increase the beauty and value of the piece as well as its appreciation by others. The work's inherent value could not be overridden by obvious imperfections that might be brought to greater prominence by the refinishing process. Refinishing ultimately had two meanings for Frank: improving his presentation to others so valuable relationships could develop and creating a different sense of closure for his very difficult series of life experiences.

REFERENCES

Ball SA: Manualized treatment for substance abusers with personality disorders: dual focus schema therapy. Addict Behav 23:883–891, 1998

Ball SA: Treatment of personality disorders with co-occurring substance dependence: dual focus schema therapy, in Handbook of Personality Disorders: Theory and Practice. Edited by Magnavita JJ. New York, Wiley, 2003, pp 398–425

Beck AT, Freeman A, Associates: Cognitive Therapy of Personality Disorders. New York, Guilford, 1990

Cecero JJ, Ball SA, Tennen H, et al: Concurrent and predictive validity of antisocial personality disorder subtyping among substance abusers. J Nerv Ment Dis 187:478–486, 1999

Costa PT, McCrae RR: Revised NEO Personality Inventory and NEO Five-Factor Inventory. Odessa, FL, Psychological Assessment Resources, 1992

First MB, Spitzer RL, Gibbon M, et al: Structured Clinical Interview for DSM-IV Axis II Personality Disorders. Washington, DC, American Psychiatric Association, 1997

Kadden R, Carroll K, Donovan D, et al: Cognitive-Behavioral Coping Skills Therapy Manual: A Clinical Research Guide for Therapists Treating Individuals With Alcohol Abuse and Dependence. NIAAA Project MATCH Monograph Series, Vol 3 (DHHS Publ No ADM-92-1895). Edited by Mattson ME. Rockville, MD, National Institute on Alcohol Abuse and Alcoholism, 1992

Rounsaville BJ, Kranzler HR, Ball SA, et al: Personality disorders in substance abusers: relation to substance use. J Nerv Ment Dis 186:87–95, 1998

Young J: Young Parenting Inventory (YPI). New York, Cognitive Therapy Center, 1994

Young J: Young Compensation (YCI-1). New York, Cognitive Therapy Center, 1995

Young J, Brown G: Young Schema Questionnaire—Short Form (YSQ-S1). New York, Cognitive Therapy Center, 1994

Young J, Rygh J: Young-Rygh Avoidance Inventory (YRAI-1). New York, Cognitive Therapy Center, 1994

Young JE, Klosko JS, Weishaar ME: Schema Therapy: A Practitioner's Guide. New York, Guilford, 2003

CHAPTER 6

Double the Trouble

Treatment of a Dual-Diagnosis Patient

Mary Brunette, M.D.
Robert Drake, M.D., Ph.D.

Mary Brunette, M.D., is Assistant Professor of Psychiatry at Dartmouth Medical School. She has provided clinical care to patients with mental illness and co-occurring substance use disorders for over 15 years as well as to patients in integrated dual-disorder treatment programs. She has consulted nationally to public mental health providers and organizations regarding the care of people with co-occurring disorders. In addition, Dr. Brunette has participated in research related to the care of people with schizophrenia and a substance use disorder and has authored publications in the areas of psychosocial treatment for people with schizophrenia and a substance use disorder, programs to address infectious disease in people with dual disorders, parenting programs for people with severe mental illness, and medications to treat substance use disorders in people with schizophrenia.

Robert Drake, M.D., Ph.D., is the Andrew Thomson Professor of Psychiatry and Community and Family Medicine at Dartmouth Medical School and Director of the New Hampshire–Dartmouth Psychiatric Research Center. While actively working as a clinician in community mental health for 25 years, he has been developing and evaluating innovative community programs for individuals with severe mental disorders. He is well known for his work in rehabilitation and health services research and has been instrumental in developing, testing, and disseminating an integrated model of care for patients with dual disorders of severe mental illness and co-occurring substance abuse as well as an effective model of vocational support for people with severe mental illness.

HISTORY

Lydia was a 45-year-old, divorced mother of two grown children whom I (M.B.) evaluated and then cared for during a research study. The first time we met, I noted that she was a petite woman dressed in a black sweatsuit who had disheveled, long, dark hair; pale skin; and unfashionably large eyeglasses. She said hello in a surprisingly booming voice that was deep, hoarse, and monotone. She smiled in a stiff but friendly way and moved awkwardly. Her jaw occasionally moved laterally as we talked.

Lydia reported that she had had a rough life, troubled by poverty, drinking, and difficulties with men. She had been in many hospitals many times. The most recent hospitalization was a lengthy involuntary stay at the state psychiatric hospital after a "bender" during which the authorities said she lit her apartment building on fire. She did not remember what happened at all. She said, "To tell you the truth, Doctor, I lied." She explained that she had lied to officials and told them that she had been hearing voices so she could escape criminal charges. She spent several years in the state hospital and then lived for several more years in a group home.

At the time of our first meeting, Lydia had just moved into her son's small apartment. She claimed to be fine except for feeling anxious about her son's welfare and depressed about how things were going between herself and him. She believed her son's apartment was inhabited by ghosts (no angels or devils) but reported that this did not bother her. Her expression of emotion with her face and hands was diminished, and she did not appear anxious or depressed. She denied having any hallucinations and did not have suicidal or homicidal ideation. Her memory was impaired, she said, possibly by all the drinking she had done, but she performed perfectly on Folstein's Mini-Mental State Examination and her results indicated no gross cognitive impairment. She had one old friend who she liked to visit once a week, but otherwise she lived a quiet and reclusive life, spending approximately 8 hours a day watching television and smoking cigarettes. She and her son smoked "just a little bit" of marijuana each night before she went to bed. In Lydia's view, her problems were related to her depressed mood and her past drinking, for which she believed she received Social Security benefits, although, according to her mental health center records, she received them under the diagnosis of schizoaffective disorder, bipolar type.

A further review of Lydia's records revealed a long history of multiple hospitalizations, some during times of despondent depression with suicidal ideation, others during times of extreme agitation, disorganization, hallucinations, grandiosity, and bizarre behavior. Whenever she presented to the hospital, she usually had been drinking. Since age 17, she drank alcohol and smoked marijuana and tobacco regularly and to excess, and it was difficult to disentangle the psychiatric symptoms from the effects of her substance use because both seemed to have occurred frequently and chronically. During her 20s and 30s, she was prescribed psychotropic medications during hospital stays, but after leaving the hospital, she attended only a few appointments and then dropped out of treatment and did not take the medications regularly. When she was age 28, her husband divorced her. She lost custody of one of her children after a period of heavy drinking and hospitalizations. The other child spent much of the time with relatives. Lydia was never gainfully employed.

According to Lydia's involuntary hospital records, police reports indicated that she was charged with arson for allegedly lighting a fire in her building during what appeared to be a psychotic episode with manic and delusional symptoms. At that time, her hospital records showed that she was extremely guarded and acted as though she were hearing voices. When asked about the fire, she had spoken briefly of battles between angels and the devil and stated that she had been lighting the way for angels. Her speech had been loud and pressured. She had paced in her room all night and day and was hostile and obstinate with staff. While hospitalized, she continued to have the symptoms and was therefore treated with risperidone (an antipsychotic medication), lithium (a mood stabilizer), and diazepam (a sedating antianxiety medication). The symptoms of psychosis and mania gradually improved. Within 2 weeks, however, she became severely depressed. She was tearful and despondent, believing the devil had taken over her soul. She would not get out of bed or eat any food. Sertraline, an antidepressant, and trazodone, an antidepressant often used in low doses to help with sleep, were added to her medication regimen. The anxiety and depression improved over the next few weeks. A court found her incompetent to stand trial, presumably because of her ongoing disorganized thinking and memory problems. The delusions and possible hallucinations were no longer evident, but her mild-to-moderate anxiety, sleep problems, disorganization, and lack of initiative persisted. She remained in the hospital for an unusually long period of time because she was felt to be a danger to society.

At the time Lydia was admitted to the state psychiatric hospital, routine testing detected elevated liver enzymes. A further evaluation uncovered a chronic hepatitis C virus infection with a moderate level of liver disease. Lydia was unable to identify a cause of infection, denying past intravenous drug use, cocaine use, and unprotected sex. With consultation from the staff internist and a hepatologist in the community, she was treated with interferon and ribavirin over the following year, after which her hepatitis remitted. Lydia also had a history of untreated hypertension. At the time I evaluated her, Lydia's main concern was a painful bunion on her foot. She had not seen an internist since her discharge from the group home 3 months earlier.

DIAGNOSIS

Lydia presented to the state psychiatric hospital with symptoms characteristic of schizophrenia, including delusions, possible hallucinations, and disorganized speech. As she spent time in the hospital and took medication, these symptoms improved, but she continued to have negative symptoms of flattened affect and avolition. While experiencing the psychotic symptoms, she also had periods of manic symptoms (elevated mood, increased energy, decreased need for sleep, psychomotor agitation, and increased sexual activity) as well as depressive symptoms (low mood, decreased interest in life, low appetite with weight loss, low energy, and suicidal thoughts). This pattern suggested the diagnosis of schizoaffective disorder, bipolar type.

Lydia appears to have experienced alcohol dependence in the past, characterized by continued use of alcohol resulting in persistent problems, tolerance (she was able to drink very large amounts of alcohol), withdrawal symptoms (while hospitalized), use of alcohol for long periods of time, and use of alcohol instead of engaging in other activities. By the time I met her, her alcohol use disorder was in full, sustained remission, as she had not had a drink for over 3 years. Lydia did, however, continue to smoke marijuana regularly and experience difficulties in functioning related to the marijuana use. She spent money on marijuana instead of on needed items, including food and simple household necessities. Her only friendship focused on marijuana use. She continued to smoke cannabis despite having medical problems that were worsened by her smoking. Her behavior met criteria for marijuana abuse because she exhibited a maladaptive pattern of use whereby she appeared to reduce other activities in favor of smoking cannabis and continued her cannabis use despite related medical problems (her cough). A diagnosis of cannabis dependence was not warranted because she did not exhibit three or more of the multiple DSM-IV-TR criteria and also did not exhibit tolerance to cannabis.

When Lydia presented for care at the hospital, her treating clinicians had to distinguish between a substance-induced psychotic disorder and separate psychotic and substance use disorders. To accomplish this, they needed to establish that the psychotic symptoms occurred when Lydia was not intoxicated with or in withdrawal from a substance. The clinicians determined whether the psychiatric symptoms occurred chronologically before the substance use disorder began or during periods of sobriety or relatively low levels of substance use. Because this type of history can be very difficult to obtain from an individual presenting with significant psychotic, manic, or depressed symptoms, interviews with family or friends and a thorough review of records of past presentations and treatment become important components of these patients' assessment. If a patient is presenting for care for the first time, continuous assessment over the next months is usually necessary to confirm the diagnosis is correct. In this case, while Lydia was at the hospital and therefore not drinking alcohol or smoking marijuana, she continued to have symptoms of schizoaffective disorder, indicating that she had co-occurring psychotic and substance use disorders (*dual disorder*).

TREATMENT

After moving out of the group home, Lydia began receiving care at a mental health center, where she was assigned to a multidisciplinary team that provided integrated treatment of her mental illness and substance use disorders. Her clinical case manager initially developed a relationship with her by talking with her about her own concerns and goals. Lydia's most pressing concern was her son, whose crack addiction drove him to steal her money and possessions. This behavior resulted in a tumultuous relationship that was the cause of much anxiety for Lydia. Lydia was not concerned about her own substance use at the time, and the case manager did not press the issue, wanting instead to focus on building a relationship with Lydia and assist her in developing some immediate stability.

Lydia continued to take risperidone, lithium, sertraline, and trazodone. She told her psychiatrist that she did not see the point of taking risperidone or lithium but thought that it was a good idea to continue the sertraline and trazodone. She continued to take all of her medications, however, in part because her team of providers helped her to understand their benefits, but mostly because she understood that she was now under an outpatient commitment to treatment that required her to take her medications as prescribed.

During the 6 months that I (M.B.) knew Lydia, she made considerable progress. Her early counseling discussions with her case manager helped her decide to try to get her own apartment and live separately from her son. Once in her own apartment, she reported that she felt much calmer. She felt this apartment was free of ghosts. She continued to smoke cannabis each night, however, despite her initial claims that she smoked only to calm her nerves and reduce the stress she experienced in relation to her son. Even when her son was "safely away in jail," she continued to smoke cannabis daily, stating that she enjoyed it and had no intention of quitting. She recognized, however, that alcohol was "the kiss of death" for her and stated that she could never drink again.

Lydia became worried that her finances "were a mess." She decided that, despite a long history of not working and experiencing anxiety about getting a job, she really needed more money. She started looking for part-time work with the help of a vocational specialist who collaborated with the mental health team. Over several months she filled out applications at half a dozen places, and finally landed a part-time job at a coffee shop. She began on-the-job training.

By this time, Lydia had been in treatment for approximately 4 months and had developed a good relationship with her case manager. Lydia's case manager knew it was time to talk with her more about her substance use. In these discussions, she learned that Lydia continued to smoke cannabis in addition to two packs of tobacco cigarettes a day. The case manager helped Lydia look at the pros and cons of ongoing cannabis and tobacco use. Lydia's main concern was her health. She had a daily cough and contracted frequent colds that quickly turned into lung infections. Her case manager helped her link these symptoms with her smoking tobacco and cannabis and assisted her in making a medical appointment. As her psychiatrist, I also helped her review the pros and cons of smoking cannabis. Because Lydia's main concern was that she needed to smoke to fall asleep, I proposed that we use other strategies to calm her nerves and help her fall asleep at night. We discussed a list of options, including exercise during the day, herbal teas in the evening, relaxing reading in the evening, and an increased dose of trazodone 1 hour before bedtime. She chose to try the herbal tea and trazodone. Over the next few weeks she continued to smoke cannabis each night, but she did abstain one night after her case manager challenged her to just see if she could sleep without it. She did sleep.

When Lydia went to her medical appointment, her new internist was also concerned about her chronic morning cough and diagnosed her with early chronic obstructive pulmonary disease. She recommended that Lydia stop all smoking. Lydia expressed a willingness to stop smoking tobacco, so the internist prescribed a nicotine patch. After using the patch, her blood pressure went up. Her internist then prescribed a medication for hypertension. A week later, Lydia did not show up for an appointment with her case manager and did not return the team's phone calls. When the case manager dropped by the coffee shop to look for her there, her boss reported she had missed work as well. The team became concerned. After 5 days, her case manager called the police for help in entering Lydia's apartment to check on her. She was found dead in her bed. No evidence of suicide or foul play was present in her apartment and no autopsy was completed. Her death certificate reported that the cause of death was unknown. Her team felt sad and discouraged that Lydia had died just as she seemed to be making so much progress.

DISCUSSION

The Impact of Dual Diagnosis

The lifetime prevalence of an alcohol or drug use disorder in patients with schizophrenia is approximately 50% as compared with 16% in the general population (Kendler et al. 1996; Regier et al. 1990). In addition, most people with schizophrenia are dependent on nicotine (58%–90%) (Covey et al. 1994), a rate approximately three times that in the general U.S. population. Lydia exemplifies how co-occurring substance use disorders complicate the course of illness and treatment of patients with psychotic illnesses. Although her course of illness was more severe than that of many persons with the dual severe mental illness and substance use disorders, each of the problems she experienced was typical for this population. In these patients, substance use is associated with treatment nonadherence, suicidality, victimization, violence, hospitalization, homelessness, incarceration, and increased risk for HIV and hepatitis B and C infections. Lydia experienced every one of these problems and more over the last 20 years of her life. Her story exemplifies how difficult dual-diagnosis patients can be to engage in treatment and how, without effective treatment, the dual diagnoses wreak havoc and catastrophe on the lives of these patients and their families.

Although Lydia's untimely death surprised and saddened her treatment providers, the more experienced providers on her team knew that patients with schizophrenia experience higher levels of morbidity and early mortality due to respiratory, cardiovascular, infectious, endocrine, gastrointestinal, and other illnesses than people without psychotic disorders. Overall, their life expectancy is about 10 years shorter. The team wondered if Lydia had had a heart attack, as she had experienced some of the risk factors for heart disease, including smoking and hypertension, or whether she had developed pneumonia and respiratory failure. They also wondered if she had committed suicide, which is the cause of death in approximately 10% of people with schizophrenia and schizoaffective disorders (Inskip et al. 1998). They thought it was unlikely that she had somehow used hard drugs and accidentally overdosed.

Although we do not know for sure why people with schizophrenia experience such poor physical health, their lifestyle factors and poor access to and use of medical care may contribute to such a prognosis. A sedentary lifestyle can lead to obesity, which can then increase the risk for diabetes and heart disease. Decreased pain sensitivity may lead to a delay in seeking health care, thereby worsening the course of illness. The high rate of nicotine dependence in people with schizophrenia also contributes to the development of pulmonary and cardiovascular diseases. Co-occurring substance use disorders lead to risk for deadly infectious diseases such as HIV and hepatitis C through sexual and drug use behaviors (Rosenberg et al. 2003). Medication side effects may also be problematic, as many of the second-generation antipsychotics are associated with weight gain and elevated risk for high blood glucose, cholesterol, and triglyceride levels. Recent expert recommendations suggest that mental healthcare providers monitor weight, plasma glucose levels, lipid profiles, and signs of prolactin elevation, a problem due to the dopamine 2 receptor blockade of antipsychotic medication, which can lead to sexual dsyfunction and other problems (Marder et al. 2004). Patients also should be examined regularly for extrapyramidal symptoms and tardive dyskinesia. Patients with a co-occurring substance use disorder should be tested periodically for infectious diseases and be immunized against hepatitis A and B.

Integrated Treatment of Dual Diagnosis

Effective treatment of patients with dual disorders requires the integration of the treatment of both disorders. Important components of integrated treatment include 1) staged interventions that are tailored to the patient's motivation for change (e.g., assertive outreach and motivational interviewing when the patient is not yet motivated to make changes in their substance use), 2) comprehensive services (e.g., medication management, rehabilitation, social support interventions), and 3) a long-term perspective (Mueser et al. 2003). Multidisciplinary mental health teams with additional addiction treatment training are best able to deliver the components of integrated care by using case management, individual counseling, treatment groups, and family interventions. Because these patients have such difficulty maintaining safe housing, access to residential services is also extremely important. If Lydia had been treated with an integrated program earlier in her life, she might have been able to avoid many of the difficulties she experienced: loss of custody of her children, infection with hepatitis C, dangerous behavior, criminal and involuntary interventions, and early death.

When individuals present with symptoms of psychosis and a substance use disorder, it is important to treat the psychotic symptoms immediately and fully. Withholding effective antipsychotic medications because a patient is using substances is not warranted because the active psychosis interferes with the treatment of the substance use disorder as well as causes a host of other problems. Rather, clinicians can treat the psychosis and the substance use disorder, monitor the symptoms of both over time, and consider gradual removal of the antipsychotic medication if the patient appears to fully and completely recover from the psychotic symptoms and is no longer abusing substances.

When they come to treatment, most people with co-occurring disorders are not aware of the difficulties that substance use creates for them and are not yet ready to change their substance use behavior. Clinicians, however, may expect them to be ready for change and then become discouraged. In addition, patients do not like it when clinicians focus on their substance use right away rather than on the issues that the patient feels are more pressing. Lydia likely experienced this mismatch of treatment focus over the first 20 years of her intermittent contact with clinicians, resulting in her dropping out of treatment over and over again. She was consequently unable to gain control over her psychotic symptoms and substance use disorder; this pattern continued until she was involuntarily hospitalized and required to take medications for a long enough period of time that she could experience the benefits of sobriety and reality-based thinking. When hospitalizations or involuntary interventions are necessary, they may help patients with a dual diagnosis gain control of their illness symptoms and attain sobriety, which then allows clinicians to develop a working relationship with them. Despite experiencing much more stability in her life with treatment (improved housing, health, and financial status), Lydia had minimal insight into her addiction to cannabis or her mental illness and the usefulness of medication to manage the illness. In addition, she appeared to not remember the symptoms she had experienced during her psychotic episode prior to and during the beginning of her involuntary hospitalization. These phenomena are not uncommon and can be gently addressed once a trusting relationship is established.

It is important for clinicians to understand the process by which people change, which occurs in stages, and the techniques they can use to facilitate change. In the early stages of treatment, dual-diagnosis patients benefit most from receiving the concrete assistance and outreach services that help to stabilize the patient and engage them in treatment. Lydia's case manager used these techniques as she helped Lydia address the concerns that Lydia identified as being most problematic for her and most likely to prevent her from achieving stability rather than confronting her about her substance use or mental illness symptoms. This kind of assistance helped Lydia to develop trust in her case manager so that they were able to develop a working alliance. Once a trusting relationship is established, the counselor can then begin to talk with the patient more about his or her symptoms of mental illness and/or substance abuse. Motivational interviewing is a counseling style proven to be effective in helping people take responsibility for and become motivated to change their substance use or manage their mental illness symptoms (Miller and Rollnick 2002). In the treatment of patients with a substance use disorder, this counseling style involves focusing on the patient's perspective of the pros and cons of using substances and helping the patient become more aware of how the substance use interferes with his or her own life goals. Lydia's clinicians used this counseling style with her once they had established a good relationship with her. Once a patient is interested in changing the substance use, the clinician can use cognitive-behavioral substance abuse counseling methods (Mueser et al. 2003) to help patients learn the skills to reduce substance use. In this case, Lydia had not quite reached the action stage, although she was close, as she had attained one night of abstinence from cannabis.

Medications also can facilitate the treatment of substance use disorders in patients with psychosis. The second-generation antipsychotic agents are generally safer and have fewer neurological side effects than older medications and may be more useful than first-generation agents in this population. Clozapine, despite its potential serious side effects (e.g., agranulocytosis, an absence of white blood cells that can be fatal if not addressed immediately), shows the most promise. Several studies have provided preliminary evidence that clozapine may reduce substance use in patients with a psychotic disorder (Brunette et al. 2005). Risperidone has not been shown to be helpful in similar studies. The second-generation antipsychotics have also been associated with improved rates of smoking cessation when used in combination with the nicotine patch and behavioral smoking cessation programs. Although risperidone helped control Lydia's symptoms of psychosis, she continued significant cannabis use.

Lydia also exhibited signs of perioral tardive dyskinesia. Her related facial movements were subtle and went unnoticed by Lydia and most people around her. They may have been caused by the use of risperidone or the first-generation antipsychotics she had taken, albeit briefly, in the past. Clozapine, a unique second-generation antipsychotic, does not cause or exacerbate tardive dyskinesia. Similar to all of the other second-generation antipsychotics, risperidone causes tardive dyskinesia at a rate of approximately 1% per year, which is lower than the rate for some of the first-generation antipsychotics, which cause tardive dyskinesia at a rate of approximately 5% per year.

The doctors had appropriately discontinued Lydia's lorazepam prescription when she was discharged from the hospital into independent community living. This is important, as prescription benzodiazepine use is controversial in individuals with a primary substance use disorder, but prescription of benzodiazepines is common for people with dual disorders of psychiatric illness and substance abuse. Because these medications do not appear to improve outcomes and are associated with the development of benzodiazepine use disorders (Brunette et al. 2003), they should be avoided in the outpatient treatment of dual diagnosis patients.

Lydia had important strengths. She wanted to function well in her role as a parent and to work, but both roles can be significantly impaired by substance abuse or mental illness. Working and parenting are normalizing experiences for adults in our society that clinicians should support and facilitate through skills training and interventions to control symptoms of psychosis and substance abuse. For parents of young children, parenting supports and training can result in improved skills and outcomes for the parent and the child. Vocational supports can help patients obtain and keep jobs. In people with a substance use disorder, the substance use often replaces meaningful daytime activities, such as working, parenting, and pursuing hobbies, important life roles that can help patients become sober and maintain their sobriety (Becker and Drake 2003). Lydia's case manager was doing the right thing when she helped her look for work. If Lydia had been parenting young children, her case manager might have offered assistance around parenting issues in addition to or instead of vocational supports.

REFERENCES

Becker DR, Drake RE: A Working Life for People With Severe Mental Illness. New York, Oxford University Press, 2003

Brunette M, Noordsy DL, Xie H, et al: Benzodiazepine use and abuse among patients with severe mental illness and co-occurring substance use disorders. Psychiatr Serv 54:1395–1401, 2003

Brunette MF, Green AI, Noordsy D, et al: Pharmacologic treatments for co-occurring substance use disorders in patients with schizophrenia: a research review. Journal of Dual Diagnosis 1:41–55, 2005

Covey L, Hughes DC, Glassman AH, et al: Ever-smoking, quitting, and psychiatric disorders: evidence from the Durham, North Carolina epidemiologic catchment area. Tobacco Control 3:222–227, 1994

Inskip HM, Harris EC, Barraclough C: Lifetime risk of suicide for alcoholism, affective disorder and schizophrenia. British Journal of Psychiatry 172:35–37, 1998

Kendler KS, Gallagher TJ, Abelson JM, et al: Lifetime prevalence, demographic risk factors, and diagnostic validity of nonaffective psychosis as assessed in a US community sample: the national comorbidity survey. Archives of General Psychiatry 53(11):1022–1031, 1996

Marder SR, Essock SM, Miller AL, et al: Physical health monitoring of patients with schizophrenia. Am J Psychiatry 161:1334–1349, 2004

Miller WR, Rollnick S: Motivational Interviewing. New York, Guilford, 2002

Mueser KT, Noordsy DL, Drake RE, et al: Integrated Treatment for Dual Disorders: A Guide to Effective Practice. New York, Guilford, 2003

Regier DA, Farmer ME, Rae DS, et al: Comorbidity of mental disorders with alcohol and other drug abuse. Results from the Epidemiologic Catchment Area (ECA) Study.[comment]. JAMA 264(19):2511–2518, 1990

Rosenberg SD, Swanson JW, Wolford GL, et al: Blood-borne infections and persons with mental illness: the five-site health and risk study of blood-borne infections among persons with severe mental illness. Psychiatr Serv 54:827–835, 2003

CHAPTER 7

"I Gotta Get Clean"

Network Therapy for Opioid Dependence

Marc Galanter, M.D.

Marc Galanter, M.D., is Professor of Psychiatry at New York University (NYU), Founding Director of the Division of Alcoholism and Drug Abuse at NYU and Bellevue Hospital, and Director of the NYU Fellowship Training Program in Addiction Psychiatry. He is also a Division Director at NYU's World Health Organization Collaborating Center and Director of its Center for Medical Fellowships in Alcoholism and Drug Abuse. He is Editor of the journal *Substance Abuse* and the annual book series *Recent Developments in Alcoholism* and is coeditor of the *Textbook of Substance Abuse Treatment*. His studies funded by the National Institutes of Health and various foundations have addressed network therapy for substance abuse, pharmacological treatment for narcotic addiction, self-help treatment for those who abuse substances, and spiritually oriented recovery.

Dr. Galanter attended Albert Einstein College of Medicine, where he did his residency in psychiatry. Afterward he was a Clinical Associate at the National Institute of Mental Health and then a National Institutes of Health Career Teacher. He later served as President of the Association for Medical Education and Research in Substance Abuse (1976–1977), the American Academy of Addiction Psychiatry (1991–1992), and the American Society of Addiction Medicine (1999–2001). Among his awards are the Gold Achievement Award for innovation in clinical care and the Seymour Vestermark Award for Psychiatric Education, both from the American Psychiatric Association; the McGovern Award for medical teaching from the Association for Medical Education and Research in Substance Abuse, and the New York State Award for Psychiatric Research.

JOHN LEFT A MESSAGE ON MY answering machine asking if he could make an appointment. On my return call he said he was referred by a patient I had seen the year before. They were both members of a circle of young artists and musicians, each of whom had achieved a measure of success living and working in New York's East Village. He wanted help in addressing his heroin habit, saying, "I gotta get clean." In response to a few questions, he described himself as a 30-year-old single artist who clearly had aspirations to achieve wider recognition. He had been using heroin intranasally on and off for 3 years, but for the past 6 months was sniffing large doses at least twice a day. Hoping to take advantage of his motivation of the moment and realizing how quickly it could flag, I had him come to see me the next evening. Here is his story as it unfolded over a number of sessions.

HISTORY

John was born into a well-to-do family living on New York City's Park Avenue and grew up with his parents and a younger brother and sister. John's family felt little economic pressure or uncertainty of social status, but his mother was a forbidding woman with little empathic connection to her boys, and his father's pattern of drinking heavily on a daily basis met criteria for alcohol dependence.

John was diagnosed by psychologists with dyslexia and hyperactivity in grade school for which he received tutoring, but he complied with the prescribed methylphenidate regimen only occasionally. He was provocative toward his teachers, and, on the advice of the school psychologist, his parents transferred him to a school for problem children.

While his sister, the "good child," and his brother, who was performing adequately, remained at home, John was sent to a boarding high school for the learning disabled during a period when his parents were considering divorce. At this point he felt banished from the family. His behavior did improve somewhat while at the school, enough so that he could enter a college where he focused on art and design. His apparent talent for painting large and compelling abstract canvases and his engaging personality allowed him to move into a circle of artists who were showing their work with some success, and the trust fund left to him by his grandfather gave him the opportunity to pursue his painting career while living comfortably. His charm and good looks led to a number of relationships with women who, in the end, were left frustrated and emotionally starved.

John fell into a downtown club scene soon after leaving college in which he dabbled in cocaine, occasionally drank to excess, and was introduced to heroin. Although he found that cocaine relaxed his edgy personality, as is typical of people with attention-deficit/hyperactivity disorder, the heroin he tried with his friends eventually became a daily habit he could not break.

DIAGNOSIS

John clearly met the DSM-IV-TR criteria for opioid dependence. He manifested five of seven characteristics at the time of his presentation (three are required): he had developed tolerance to the drug, experienced withdrawal signs and symptoms at times, used heroin in larger amounts than he had intended, had been unsuccessful in efforts to control its use, and had given up activities because of its use.

TREATMENT

Initial Encounters

At our first session, I told John that it would be best to begin with a brief inpatient detoxification, but he was averse to going into a hospital. The option of detoxifying him on an ambulatory basis with buprenorphine did not arise, as the drug was not yet available.

This initial encounter had taken place late on a Thursday night, and I had no time to meet with him again until the following Monday evening. I was concerned about his reliability in returning and wanted to engage collateral support, so I asked him if we could speak on the phone with a friend or a close family member who could be a resource for him over the weekend. Although he was somewhat wary, he agreed to our calling his cousin, Andy, with whom he had a close relationship and who had repeatedly expressed concern over John's drug use. However, Andy was to be out of town until Monday, so we agreed that he would meet John for dinner Monday evening and come with him to his next appointment.

John did show up with his cousin that Monday. He was somewhat tremulous and reported that he and a friend, also addicted to heroin, had decided late Thursday night to detoxify themselves abruptly with some naltrexone that his friend had acquired. They supported each other, suffering miserably over the weekend. John had used no heroin since our last session. I complimented him on his fortitude but also made clear to him and his cousin that his vulnerability to relapse was very high. He needed a structured plan to ensure a stable abstinence, so we sat down to work on how to proceed.

Network Therapy

The approach we used was one that I began to formulate back when the subspecialty of addiction psychiatry was in its infancy and that I continued to develop over years of dealing with substance-dependent people (Galanter 1993). When I first began working on this approach, there was virtually no literature on the ambulatory management of addictive disorders other than referral to Alcoholics Anonymous (AA), use of disulfiram (used because a patient taking it on a daily basis experiences considerable dysphoria if he or she drinks alcoholic beverages), methadone maintenance, and failed psychoanalysis (Bean and Zinberg 1981). But there were certainly many mental health professionals who were conducting individual therapy who could be a resource for treating addicted people, if they had competency in managing them.

The defense mechanism of denial is, of course, characteristic of people addicted to substances. No matter how well-intentioned these individuals might be, important aspects of how their substance use has compromised their lives and those of family members are inevitably withheld in the treatment context or simply repressed. Therapists are typically left at a loss when these patients run into problems in their daily lives or have minor relapses to their abused substance, as the succor offered by the substance is usually greater and more compelling than the clinician's best efforts. As a consequence, patients who slip often use their drug covertly while in therapy or rationalize termination of the treatment, as attested to by many people speaking at AA meetings.

The treatment outcome for a major mental illness in its acute stages is usually enhanced by collaboration of the therapist, patient, and other supportive figures. In my experience, this model seemed to hold advantages for substance-dependent people as well, who are liable at any point to develop an acute problem. So I developed a technique over time in which new patients would work with me in choosing from among their family and good friends a few people who did not abuse substances. These collaborating individuals could help patients undercut their denial, support their motivation for recovery, and, if need be, provide them with material support such as going to dinner together or meeting with them if I was out of town.

John was a good candidate for network therapy: he had been continuously dependent on heroin for less than a year, following his previous pattern, and so he met criteria for abuse only and not dependence. He also did not meet the criteria for methadone maintenance, which require the patient to have previously failed in treatment attempts and be addicted for longer than 1 year. In any case, it was preferable to avoid his developing a long-term dependence on opioid maintenance for an open-ended period and John himself was not interested in methadone treatment. Instead, it was felt that if he could be sustained in an abstinent state with the network's help, he could also engage in individual therapy to address the adaptive problems that demanded attention.

I knew enough to appreciate that John was quite vulnerable to a relapse; to avoid this eventuality as well as his vulnerability to falling into other substance use, a number of steps were required.

Engaging the Network

John's network ultimately included three people: Andy, John's cousin; Bill, a close friend; and Sam, a man who was 20 years John's senior and whom John viewed as a mentor and friend. The network sessions were arranged with the frequency necessary to protect John's abstinent state.

John and I initially met twice a week. For the first 3 weeks, his network joined him for one of those sessions and he and I met individually for the other. Over the ensuing weeks, I decreased the frequency of network meetings relative to my sense of John's stability in treatment, so that after 6 months he was coming once a week and his network attended a session only once every month or two.

The network members were instructed that their role was to be supportive of John and that any difficulties he might encounter in sustaining his abstinence should be viewed through an understanding of the nature of addictive disorders rather than through a judgmental stance. It is essential to this technique that network members maintain a positive and forward-looking approach to sustain the patient's morale and allow him or her to experience relief from the self-blame that he or she inevitably feels for any compromise caused to the network members and people close to them. In John's case, promotion of a supportive atmosphere was important because of the ambivalence that John's cousin, Andy, felt toward him. Although the two were very close, Andy was acerbic by nature, and at times I had to explain that some of the complaints he voiced about John concerned addiction-related behaviors and that personal traits independent of John's addiction would be dealt with in John's individual therapy.

Medication Therapy

A second component of the treatment was to protect John from relapsing by having him take naltrexone, an opioid antagonist that would block the effects of heroin on the opioid receptors in the brain. Naltrexone has been found to be of relatively little clinical value because patients typically "forget" to take it at some point and thus become vulnerable to relapse. On the other hand, a reasonably well-motivated patient will take naltrexone (as a similarly motivated alcoholic patient will take disulfiram) when the self-administration is observed by a network member. This procedure is most easily carried out if the patient is living with a spouse who can observe the patient taking the medication each morning. However, in John's case that was not possible, so we formed an understanding that he would take two 50-mg pills twice weekly (on Monday and Wednesday) and three on a third occasion (Friday). He would do this in front of Bill, his older friend, who lived only one block away.

Bill's role was not to go to John's house to ask him to take the pills or admonish him if he did not, but instead only to observe John's behavior and leave me a phone message if he did not see John take the pills on a given occasion. It is the patient's responsibility to take the pill so that the observer can see that it has been swallowed. To ensure that Bill kept up with the regimen, he was expected to mark on a calendar each time John took the pills. We continued with this naltrexone regimen over the course of the ensuing 10 months and after that on John's own recognizance for 4 more months.

Avoiding Other Substances

At the outset of treatment, I also stipulated that John was not to use marijuana, alcohol, or other drugs, explaining to him and the network how any of these could easily lead to a relapse. I asked him at random times to give a urine sample for toxicology to ensure his compliance with this requirement. At one point in treatment, John said that his desire to avoid a positive urine toxicology supported him in his efforts to avoid marijuana. He was implicitly acknowledging that he would be disappointing the network members in addition to himself if he relapsed.

AA is certainly a valuable adjunct to securing a patient's abstinence, and I asked John, as with other patients, that he attend at least four AA meetings, so that we could discuss his views—which were not very positive—of the fellowship. John did, in fact, attend the meetings, as I pressed him to do so in the individual and network sessions. He later went to some meetings over the ensuing year with a friend who was in recovery, but concluded that he did not want to attend AA on a regular basis.

After 3 months, John told me that he had "never bargained for not drinking at all" and that he did not quite see himself as being abstinent from alcohol for the long term. As we discussed this, I said it was best that he stay abstinent for at least a year and that toward the end of that time we would discuss his options. In the ninth month of treatment we began to consider the issue. It seemed clear that John was not committed to remaining abstinent from alcohol after the treatment ended. It seemed better that he try to drink in a moderate way while in treatment so that we could discuss the decision, rather than his beginning to drink after treatment ended and leave him with no opportunity to examine how it went. We discussed this with the network members, who were quite wary of John embarking on something other than total abstinence, but they responded to the "better during treatment than afterward" approach. John fancied himself an expert on various brews, so with the network's agreement, he and I agreed on a plan whereby he could have up to two beers on a given day, then later three, while keeping a log of his use that we could discuss together and in network sessions.

I had often discussed with John the issue that, given his family history, he was vulnerable to alcoholism. Alcohol was a blight on his family because his father always drank heavily in the evening, putting John in an uncomfortable position during his occasional visits home. At one point during his treatment, tragedy befell the family: John's younger brother, who occasionally drank abusively (although he was not dependent on alcohol) had an automobile accident while he was drunk and was gravely injured. John was profoundly upset and felt guilty that he had not done more to intervene with his brother beforehand.

John continued to keep his drinking diary and after 3 months of this regimen, a month after his brother's accident, he decided that he was better off remaining abstinent. A few years after the termination of his treatment when we met for several 45-minute sessions to deal with an issue that had arisen between him and the woman he was to marry, he said he was still not drinking. This did seem to be the case, although I was not in a position to verify his statement.

Individual Therapy

Throughout the period of his treatment, I conducted a psychodynamically oriented therapy with John while addressing the potential triggers to drug use through a cognitive-behavioral approach. One important issue we dealt with was the nature of his relationships with women, as he seemed to be unable to establish a stable and lasting bond with any of his girlfriends. It was clear that he was greatly conflicted about the possibility of being intimate with a woman whom he regarded as an equal, and complained that he had never come across one who might be a potential mate. After this issue had been dealt with at length in therapy, he turned to a more appropriate relationship that eventually did end in marriage. Such personal issues, ones not directly related to his abstinence, were not discussed in network meetings.

Individual therapy directed at achieving the goals patients set for themselves is a key factor in their recovery and commitment to treatment. It is important that the treatment of addicted patients carry with it more than an injunction against their abusing a substance that is compromising their life. Because these patients are expected to go through the difficult process of relinquishing an agent that paradoxically gives them comfort in times of difficulty, they need to have a sense that there are positive changes they can anticipate. For John, his relationship with women and a number of other areas of conflict, such as his pursuit of his work as an artist, offered this opportunity.

DISCUSSION

The clinician has to approach the treatment of opioid addiction with humility, as the course of treatment is fraught with ongoing risk of relapse. I was heartened that John, at his own initiative, had detoxified himself over the course of the weekend after we first met and that he was willing to accept the regimen we had laid out with the support of his network. My relationship with him was a congenial one during which I was active in engaging him over issues relevant to his life. It was clear that the transference was such that he found solace in a relationship with a paternal figure that could replace, in some measure, a father whose drinking had left John in need of support and a mother who had not been empathic or demonstrative of affection toward him.

The treatment of substance dependence (but not necessarily substance abuse) can be problematic if it is conducted with a relatively passive psychodynamic stance, as patients need to be effectively guided through the many pitfalls that may arise. Other approaches, be they cognitive or AA oriented, are facilitated by a supportive relationship being developed between the person who must face the very difficult tasks of establishing a pattern of recovery and another individual. There is little advantage to allowing addicted people to be left to blame themselves or respond defensively, given their existing burden of guilt over their prior actions and their internal pressure to return to their addictive drug. It is also important to maintain a similar stance in the network sessions, and I felt comfortable in John's network meetings because we were able to maintain a friendly atmosphere.

Some networks can be fraught with tension and require a carefully framed approach to keep them going, particularly if the patient has slips during the treatment. The atmosphere a therapist establishes in this context is not unlike that maintained by a treatment team in a nursing station, where fostering positive morale in the face of potential difficulties is important. One objective therefore is to steer away from interpreting any failings or problematic character traits in any of the network members because their attendance is clearly voluntary and they must feel safe from the scrutiny of other members or the therapist. In this regard, the network meetings are quite different from those in systemic family therapy (Steinglass et al. 1987), where one tries to reconstruct and reorder relationships among members of a family to address the presenting person's symptoms. In the network approach, it is clearly acknowledged that the patient is the focus of attention, and each member of the network, the therapist included, has a role in helping with this endeavor.

At the same time, it is important for the therapist to maintain a certain emotional distance from events to ensure objectivity, particularly given the complexity of interactions among a group of four to six people (therapist and patient included). This means maintaining a certain degree of authority, based primarily on an acknowledgement of the therapist's expertise and a realization on the network members' part that the therapist will be supportive of both their efforts and the patient's well-being for the long term. As things settle down, therefore, the therapist can ask the patient if it is okay for network members to speak with the patient himself or herself or with the therapist too if they become concerned that the patient may be vulnerable to relapse. It is understood that the network can reconvene, even a long time later, if the patient runs into trouble.

Alternatives to the Network Approach

Opioid Maintenance

As indicated above, John did not meet criteria for methadone maintenance. In addition, few middle-class people feel comfortable attending methadone maintenance clinics, at least in New York City, where the patients are typically economically disadvantaged and often involved in antisocial activities. Among these activities is the use of secondary drugs, particularly alcohol, but also cocaine and benzodiazepines. Involvement in a methadone clinic environment is often associated with acculturation into a variety of antisocial and drug-related behaviors that may compromise an individual's adjustment to general society. A pattern can emerge, not unlike that in the penal system, where inmates model their behavior on that of hardened criminals.

Buprenorphine, a partial agonist, is available for use in office-based treatment by physicians trained in addiction psychiatry or addiction medicine (Fudala et al. 2003). The initiation of buprenorphine use at the hands of an experienced physician is relatively easy; however, the patient must be free of heroin for at least 16 hours, and preferably 24 hours, before taking buprenorphine because the drug is competitive with heroin for opioid receptor sites and can precipitate acute drug withdrawal in a person who still has significant blood levels of heroin or other opioids. There is little experience, however, with the long-term outcome of buprenorphine maintenance. Withdrawal from buprenorphine does not produce the degree of symptom severity that withdrawal from heroin does, but it does create dysphoria and fatigue, which, in the recovering addict, can serve as a trigger for reestablishing a heroin habit. In addition, my colleagues and I, among others, have found that there is a clinically significant prevalence of the use of secondary illicit opioids among patients on buprenorphine maintenance because full blockade of opioids in high doses may not be possible (Galanter et al. 2004). Of course, buprenorphine is not an effective agent in patients who use nonopioid drugs. Nonetheless, this medication has provided a useful tool to the clinician for stabilizing a heroin addict who is engaged in ongoing psychosocial treatment.

Inpatient Rehabilitation

Acute detoxification on an inpatient basis without adequate follow-up has long been found to precede a relapse to opioid use in almost all cases. On the other hand, when a patient like John is discharged from long-term residential care and given intensive follow-up, inpatient detoxification can be a valuable tool. For a clinician with limited experience in the addiction field, residential rehabilitation may be the best choice.

Virtually all residential rehabilitation programs are organized around the 12-step philosophy, with intensive involvement in AA or other similar anonymous-profile groups. Although acculturation into a 12-step orientation is very helpful to individuals addressing addictions, it should be appreciated that the person entering a residential treatment built around this approach may have difficulty in establishing a stable abstinence and that concomitant psychotherapy in addition to AA can be important for ensuring a safe recovery and an improved social adaptation.

Dialectical Behavior Therapy

The network approach bears certain salient similarities to the dialectical behavior therapy approach, which was developed for the treatment of severe personality disorder (Linehan et al. 1999). Both rely on authenticity, even equality, in the caregiver's approach to the patient and allow for therapeutic contacts between sessions. Network therapy, however, involves family and peer interactions in this way, thus relieving the therapist of many of the burdensome aspects of this role as well as the countertransference that may weigh heavily on one called to treat the difficult problem of addiction. Both also use a careful cognitive analysis of those events or triggers during treatment that might have set off a relapse to pathological behavio—for example, a suicide attempt in dialectical behavior therapy setting or a slip into drinking in the network approach.

Conclusion

John's case illustrates the value of a variety of community reinforcements (Hunt and Azrin 1973) and the compelling nature of personal ties with people close to the patient in shaping behavior. When properly orchestrated, these ties can be used in a more effective way than if individuals close to the patient act separately. John's case also suggests a way in which classical "interventions" (Johnson 1986) for the addict, popular in the media, may be tempered and integrated into subsequent care.

Network therapy leans heavily on a cognitive-behavioral approach to avoiding relapse, wherein triggers for drug-seeking behaviors can be examined with the patient individually as well as with their network. Psychopharmacology can also be initiated when indicated. Clinicians should feel free to apply the concept of network support with whatever modalities they find helpful and effective in the emerging area of psychotherapy for addictive disorders.

REFERENCES

Bean MH, Zinberg NE (eds): Dynamic Approaches to the Understanding and Treatment of Alcoholism. New York, Free Press, 1981

Fudala PJ, Bridge TP, Herbert S, et al: Office-based treatment of opiate addiction with a sublingual-tablet formulation of buprenorphine and naloxone. N Engl J Med 349:949–958, 2003

Galanter M: Network therapy for addiction: a model for office practice. Am J Psychiatry 150:28–36, 1993

Galanter M, Dermatis H, Resnick R, et al: Short-term buprenorphine maintenance: treatment outcome. J Addict Dis 23:39–49, 2004

Hunt GM, Azrin NH: A community reinforcement approach to alcoholism. Behav Res Ther 11:91–104, 1973

Johnson VE: Intervention: How to Help Someone Who Doesn't Want Help. Minneapolis, Johnson Institute, 1986

Linehan MM, Schmidt H III, Dimeff LA, et al: Dialectical behavior therapy for patients with borderline personality disorder and drug dependence. Am J Addict 8:279–292, 1999

Steinglass P, Bennett LA, Wolin SJ, et al: The Alcoholic Family. New York, Basic Books, 1987

CHAPTER 8

Vietnam Junkie

What He Taught Me About Opiate-Dependence Treatment

Thomas Kosten, M.D.

Thomas Kosten, M.D., is Professor of Psychiatry and and Neuroscience at Baylor College of Medicine and former Professor and Chief of Psychiatry at Yale's VA Connecticut. He is the Director of the Baylor Division of Substance Addictions and founding Director of the Yale Division of Substance Abuse in 1994. He has directed the NIDA Substance Abuse Medications Development Research Center at Yale and now Baylor since 1990. He is President of the College on the Problems of Drug Dependence, Past President of the American Academy of Addiction Psychiatry, a Distinguished Fellow of the American Psychiatric Association, and a Fellow of the American College of Neuropsychopharmacology. Dr. Kosten is the founding Vice Chair for Added Qualifications in Addiction Psychiatry of the American Board of Psychiatry and Neurology

---

This work was supported by National Institute on Drug Abuse Grant K05-DA00454, P50-DA12762, R01-DA05626, and Department of Veterans Affairs, New England Grant MIRECC.

and has served on the National Academy of Sciences.

Dr. Kosten has won several major clinical research awards, is Deputy Editor of two major journals in substance abuse, has served on the *American Journal of Psychiatry* editorial board, and has published over 450 papers, books, and reviews. His pharmacotherapy contributions include a cocaine vaccine, disulfiram for cocaine dependence, vasodilators for cocaine-induced cerebral perfusion defects, and buprenorphine for opioid dependence. In addition to these pharmacotherapies, he has advanced medicine's understanding of opiate and cocaine dependence mechanisms and treatment using single-photon emission computed tomography and functional magnetic resonance neuroimaging.

JIM, WHO WAS BORN IN 1954, is a few years younger than I am. I first met him when I was a psychiatric resident at Yale University School of Medicine 25 years ago. Since then, I have maintained contact with Jim and his various family members.

HISTORY

We first engaged in treatment after he had completed his fifth or sixth detoxification from intravenous heroin. He could not remember the number of detoxifications or all the places he had gone to for treatment. Despite his being entitled to free care because of his service in Vietnam, most of his treatment had not been at the U.S. Department of Veterans Affairs (VA) hospitals. He had been dishonorably discharged because of his opiate smoking in Vietnam. He had used other drugs and alcohol before going into the Army, but had never tried opiates until he started "chasing the dragon" by smoking opium in Vietnam. The clinical staff called him one of the Vietnam junkies.

While in Vietnam, he smoked opium (which is in the same drug class as heroin and has the same effects) mostly on weekends; he simply stopped smoking opium, after which he experienced minimal withdrawal symptoms. This restrained use in Vietnam had not prepared him for the significant unpleasantness of opiate withdrawal. When he returned to the U.S., he obtained heroin and for several months snorted it on weekends (called "chipping"); however, the heroin use escalated to daily use and dependence. Because he was dependent, the first few times he tried to stop his three times daily use of heroin on his own he became sick with all the classic symptoms of opiate withdrawal. Within 24 hours of his last use, he developed rhinorrhea (runny nose), lacrimation (tearing), goose bumps, nausea, and diarrhea. He became more anxious over the next 48 hours, and his posttraumatic stress disorder (PTSD) symptoms were exacerbated as he began vomiting on the third day of abstinence. He had shaking chills, sweating, and what he considered the worst case of influenza in his life. He could not sleep, could not sit still, and was angry with everyone and paranoid about the police coming to get him. He hid in his room for those 3 days, drinking juice and beer but not being able to eat anything. After that grueling 3-day experience, his symptoms began to improve and after a week he felt drained, exhausted, and fairly intoxicated from all the beer. He thought that he might die or at least have a seizure, as he had seen his alcoholic father do once; however, seizures do not occur from opiate withdrawal.

Jim had returned to drug use within a few months of coming back to the United States from his Vietnam tour because the alcohol and drugs reduced his PTSD symptoms and made him feel good. He initially returned to using alcohol as he had before he went into the Army, but his usage escalated to daily alcohol abuse and finally developed into alcohol dependence, with Jim experiencing significant withdrawal symptoms when he tried to stop using alcohol. He detoxified himself from alcohol several times but initially did not seek professional treatment

After he detoxified himself several times from alcohol and heroin, his ability to endure the withdrawal symptoms weakened. He then entered detoxification facilities when he ran out of money and had to stop using heroin. These treatments did not help as much as he wanted, but they were better than enduring untreated withdrawal.

TREATMENT

Starting a Therapeutic Relationship

Just prior to our beginning outpatient treatment, Jim had been detoxified with clonidine (an α_2-adrenergic agonist that reduces adrenergic activity by feedback inhibition of brain locus coeruleus neurons). He was one of the early successes on our research unit at the Connecticut Mental Health Center (CMHC). He had endured 7 days of first increasing and then decreasing doses of clonidine and, to the delight of all the faculty and residents, he became free of opiates, medically stable, and more or less symptom free. I add "more or less" because he still told me that he really was not sleeping well but did not want to tell the "head docs, 'cause they might throw me out." I kept his confidence, but this was probably a mistake made as a naïve therapist on a biological research unit. It is always critical to let the substance-dependent patient know that you are not keeping any secrets that may be important for others to know. Without this disclosure to important figures in the patient's life, you end up being isolated with a failing patient. I later found this out the hard way, when I began working with Jim and his family as an outpatient.

Preventing Outpatient Relapse After Detoxification

What was I going to do for Jim now that he had successfully detoxified from heroin? It seemed to me that the options were limited. However, my mentor, Dr. Herb Kleber, had introduced me to naltrexone—a long-acting, oral, competitive opiate antagonist typically taken two to three times per week—as an experimental treatment option. It sounded perfect. Unlike methadone, which is an opiate agonist (it acts like heroin in terms of stimulating the opioid receptors), naltrexone is an opiate antagonist in that it blocks the receptors. Patients do not become addicted to naltrexone like they do to methadone, making its easy for the patient to stop receiving it. Furthermore, it produces a complete blockade of heroin, preventing a heroin high if the patient uses any. One significant issue in using naltrexone is that it must be taken regularly for it to work. Dr. Kleber had successfully addressed this adherence challenge in treating populations who faced significant consequences for noncompliance with naltrexone, such as physicians who were liable to losing their medical license or criminals on work-release programs who faced being reincarcerated: the key was some type of monitoring and powerful contingencies for nonadherence.

At the time when I was seeing Jim, Dr. Duke Stanton had written about using family members of patients in methadone programs to improve treatment outcomes (Stanton 1978). I called him and asked about using his program for naltrexone in an opiate-dependent patient. He was encouraging and supportive and sent me his book. Because Jim had recently been divorced, a couple's model of family treatment was not an option. However, it seemed that the adolescent family model of working with Jim's parents was the way to approach family therapy. I therefore arranged to meet with Jim, his mother, and his younger sister (the one closest to his age). His father would not come in to see me, and the rest of the family "did not know about Jimmy's problem with drugs" and so would not be coming in for a meeting. It was a start at least.

We first worked on the thrice weekly naltrexone dosing. Jim was to take the naltrexone on Monday (100 mg), Wednesday (100 mg), and Friday (150 mg). I would meet with him alone once a week and in conjunction with the family once a week, and if things were going well after 6 months, I would then meet with the family monthly but continue weekly with Jim. The next week, after my initial meeting with Jim and his mother and sister, his mother called to say that Jim would not be coming in, but that she was willing to come see me. Jim had already come in to the clinic for the naltrexone twice that week. I asked to speak to him, but she said she did not know where he was. ("Jimmy stormed out of the house, and I think he left town.") Jim had never left town since his discharge from the Army 6 years earlier. Even when he was married, he lived upstairs from his parents in their multifamily house. These close quarters with his mother had been one of the precipitants of Jim's failed marriage, but Jim's PTSD symptoms from Vietnam were also significant contributors to the breakup.

Jim did not show up for his next naltrexone dose or for therapy with me, but I was to meet with his mother alone and had some questions to resolve. How could I determine her motivation for supporting Jim's abstinence, and how could I persuade her that Jim's taking naltrexone was the key to his successfully stopping his drug abuse? As I listened to her, she said that she could easily find Jim. Her motivation for helping him sustain abstinence was that she wanted him to obtain an honorable discharge from the Army. She really did not see the drugs as important because Jim's dad, her husband, was an alcoholic and went to work, took care of the family, and had raised a son who had served his country in the Army. In her opinion, Jim's father was successful because he had been in the Army in World War II and had come home a hero, not a bum. Jim, her son, was a bum who was thrown out of the Army. The task that could unite us was obtaining an honorable discharge from the Army for Jim. I indicated that I now worked at the VA, where I could work on this issue with Jim, but that he had to remain free of drugs and show up to see me. The next day, Jim came in to take his naltrexone and to see me.

Psychiatric Comorbidity: Establishing a Diagnosis

Establishing a diagnosis of PTSD allowed Jim to obtain the type of military discharge that made him eligible for treatment services at the VA. He eventually also obtained a status of partial disability for PTSD. His PTSD symptoms had been present for over 5 years, but he had not admitted to any of these symptoms when he entered the inpatient clonidine detoxification protocol for heroin. Over the first few months of our therapy, he gradually revealed a wide range of PTSD symptoms. He had insomnia and nightmares about his combat experience; he reported experiencing easily provoked startle reactions and flashbacks that occurred when he heard helicopters or smelled diesel fuel (it reminded him of napalm); he was also irritable, which came with being constantly on guard for the cues that might lead to flashbacks. These symptoms had increased over the years since he had returned home and were associated with his attempts to self-medicate with alcohol and drugs.

Jim's PTSD and military discharge status were clearly relevant to his treatment for addiction, because it was the hook that kept him, his mother, his sister, and eventually his father returning to the treatment sessions for a year. His PTSD treatment was a series of successes and failures and, like his substance dependence, it was a chronic relapsing disorder. Entering into the VA system provided the setting for Jim to receive appropriate treatment for his PTSD in conjunction with his substance dependence. In addition, Jim's care at the VA and his military discharge status changed his father's life. His father gave up drinking, and both his father and mother had a brief evaluation with me for couples treatment. The couple then went to Catholic Family Services, where they saw a social worker for a few months. The parents did not live happily ever after, but Jim did move out of the house (two houses away) and began an independent life.

A Chronic Relapsing Disorder

Jim became heavily involved in self-help support and felt sufficiently secure in his abstinence that he stopped the naltrexone about 4 months before transferring his care from the CMHC to the VA. During his time at the CMHC, he was abstinent while on naltrexone for about 6 months. Jim became very excited about his sustained abstinence and wanted to share his program of recovery with others. This desire led him to develop a chapter of Narcotics Anonymous (NA) in New Haven, which supplemented Jim's professional contacts with the CMHC naltrexone treatment program. When he transferred from the CMHC program, he was having twice-weekly urine monitoring and had been abstinent from heroin for over a year. During the last 4 months at the CMHC, he remained abstinent without the aid of naltrexone. We considered this 4 months of abstinence an indication that it would be appropriate to further reduce his therapy and urine-monitoring visits. He therefore reduced the frequency of his treatments at the VA to monthly. He also became active with his fellow veterans and set up a new Narcotics Anonymous group at the VA for veterans who were in a month-long residential and day treatment drug program.

Jim was also succeeding in his psychosocial rehabilitation. He was working in the family's business of installing flooring and had taken on increasing responsibility. His father now viewed Jim as his successor in running the business, and after 3 years of their steadily working together, his father even began to talk about retirement. However, at this point, Jim was injured on the job. His injuries led to chronic back pain, surgery, and Jim's being placed on oxycodone (OxyContin), a slow-release, oral opiate analgesic, for pain relief. At this stage, Jim had been free of illicit opiates for over 4 years and had remarried. However, the temptation to use opiates for more than just pain relief became overwhelming. He began by simply crushing the OxyContin tablets and taking them orally, but he returned to intravenous heroin within months. He was soon back in his parent's house. His mother called me and told me that Jim was not going to work, had been thrown out by his new wife, and was in need of help.

Jim saw me at the VA and asked for help, but he thought that inpatient detoxification at the VA was going to be a problem. He considered himself a role model for the other veterans who had used heroin and felt he could not disappoint them. So he refused inpatient detoxification, and we arranged for a rapid clonidine and naltrexone detoxification in a day-hospital setting. Jim began receiving clonidine the next morning at 9:00 A.M. and was given his first 12.5-mg dose of naltrexone (a quarter of a tablet) at 11:00 A.M. He was sick but sedated. He continued taking the clonidine on a thrice daily schedule. He came back the next day and obtained 25 mg of naltrexone and more clonidine. His 24-hour total clonidine dose was 1.2 mg, and he needed chloral hydrate at night to sleep. On day 3 he was given 50 mg of naltrexone, and he continued the clonidine for a week while taking naltrexone at 50 mg/day. The next week he began naltrexone at 100 mg on Monday and Wednesday and 150 mg on Friday along with urine monitoring and weekly individual counseling. Life returned to normal for him, and he entered into a VA pain management program that did not use opiate medications.

Over the next few years he went on and off naltrexone, but could not maintain opiate abstinence and eventually enrolled in the VA methadone program. Methadone is an oral, long-acting opiate given once daily at a dose of 60–150 mg to prevent opiate withdrawal, reduce craving, and block the effects of abused opiates by cross-tolerance. He was remarkably stable on the program and was considered a model patient. After 3 years of drug-free urine tests, he earned the privilege of having six bottles of methadone to take home each week. Normal practice at the methadone program would be to attend the clinic every day to get the methadone, and the privilege of take-home bottles for 6 of the 7 days each week reflected his outstanding performance in the clinic, including his remaining free of all abused drugs and alcohol. I would see him informally in the hallways of the VA, not in the methadone clinic, which he attended once a week at 7:00 A.M. before he went to work. Jim told me that he had developed diabetes, which was under treatment at the VA primary care clinic. Even with the diabetes, he was a compliant patient in taking his daily insulin injection to control his blood glucose levels. He had relatively few complications, but did develop diabetic neuropathy and pain that again became difficult to manage. He was given various nonopiate medications for the pain, including antidepressants (such as the tricyclic imipramine, which is effective in low doses for pain), and gabapentin and valproate (both antiseizure agents and enhancers of γ-aminobutyric acid neurotransmission that are also effective for treating pain). These medications were marginally successful, and when he stopped me in the hallway, he would tell me not only about his diabetes but also about his parents and his family business. He never spoke about his past opiate abuse. I wondered whether Jim had matured out of opiate dependence and abuse, as has been described for many former addicts as they reach age 40 years.

However, it turned out he had not ended his career in drug addiction and his love affair with heroin. He started looking for doctors outside of the VA health care system to obtain opiates for his various pains. He used synthetic opiates such as oxycodone that are difficult to detect on urine toxicologies and supplemented his methadone doses with supplies from other sources besides the methadone program. He then returned to heroin and his urine toxicologies became positive for morphine. His take-home methadone privileges were taken away, and he went back to daily visits to the methadone program and eventually was restabilized. However, he wanted a different life than what his daily ties to methadone offered.

Treatment With Buprenorphine

The opportunity for a different approach to Jim's treatment came a few years later. He was again stable on methadone, going to the clinic once a week and receiving take-home bottles of methadone. His methadone dosage had been reduced to 50 mg/day, but he wanted his dosage to be tapered lower and to eventually stop taking methadone completely. He seemed ready for a change. I had been working with buprenorphine as an alternative to methadone. Buprenorphine was appropriate because he was socially stable, was taking relatively low dosages of methadone, and had a positive relationship with a primary care medical setting.

Buprenorphine is a partial opiate agonist that acts like the agonist methadone at sublingual dosages (below about 4 mg/day) but at higher dosages (8–32 mg/day) acts more like the antagonist naltrexone. This antagonist action can precipitate opiate withdrawal if given to a patient who is maintained on the usual methadone dosages of 60–150 mg/day.

Jim met all criteria for office-based buprenorphine in the primary care clinic. The clinic had a physician who wanted to work with me to pilot office-based buprenorphine in the clinic. We initially scheduled weekly visits for Jim at the primary care clinic to give Jim a week's supply of buprenorphine rather than the methadone that he had been receiving. During these visits he met with a nurse who provided brief drug abuse counseling, obtained a urine toxicology, and checked his diabetes. Jim was also having follow-up visits for the pain management, with all the medications being supplied by his primary care physician. He loved this new setting for his medical and addiction care and said that he felt like a human being again, not a herded animal. Although Jim's story is not meant to be an indictment of methadone maintenance and its legislated constraints, it does show that stable patients can move beyond regimented methadone treatment to medical maintenance with either methadone or buprenorphine. Treatment of opiate dependence can be like the treatment of other chronic diseases, where office-based therapy is the norm. Opiate maintenance is effective treatment, not a moral statement.

Jim became insulin dependent and took insulin just as he took his buprenorphine. He maintained his medication regimen religiously and adhered to his diabetic care considerably better than many veterans do. He visited his primary care physician monthly for the buprenorphine and updated his care providers on his medical and psychological condition. He also remained in treatment for his PTSD and took antidepressants consistently (switching to sertraline, a serotonin reuptake inhibitor, because of its fewer side effects and lower overdose risk than imipramine) and used other medications for brief periods. He obtained weekly group counseling at the VA's center in West Haven and was provided medications by his psychiatric consultations in the VA substance abuse program.

DISCUSSION

I consider Jim a success story in the treatment of his opiate addiction, a chronic relapsing brain disease. At many points in his career, he appeared to be a failure, particularly when he showed up in the emergency department intoxicated, overdosed, or suicidal due to some combination of PTSD symptoms and drug intoxication or withdrawal. These events are discomforting to any clinician, no matter how many years you are in practice. Nevertheless, because of the rewards, personal insight, and the expansion of your capacity for empathic treatment that can be attained with patients like Jim, I hope you are able to find your own substance-abusing Jim. If such a patient has not entered your practice yet, it is worthwhile to keep searching for that patient. The world is filled with young and old patients like Jim.

As one of my earliest substance-dependent patients, Jim's treatment was a very fortunate initiation for me because he seemed to be a lot like me, yet so different. Both of us are white men who came from blue-collar communities in the northeast, not far from New York City. We both had relatively large families and younger sisters for whom we felt some, almost parental, responsibility. Both of us had been in the Army. He had been a private who was shot at in Vietnam, while I had been in the Reserve Officer Training Corp and had avoided combat through multiple deferments until the end of the military draft. This military connection soon became the basis for a longer-term relationship not only with Jim but also with the rest of his family.

The fundamental humanity of the opiate-dependent patient is most important to find and to bond with, because successful treatment will be a long haul of relapses as the clinician manages a chronic relapsing disease. The diagnosis of opiate dependence is usually easy to make, and detoxification is a minimal clinical challenge. As Mark Twain said about addictions, "Stopping is easy, I have done it hundreds of times." The statement that recovery is lifelong work has become almost a trite saying because of the work that Alcoholics Anonymous has done for over half a century. Nevertheless, the work of avoiding relapse after stopping drug use is lifelong for the 10% of adolescents who start using various drugs and just cannot stop. Every addict had been urged to "just say no" long before Nancy Reagan came around with that saying as a national policy statement on drug abuse–relapse prevention. The addicted population includes people like you, the reader, and finding even one addict who touches your life experience in some way will help more than any amount of knowledge about psychopharmacology or behavioral therapy, even with every word scripted for you.

Opiate dependence is a brain disease for which there are some of the most effective treatments available for any disorder in psychiatry. We have pharmacotherapies that are agonists (methadone), antagonists (naltrexone), and partial agonists (buprenorphine) as well as various detoxification agents (clonidine). A soon-to-be-available innovation is depot naltrexone, which provides a month of heroin blockade after a single injection. (A depot medication is typically encapsulated in thousands of little pellets that slowly break down and deliver sustained release amounts of medication over a long time period.) We also have developed behavioral therapies targeted to substance-dependent patients, including couples and family therapies, relapse-prevention therapies, cognitive therapies, and 12-step therapies based on the principles of Alcoholics Anonymous but applied to opiate dependence. Opiate addiction usually begins at a young age, but the number of older patients abusing prescription opiates has been rising in a similar way to Jim's relapse into opiate use when he experienced various painful syndromes. Oxycodone (OxyContin) is one substance that is increasingly abused by adolescents as well as by older patients being treated for chronic pain. Nevertheless, we have effective treatments for all of these patients including long-term residential treatment in places like Daytop or Phoenix House, where patients make a gradual reentry into the community over a period of 6–18 months.

This case report also illustrates comorbid psychopathology, which is quite common among opiate-dependent patients. The most common disorder is depression, but PTSD is also common, and both can be quite responsive to antidepressant medications such as the selective serotonin reuptake inhibitors (e.g., sertraline). Antisocial personality disorder is not uncommon among these patients, and the most severely antisocial patient may respond only to residential treatment with strong behavioral controls.

Although in this case report I did not emphasize the comorbid substance dependence among opiate addicts, alcohol, cocaine, and marijuana are relatively frequently abused among those entering methadone maintenance, with rates of 25%–50%. This codependence may require medical detoxification in the case of alcohol and benefit from additional pharmacotherapies as well as behavioral contingency interventions. For example, naltrexone can be useful for reducing relapse in both alcohol and opiate dependence in some alcoholic opiate-addicted patients who are detoxified from both drugs. As an alternative to naltrexone, many patients are treated with methadone, and if alcohol is a significant problem for these patients, daily breath alcohol levels are typically obtained as a medical safety consideration. A behavioral intervention is thereby set up in which patients are not given their dose of methadone until their alcohol breath levels drop below legal intoxication limits. If their breath alcohol levels are repeatedly above legal intoxication levels, then the treating staff often consider mandating disulfiram use as a condition of the patient continuing in methadone maintenance. (Disulfiram [Antabuse] is an inhibitor of aldehyde dehydrogenase, the enzyme that coverts aldehyde to water and carbon dioxide. Aldehyde is formed in the first step of the conversion of alcohol to water and carbon dioxide. However, aldehyde at high levels is quite toxic and makes people sick. Thus blocking its conversion makes people sick when they drink alcohol.) In this way, a comprehensive program can be enforced for alcohol and opiate abstinence. Overall, behavioral contingencies are widely used in opiate-dependence treatment and can be quite effective.

My review of Jim's case has covered many treatment interventions that might be needed in managing the long-term care of patients with this chronic relapsing disorder. The treatment options are broad and effective. The pharmacotherapies are frequently complemented by well-targeted behavioral therapies that enhance medication compliance, reinforce abstinence from illicit opiates, and promote prosocial behaviors. I hope this case has left you with enthusiasm for learning more about treating opiate-dependent patients and particularly for exploring the use of office-based buprenorphine in a disorder that afflicts an estimated 1 million people from heroin and 3.5 million from prescription opiates like OxyContin.

REFERENCES

Stanton MD: Structural family therapy with heroin addicts, in The Family Therapy of Drug and Alcohol Abusers. Edited by Kaufman E, Kaufman P. New York, Gardner, 1978

SUGGESTED READING

Amass L, Kamien JB, Mikulich SK: Thrice-weekly supervised dosing with the combination buprenorphine-naloxone tablet is preferred to daily supervised dosing by opioid-dependent humans. Drug Alcohol Depend 61:173–181, 2001

Center for Drug Evaluation and Research, U.S. Food and Drug Administration: Subutex and Suboxone tablets. Available at: http://www.fda.gov/cder/drug/infopage/subutex_suboxone/default.htm

Center for Substance Abuse Treatment, Substance Abuse and Mental Health Services Administration: Buprenorphine. Available at: http://buprenorphine.samhsa.gov/

Fudala PJ, Bridge TP, Herbert S, et al: Office-based treatment of opiate addiction with a sublingual-tablet formulation of buprenorphine and naloxone. N Engl J Med 349:949–958, 2003

Hulse G, Basso MR: Reassessing naltrexone maintenance as a treatment for illicit heroin users. Drug Alcohol Rev 18:263–269, 1999

Kleber HD, Riordan CE, Rounsaville B, et al: Clonidine in outpatient detoxification from methadone maintenance. Arch Gen Psychiatry 42:391–394, 1985

National Consensus Development Panel on Effective Medical Treatment of Opiate Addiction: Effective medical treatment of opiate addiction. JAMA 280:1936–1943, 1998

Novick DM, Pascarelli EF, Joseph H, et al: Methadone maintenance patients in general medical practice: a preliminary report. JAMA 259:3299–3302, 1988

O'Connor PG, Kosten TRL: Rapid and ultrarapid opioid detoxification techniques. JAMA 279:229–234, 1998

O'Connor PG, Carroll KM, Shi JM, et al: Three methods of opioid detoxification in a primary care setting: a randomized trial. Ann Intern Med 127:526–530, 1997

Rosenheck R, Kosten T: Buprenorphine for opiate addiction: potential economic impact. Drug Alcohol Depend 63:253–262, 2001

Rounsaville BJ, Kosten TR: Treatment for opioid dependence: quality and access. JAMA 283:1337–1339, 2000

CHAPTER 9

Free At Last

Natural and Conventional Treatment of a Patient With Multiple Comorbid Psychiatric Disorders

Sharon Sageman, M.D.
Richard Brown, M.D.

Sharon Sageman, M.D., is an Assistant Professor of Psychiatry at Columbia University College of Physicians and Surgeons and New York University Medical School. She is also the Medical Director of the Women's Health Project, a program for the treatment of women who are in recovery from severe trauma and comorbid conditions (including substance abuse and affective disorders) at St. Luke's-Roosevelt Hospital Center in New York City, a teaching hospital center for Columbia University. Dr. Sageman is board certified in adult psychiatry, addiction psychiatry, and geriatric psychiatry as well as being certified in holistic medicine by the American Board of Holistic Medicine. Dr. Sageman is the author of numerous articles in the fields of trauma, alternative approaches in mental health, and psychotherapy, including "Women With PTSD: The Psychodynamic Aspects of Psychopharmacologic and 'Hands-On' Psychiatric Management," "The Rape of Boys and the Impact of Sexually Predatory Environments: Review and Case Reports," "How Sudarshan Kriya Can Treat the Cognitive, Psychodynamic, and Neuro-Psychiatric Problems of Post Traumatic Stress Disorder," and

"Breaking Through the Despair: Spiritually Oriented Group Therapy as a Means of Healing Women With Severe Mental Illness." She is also author of "Group Therapy for Patients With AIDS," a chapter in *Group Psychodynamics: New Paradigms and New Perspectives.*

Richard Brown, M.D., is an Associate Clinical Professor of Psychiatry at Columbia University College of Physicians and Surgeons. He received his medical degree in 1977 from Columbia University College of Physicians and Surgeons and completed his residency in psychiatry and fellowship in psychobiology and psychopharmacology at New York Hospital. In 1999, Dr. Brown introduced S-adenosylmethionine (SAM-e) at the New York Academy of Medicine and the American College for Advancement in Medicine. He coauthored *Stop Depression Now (2000),* a holistic approach to depression that includes SAM-e. Dr. Brown wrote the chapters "Complementary and Alternative Treatments in Psychiatry" in *Psychiatry,* 2nd Edition (2003), and "Alternative Treatments in Brain Injury" in *Neuropsychiatry of Traumatic Brain Injury (2004).* The American Botanical Council published his article "Rhodiola rosea: A Phytomedicinal Overview" in 2002. In 2003 he lectured on Rhodiola rosea at the Columbia University Botanical Medicine course and in 2004 coauthored *The Rhodiola Revolution.*

I (S.S.) EVALUATED HOPE AT THE request of her cognitive-behavioral therapist after she was abruptly thrown out of treatment by her prescribing clinician from another program, who stated that it was too dangerous to prescribe medications while the patient was still drinking. Our program is an outpatient treatment center serving women with a history of childhood abuse and/or adulthood trauma who may also be struggling with an addiction.

HISTORY

Hope had come to our program several months before with the chief complaint "I've got to stop drinking." She admitted to having engaged in frequent binge drinking and marijuana use since age 15 years. Her history included one inpatient admission for alcoholism and three emergency department visits in the past 5 years for alcohol-related injuries, including injuries she once received after falling out of a window while she was drunk.

Hope was an attractive 37-year-old, unemployed acting teacher and stage director with a history of very severe childhood physical abuse and adult sexual assault. Despite the efforts to protect her by a nanny that Hope had when she was young (ages 2–5 years), Hope remembered being repeatedly tortured by her two older brothers between ages 3 and 10. They tied her up and whipped her, killed her beloved pets in front of her, forced her to swallow LSD, and put lizards and snakes on top of her which bit her while she lay tied up and helpless. Hope said, "I was brought up like Strindberg's Miss Julie." She was enraged at her parents who failed to protect her and always found fault with her, making her feel defective, unwanted, and abandoned. She admitted to feeling a severe distrust of authority and said she became enraged whenever she sensed any abuse of power.

DIAGNOSIS

In her first session, she refused to take any conventional psychiatric medication, saying that at this point she would accept only natural remedies. Her record indicated that she had made no improvement on depakote, lamotrigine, or gabapentin, mood stabilizers that had been tried during the previous 3 years. Nevertheless, she wanted help with her symptoms, which she said had plagued her since early adolescence. Hope said she had problems with impulse control, cried several times a day, acted rageful, and had excessive sweating. She also manifested hypervigilance, poor self-esteem, irritability, emotional lability, intrusive memories, flashbacks and nightmares of being tortured, occasional grandiosity, flight of ideas, impaired concentration, and suicidal thoughts (but no plan). Hope reported having difficulty sleeping and said she often had frightening "lizard dreams" if she had not smoked marijuana that day. The "lizard dreams" were nightmares in which she reexperienced being tied up by her brothers and bitten by lizards. She also reported a history of chronic back pain.

Hope said she last used marijuana 1 week before our first session. She noted, "After smoking one joint, it made me manic. I cleaned all the windows and organized a lot of things that I would otherwise have procrastinated about."

Her symptoms were reflected in her behavior during sessions. Most of the time she appeared very depressed, was tearful and agitated, described herself as a failure, had suicidal thoughts, and felt helpless, unlovable, and unable to manage her life. She occasionally presented in a very humorous mood, brightly dressed in new clothes from thrift shops where she said she had spent more than she could afford, displaying grandiosity, laughing and speaking rapidly, and reporting racing thoughts. At times, due to her trauma symptoms, she would miss appointments because she was avoidant and fearful of leaving her home.

Because of her severe trauma symptoms and mood lability, Hope had significant impairment in the occupational and social areas of functioning. Hope was unable to hold any job. Despite her having an above average to superior intelligence, she could not focus her attention adequately to learn new information, so school was also not an option. She had excessive and inappropriate feelings of guilt and blamed herself for not being more productive.

Hope was admitted to our program with diagnoses of posttraumatic stress disorder (PTSD), bipolar I disorder, alcohol dependence, and cannabis abuse. PTSD was diagnosed because of her history of severe physical abuse; her symptoms of avoidance, reexperiencing, flashbacks, nightmares, hypervigilance, irritability, difficulty concentrating, and insomnia; and the intense psychological distress she experienced after being in situations that reminded her of her early trauma (e.g., visits with her family). Her bipolar I diagnosis was based on her history of manic episodes; current periods of grandiosity, rapid speech, talkativeness, excessive spending, and racing thoughts; and periods of depression with tearfulness, feelings of worthlessness, suicidal thoughts, insomnia, and inability to concentrate.

TREATMENT

In the first session, because Hope refused all conventional medications and would only accept natural remedies, I prescribed multivitamins, folic acid, melatonin (6-hour time-release capsules) for her problems with insomnia, and fish oil (10 capsules/day) as a mood stabilizer.

On the following visit, 4 weeks later, Hope told me she had purchased the fish oil, vitamins, and melatonin, but had not taken them every day. She was struggling to remain abstinent from alcohol and had started attending two Alcoholics Anonymous (AA) meetings every day. Hope admitted to a two-day drinking binge, triggered by a visit with her parents, after 28 days of being abstinent. She was tearful, displayed a depressed mood and affect, and was self-critical, telling me that she says to herself, "Your problem is you just don't want to deal with life."

After we discussed the pros and cons of natural versus conventional treatment, Hope agreed to start quetiapine (25–50 mg qhs), a second-generation antipsychotic and an antimanic medication that can be useful in reducing anxiety, agitation, mood swings, depression, and insomnia.

Hope's mood became less labile and agitated with the quetiapine as her dosage was gradually increased up to 300 mg qhs, but she still complained about anxiety, depression, and chronic pain. Gabapentin (an anticonvulsant used to treat anxiety and pain) at 300 mg tid was added, which helped reduce her anxiety and chronic pain, but Hope continued to ask for an antidepressant. She also reported waking up to eat four times each night since starting quetiapine, saying the drug had increased her appetite. Melatonin (6-hour time-release capsules, 6 mg qhs) was added to help her stay asleep through the night.

A week later, Hope requested an extra visit because she was having strong cravings to drink. This was actually the first time she had asked for help in coping with her cravings and mental anguish instead of turning to alcohol or marijuana. She said that the melatonin helped her sleep with fewer awakenings, and that she now experienced only two awakenings each night instead of four. She was sad and tearful.

Hope was given venlafaxine (an antidepressant) at 75 mg every morning. A week later she reported feeling less depressed and crying less. She was calmer with less mood lability and a more positive attitude. The content of the session was less about problems and more about her career goals and interests in acting and directing. She did report having a slip and drinking 4 days earlier after someone had hurt her feelings. Venlafaxine was gradually increased to 150 mg every morning, and Hope reported crying only once per week instead of several times a day. Hope then began to experience difficulty with swallowing while taking the quetiapine (although esophageal dysmotility and aspiration have been associated with antipsychotic drug use, difficulty swallowing is not a known common side effect of quetiapine), so her dosage was tapered and and the quetiapine was replaced with oxcarbazepine 300 mg bid, an anticonvulsant that is thought to have mood-stabilizing properties. While taking this dosage, her mood remained labile and she reported spending too much money, so her dosage was gradually increased to 300 mg bid and 900 mg qhs.

At this point in treatment, Hope had better attendance at AA and fewer slips, but she still did not feel well, still had some mood swings and suicidal thoughts, and was not able to hold a job. She continued to have episodes of binge drinking every time she visited her family or encountered other painful reminders of past abuse. Hope did not want to take disulfiram (a medication taken daily to help individuals resist the temptation to drink alcohol due to its ability to make one violently ill after having even a single drink), and since she had already gained 15 pounds, she did not want any treatment, including lithium or valproic acid, that could cause further weight gain.

I asked her if she was interested in trying yogic breathing as a means of self-soothing and treating her depression and flashbacks without having to take more medication. She was very interested and started a 5-day basic course in yogic breathing. This course includes three major forms of yogic breathing: advanced *Ujjayi* (victorious breath), *Bhastrika* (bellows breath), and a unique breathing called *Sudarshan kriya* (translated as "proper vision by purifying action"). However, Hope left the class after 2 days because she became too anxious to complete it. It appeared that she had been very outgoing, open, and self-revealing with others in the breathing course and that this made her feel too frightened, foolish, exposed, and vulnerable to tolerate staying in the class.

Hope was given instruction in doing only Ujjayi breathing for 5 minutes twice a day at home for a few months. (Ujjayi is slow yogic breathing against airway resistance created by slight contraction of the laryngeal muscles. This most basic form of yogic breathing reduces sympathetic nervous system tone and enhances vagal tone, and thus prepares the nervous system for more intense breathing work.) She was then ready to attempt taking the course again. This time Hope kept a lower profile, was less anxious, and succeeded in completing the course. After doing the daily breathing exercises, she still had nightmares and some mood lability but said she felt more balanced, adding, "I feel like I am on the precipice of hope." She continued to do the recommended breathing exercises and attend the weekly group yogic breathing sessions. A year later I asked her if she continued to have any suicidal thoughts. She said she had had none since she started to do the yogic breathing.

In an attempt to manage her mood problems, insomnia, and trauma symptoms, over the next 16 months Hope was prescribed various other antidepressants and antipsychotic medications but with only limited success. Throughout the period that I treated her, she was also treated with cognitive-behavioral therapy for her PTSD, bipolar disorder, and substance abuse. This helped her to understand her symptoms and identify cognitive distortions and triggers related to her drinking as well as to her response to trauma. After completing 2 years of treatment, she rarely attended her cognitive-behavioral therapy sessions but continued to improve with aripiprazole, oxcarbamazepine, venlafaxine, and daily yogic breathing.

The last time I saw her she had lost weight and looked slender and beautiful. She was on the brink of celebrating her first year of total abstinence since age 15 years. Hope said she no longer had flashbacks or experienced depression and that she felt centered and optimistic about her future. She was unable to attend our clinic because she was too busy attending classes in entertainment technology and lighting and holding down three part-time jobs to support herself. Hope said she loves her current field of study and has a good chance of obtaining a stable, well-paying job after graduation. She still attends AA meetings regularly, is compliant with all of her medications, and has found a new treatment source for them which is more compatible with her busy schedule. She thanked me warmly for being so patient and caring with her during our years together. Free of her feelings of self-hate, rage, and despair and no longer haunted by memories of torture, she is finally able to enjoy her life and be the active, creative, independent woman she has always wanted to be.

DISCUSSION

The issue of differential diagnosis is quite complicated in Hope's case, but her story is being presented because it is reflective of the myriad problems clinicians face in the real world in treating adult survivors of severe childhood trauma. PTSD is highly comorbid with other psychiatric disorders. According to the National Comorbidity Survey (Kessler et al. 1995), more than 50% of patients with a lifetime history of PTSD have comorbidity with three or more other mental disorders, and over 90% of persons with bipolar disorder also have at least one anxiety disorder at some point during their lifetime. Only a small number of patients with PTSD (approximately 20%) have no other psychiatric diagnosis. Patients with PTSD have much higher rates of alcohol and drug abuse, somatic symptoms, and affective disorder (Frayne et al. 2004). Hope's struggle to endure the problems of PTSD along with her efforts to cope with four other diagnoses (alcohol abuse, marijuana abuse, chronic pain, and bipolar disorder) is thus the norm rather than the exception in this population.

It is unclear whether Axis II pathology was present in Hope's case. Her symptoms could all be accounted for by her severe PTSD, bipolar disorder, and substance abuse. When she was discharged from therapy, after benefiting from treatment for PTSD and bipolar disorder and being abstinent from alcohol and marijuana, she was relieved of most of her trauma and mood symptoms. At that point she did not manifest significant problems in cognition, affectivity, interpersonal functioning, or impulse control as would be expected with a personality disorder.

The urgency for treating these comorbid psychiatric illnesses is further underscored by the serious risk for suicide seen with this kind of patient (Kessler et al. 1997). Research from the Stanley Foundation Bipolar Network indicates that a history of childhood physical or sexual abuse is a prominent risk factor for attempted suicide and results in an approximate 15% increase in lifetime incidence of suicide attempts over the baseline rate of about 25% for patients with bipolar disorder (Post 2002). Substance abuse and comorbid medical problems (e.g., chronic pain) increase the risk of suicide even further.

Without treatment, Hope was in a high risk group for attempting suicide. In our very first meeting, Hope revealed an identification with Strindberg's (2000) "Miss Julie"; this was an ominous reference to a fallen young aristocratic woman whose life ended in a tragic suicide. In the play, Miss Julie slits her own throat with a razor given to her by her male servant and lover shortly after he chops off the head of her pet finch in front of her. Hope's childhood torture included having to watch helplessly as her pets were slaughtered in front of her, and she, like Miss Julie, viewed herself as a hopeless failure. She admitted to often wishing she were dead and having recurrent suicidal thoughts.

This case also demonstrates the crucial importance of making a clear and thorough differential diagnosis to provide effective treatment. Hope's symptoms of bipolar disorder and PTSD started in early adolescence; however, she received no treatment for these disorders and instead was treated only for substance abuse for many years. Bipolar disorder and PTSD are frequently misdiagnosed, and the presence of a history of childhood physical abuse delays the appropriate treatment of bipolar disorder from an average of 8 years for those without a history of childhood abuse to 13 years for others (Leverich et al. 2002). Patients with a childhood history of physical abuse also have an earlier onset of bipolar symptoms, which is associated with a worse prognosis and an increased number of Axis I, II, and III comorbid disorders, including drug and alcohol abuse, faster cycling frequencies, and a higher rate of suicide attempts (Leverich et al. 2002).

The differential diagnosis of Hope's symptoms was further complicated by the considerable overlap in the symptoms of substance abuse, bipolar disorder, and PTSD. All three can present with agitation, insomnia, poor self-esteem, poor vocational and social functioning, emotional lability, and depression, as was seen in Hope's case. Hope also presented with symptoms such as flashbacks and intrusive memories of trauma, which are unique to the cluster of symptoms in PTSD called "reexperiencing," and flight of ideas and grandiosity, which are unique to the manic symptom profile seen in bipolar disorder. The symptoms of hyperarousal and hypervigilance that are characteristic of PTSD can be difficult to distinguish from the psychomotor agitation, sleep difficulty, and pressured speech seen in bipolar disorder. Hope presented with all of these.

In addition to clarifying the differential diagnosis of Hope's problems with PTSD, bipolar disorder, and substance abuse, it is crucial to understand the relation of each of the three in the genesis of her symptoms and the role each played in her downward spiral. Female patients with PTSD or bipolar disorder may use alcohol to self-medicate intolerable affect. Hope also used marijuana to help relieve her depression and nightmares of torture (lizard dreams). Her slips with alcohol always followed reminders of past abuse. Her substance use further exacerbated her affective symptoms, including her low self-esteem, feelings of guilt and hopelessness, depression, and mood instability. The prescribing clinician who refused to treat Hope until she stopped drinking showed a lack of understanding of the complex differential diagnosis present, the inextricable intertwining of the three diagnoses, and thus the need to treat all three simultaneously for the patient to recover.

This case also illustrates the burgeoning interest in and demand from patients for natural and alternative treatments, reflecting a major societal trend. Patients who refuse treatment with conventional agents often do so because they have had unpleasant experiences with other medications. In some cases, the insistence on natural treatments is also a reflection of specific psychodynamic issues. In our first meeting, Hope said she would accept only natural remedies. This was probably due, at least in part, to the fact that she had been disappointed with prior failed treatment attempts with depakote, lamotrigine, and gabapentin. Hope's refusal to accept any conventional psychiatric medication may also have been a manifestation of her distrust and rage at authority figures, an attitude that is frequently seen in trauma survivors (Herman 1992). It may also have stemmed from her fear of being powerless and being abused again, which she handled by insisting on being in control of the type of treatment she would accept.

My willingness to try to help Hope even though she would accept only natural treatments and even though she was still drinking conveyed a message of acceptance and respect for her feelings that paved the way for a positive therapeutic relationship with this severely traumatized woman. Alternative treatment also played an important role later in her treatment course when she committed herself to the daily practice of yogic breathing. Hope said that the breathing she practiced gave her hope and stopped her from having suicidal thoughts. She described the yogic breathing as helping her "feel light but grounded" and as "a self-soothing kind of thing" that allowed her to feel calmer and safer without having to turn to drugs.

This case also illustrates another current trend in treatment in which patients are treated simultaneously by more than one clinician. Currently, the role of the psychiatrist is often as the psychopharmacologist and not as the primary therapist. Hope developed a close and trusting relationship with me, even though I was not her primary therapist, and it may have been an important factor in her recovery. This case illustrates the role of the psychopharmacologist as not just as a dispenser of pills but also as a source of comfort, unconditional acceptance, and hope in the face of despair. This type of interaction can make a life or death difference for patients like Hope, who feel hopeless and demoralized after experiencing a lifetime of severe mental illness. The wealth of treatments available today for severe depression and trauma provide a realistic basis for optimism. The healing power of the therapeutic relationship with patients like Hope who live in a world of self-hate, dread, and despair is predicated on always conveying an attitude of unconditional love and acceptance as well as the hope that they can improve and become well.

Hope's case illustrates how patients presenting with multiple comorbid diagnoses, such as PTSD, mood disorders, and substance abuse, often require complex treatments to recover and succeed in remaining abstinent. Hope showed a reduced frequency of binge drinking and marijuana use after cognitive-behavioral therapy, daily attendance at AA, and treatment with oxcarbamazepine, gabapentin, and venlafaxine. The biggest gains, however, in her being able to maintain prolonged abstinence and becoming well enough to return to school and work appear to have occurred after the addition of daily yogic breathing and aripiprazole.

Aripiprazole is the newest of the atypical antipsychotic drugs. It has been shown to be effective in treating bipolar mania in both the manic and the mixed states and for patients with a history of rapid and nonrapid cycling (Keck et al. 2003). It also has been shown to have dopamine (D_2) agonist and antagonist activities on dopaminergic neurons of the ventral tegmental area and nucleus accumbens (Matsubayashi et al. 1999), both areas that are known to play a major role in addiction and craving. It has been approved for the treatment of mania and is currently being studied as a treatment for substance abuse. Several published studies on other atypical antipsychotics (olanzapine, quetiapine, risperidone) (Hamner et al. 2003; Reich et al. 2004; Stein et al. 2002) have shown a significant improvement in trauma symptoms, reduced scores on the Clinician Administered PTSD scale, and reduced symptoms of hyperarousal. In the author's experience with aripiprazole, it has shown improvement in PTSD symptoms similar to other atypical antipsychotics and also significant improvement in craving and addictive behaviors. Thus it is possible that aripiprazole played a key role in Hope's recovery by providing affective stabilization, reducing her cravings for alcohol and marijuana, and decreasing her hyperarousal and trauma symptoms.

Hope credited her practice of yogic breathing with enabling her to feel more balanced, giving her hope, and freeing her of suicidal thoughts. In her second attempt at the breathing course, she felt accepted without being judged. Several months of preparation, including basic yogic breathing to strengthen her system, made it possible for her to complete this course. She reported several years later that she feels "high in a good way" from breathing compared with the self-destructive high she had felt with substances of abuse. She had stopped having flashbacks and sleep problems. Hope said that for her the breathing was a means of "getting the strength back to trust people again." When asked how the breathing did that, she said that it works "by grounding you" so that "you can be light but grounded." She expressed having a sense of being "cleansed" (cleared of negative emotions) after long breathing sessions. It is notable that she has been more adherent to yogic breath practice than to medication or psychotherapy.

Patients with depression, panic disorder, and PTSD have overactive sympathetic systems and underactive parasympathetic systems. Yogic breathing corrects these imbalances and the hemispheric asymmetry that is associated with depression (Brown and Gerbarg 2005; Brown et al. 2003). Long-term practitioners of this style of yoga show improved integration of the cortical hemispheres and a brain wave pattern characteristic of both enhanced vigilance and relaxation (Bhatia et al. 2003). Levels of cortisol, the stress hormone, decrease, and prolactin, one of several antistress and social bonding hormones, is released. These yogic breathing techniques have been used effectively to treat survivors of mass disasters, rapes, and violent war crimes. (For more in-depth reviews, see Brown and Gerbarg 2005; Brown et al. 2003; Gerbarg and Brown, in press.)

Hope credited the yogic breathing with providing her with a means of self-soothing and for increasing her resilience so that she no longer became despondent and hopeless when painful triggers recurred. In yogic philosophy, one of the breathing forms she learned, the Sudarshan Kriya, serves to break the link between past trauma and negative emotions. After 2.5 years of practice, she felt free of the sense of fear and dread that had previously paralyzed her. In our last conversation she said, "I'm in a good placeæin a safe place, that safety that nothing can take away."

REFERENCES

Bhatia M, Kumar A, Kumar N, et al: Electrophysiologic evaluation of Sudarshan Kriya: an EEG, BAER, P300 Study. Indian J Physiol Pharmacol 47:157–163, 2003

Brown RP, Gerbarg PL: Sudarshan Kriya yogic breathing in the treatment of stress, anxiety, and depression, I: neurophysiologic model. J Altern Complement Med 11:189–201, 2005

Brown RP, Gerbarg PL, Muskin PR: Alternative treatments in psychiatry, in Psychiatry, 2nd Edition. Edited by Tasman A, Kay J, Lieberman JA. London, Wiley, 2003, pp 2147–2183

Frayne SM, Seaver MR, Loveland S, et al: Burden of medical illness in women with depression and posttraumatic stress disorder. Arch Intern Med 164:1306–1312, 2004

Gerbarg PL, Brown RP: Yoga in psychiatry, in Clinical Manual of Complementary and Alternative Treatments in Psychiatry. Edited by Lake JH, Spiegel D. Washington, DC, American Psychiatric Publishing (in press)

Hamner MB, Deitsch SE, Brodrick PS, et al: Quetiapine treatment in patients with post-traumatic stress disorder: an open trial of adjunctive therapy. J Clin Psychopharmacol 23:15–20, 2003

Herman JL: Trauma and Recovery. New York, Basic Books, 1997, p 111

Keck PE, Marcus R, Tourkodimitris S, et al: A placebo-controlled, double-blind study of the efficacy and safety of aripiprazole in patients with acute bipolar mania. Am J Psychiatry 160:1651–1658, 2003

Kessler RC, Sonnaga A, Bromet E, et al: Posttraumatic stress disorder in the National Comorbidity Survey. Arch Gen Psychiatry 52:1048–1060, 1995

Kessler RC, Rubinow DR, Holmes C, et al: The epidemiology of DSM-III-R bipolar I disorder in a general population survey (abstract). Psychol Med 27:1079–1089, 1997

Leverich GS, McElroy SL, Suppes T, et al: Early physical and sexual abuse associated with an adverse course of bipolar illness. Biol Psychiatry 51:288–297, 2002

Matsubayashi H, Amano T, Sasa M: Inhibition by aripiprazole of dopaminergic inputs to striatal neurons from substantia nigra. Psychopharmacology (Berl) 146:139–143, 1999

Post RM: New findings on suicide attempts, substance abuse, obesity, and more. Curr Psychiatry 1:26–32, 2002

Reich DB, Winternitz S, Hennen J, et al: A preliminary study of risperidone in the treatment of post-traumatic stress disorder related to childhood abuse in women. J Clin Psychiatry 65:1601–1606, 2004

Stein MB, Kline NA, Matloff JL: Adjunctive olanzapine for SSRI-resistant combat-related PTSD: a double blind placebo-controlled study. Am J Psychiatry 159:1777–1779, 2002

Strindberg A: Five Major Plays. Translated by Mueller CR. Lyme, NH, Smith & Kraus, 2000

PART V

Schizophrenia and Other Psychotic Disorders

CHAPTER 10

Like a Glass on the Edge of a Chair

Inpatient Treatment of Schizophrenia

Paul J. Rosenfield, M.D.
Ronald O. Rieder, M.D.

Paul J. Rosenfield, M.D., is Assistant Clinical Professor of Psychiatry at Columbia University College of Physicians and Surgeons and Attending Psychiatrist and Assistant Unit Chief of the Schizophrenia Research Unit at New York State Psychiatric Institute. He received his bachelor's degree in history from Brown University and his medical degree from Columbia University. He completed his residency at the University of California, San Francisco, where he received the Laughlin Award for excellence in therapeutic skills and dedication to the welfare of patients. His clinical and research interests include the diagnosis and treatment of schizophrenia, particularly the phenomenology of disease subtypes and issues surrounding medication adherence. He is an active clinician-educator in the medical school, teaching and supervising students at all levels of training.

Ronald O. Rieder, M.D., is Vice Chairman for Education, Professor of Clinical Psychiatry, and Director of the Schizophrenia Research Fellowship in the Department of Psychiatry of Columbia University, as well as Director of Postgraduate Education and the Adult Psychiatry Residency Program at the New York State Psychiatric Institute. He did his undergraduate and medical training at Harvard University, his psychiatric residency at Albert Einstein College of Medicine, and research training at the Intramural Research Program of the National Institute of Mental Health. Dr. Rieder's research and teaching interests have been in the area of schizophrenia, including research on the phenomenology, genetics, and neuroanatomy of the disorder. He is the recipient of two National Institute of Mental Health grants to fund research training in schizophrenia and affective and related disorders. He has served as President of the American Association of Directors of Residency Training.

ANTONIO WAS A 24-YEAR-OLD, single, unemployed, bilingual, Hispanic man living with his adoptive parents whose mother brought him for screening and subsequent admission to our inpatient schizophrenia research unit after he told her he wanted to kill himself by jumping in front of a bus. He agreed to come into the hospital as a last resort because he felt he could potentially get "energy to fight against the people controlling my body." Antonio had already been hospitalized four times over the previous 4 years for psychosis, bizarre behavior, and agitation and was repeatedly nonadherent with his medications and follow-up treatment. He was not taking any medication on admission.

Antonio was a good-looking, likable, earnest young man whose gentle demeanor was largely obscured by his anguish and intense efforts to contain his psychotic experience. He tried to minimize his distress, stating that he was relaxed and "not desperate anymore," although this was clearly not the case. He proceeded nonetheless to explain that 20–40 people had entered his body and taken his strength. Voluntarily making his arm limp, he demonstrated that the people inside him were controlling his movements and his ability to hold himself up so that he was almost like a puppet. He kept a yellow string hanging from his lips down to his chin whose purpose was to "hold" him together and focus his concentration on getting the people out. Displaying obvious disgust, he explained that these people spit their saliva into his mouth and that was why he repeatedly spit into a cup he was holding. He excused himself during the interview to go to the bathroom to loudly snort and clear his throat to rid himself of the saliva and to evade the people following him. He was convinced that the people were scratching and tearing away at his skin to enter him. His lips were "stretched" because his former boss, "a fat black man," had entered him and superimposed his lips on his. He complained that his pulse was too fast because it included beats from the people inside him. His mother reported that he sometimes turned on all the burners on the stove at home to burn the people and that he regularly went to the bridge "trying to throw the people off." She feared he would throw himself off as well.

Antonio reported experiencing persecutory auditory hallucinations. The people inside him repeatedly called him a faggot and declared to him or to each other, "We don't care about you," or "He's not a man." He asserted that the voices "freeze my face," paralyzing his facial muscles. Antonio also claimed that he could smell the people inside of him and that sometimes he saw them having sex with one another. He could taste their semen in addition to the saliva filling his mouth. He expressed concern that the voices would not let him eat and that he had lost up to 20 lb over the past 3 months. He was frequently noted to be talking loudly to himself in his room and laughing inappropriately.

Antonio complained of an intermittently depressed mood and decreased energy and concentration, such as he had for several days before his admission. He denied a sense of guilt or worthlessness but endorsed feelings of hopelessness and passive suicidal thoughts. He had no history of suicide attempts.

HISTORY

Antonio's mother reported that as a teenager Antonio had become involved with "the wrong crowd" and had started using alcohol and marijuana. He had drunk two to six beers about twice a week since age 19 years, which Antonio reported helped him cope with his problems. He stated he still did not feel a desire to cut down on his drinking, although his mother felt he should. His mother reported no evidence of alcohol tolerance or physiological withdrawal and denied Antonio's having any history of blackouts, medical complications, or substance abuse treatment. Antonio reported that he had been smoking one marijuana joint every 1–2 weeks since age 18 and that the amount had recently increased to two or more joints weekly to help him "bring [his] old person back." He reported a history of smoking one-half of a pack of cigarettes a day for 6 years, but stated he had quit smoking 1 year earlier.

Prior to his first hospitalization at age 20, Antonio was often awake at night and asleep in the day, played music loudly to distract himself from disturbing thoughts, believed that Jennifer Lopez was sending him messages on the TV and radio, and at times vomited the meals his mother prepared for him for reasons that were unclear. On one occasion, he became argumentative with his family and punched a hole in the wall, after which his family admitted him to the hospital for the first time. A urine toxicology was positive for cannabinoids, evidence of marijuana use. He was stabilized on the antipsychotic medication risperidone 3 mg/day and discharged to an outpatient treatment program, but he did not attend.

After 6 months, he started using marijuana and alcohol again. He was admitted to the emergency department several times for bizarre behavior and released to his parents. He was hospitalized for a second time at age 22 with psychotic symptoms, including religious preoccupation, auditory hallucinations, and for having made threats to kill his father. He initially refused medication but required emergency haloperidol and lorazepam after verbal altercations with peers. He was then treated with olanzapine up to 25 mg and responded fairly well, although he gained 15 pounds. During his third hospitalization for psychotic symptoms a few months later, he received ziprasidone and risperidone, both of which he said caused "shaking" side effects. He was referred to a dual-diagnosis residence for the treatment of individuals struggling with mental illness and substance dependence but returned home after 3 days. For 8 months, he reportedly abstained from substances yet continued to have mild psychotic symptoms. During his fourth hospitalization, at age 23, he was started on monthly haloperidol decanoate injections (instead of the daily oral form) but claimed the drug made him weak and caused "the people to start entering my body." He said his body had not felt the same since, and he attributed his current delusions and somatic symptoms to those injections. His mother reported that after he began taking the haloperidol decanoate he had actually been doing well and was initially able to work with his father as a forklift operator. After 3 months, however, Antonio refused the next injection and his mother reported that his symptoms returned. Within 2 months, Antonio reported that his "fat man boss" had entered his body. Antonio visualized running over him with the forklift to "stop his pulse inside my body," but he never acted on these violent thoughts.

Antonio was adopted at age 2 years after his mother, who had been renting a room from his future adoptive parents, started drinking, then neglected and eventually abandoned him. After an unsuccessful attempt to find her, his adoptive parents decided to raise him as their own child. They told him of his adoption when he was age 10, but they almost never discussed it again and never told anyone outside the family (Antonio did not want his mother to tell us either). As a child in Venezuela, Antonio was a good student and a chess player but was quiet and shy. At age 12, 2 years after moving to the United States, he dropped out of school because the other children made fun of him. He decided instead to make money doing temporary cleaning and construction jobs. By age 17, he became more angry and withdrawn to the point of losing contact with his friends, but he continued to do temporary jobs.

Antonio had no reported history of head trauma, seizures, or other medical conditions that could cause psychosis. On admission, his physical examination was unremarkable and he had a normal body mass index (a measurement of weight that adjusts for height) of 24. There were no signs of tardive dyskinesia, a movement disorder related to long-term antipsychotic medication use. The results of his electrocardiogram and laboratory tests, including an HIV test, were all within normal limits except for the presence of cannabinoids in his urine toxicology screen. A magnetic resonance imaging (MRI) scan, which produces detailed images of the brain to allow identification of any abnormalities, showed no signs of bleeding, mass, or infarct and no significant enlargement of ventricles (although mild brain matter loss and subsequent ventricular enlargement are common findings in schizophrenia). An electroencephalogram was normal and provided evidence to rule out a seizure disorder.

DIAGNOSIS

Antonio's primary diagnosis was schizophrenia, undifferentiated type. He had multiple bizarre delusions, auditory and gustatory hallucinations, disorganized behavior and speech, inappropriate affect, persistent signs of illness for several years, and significant decline and ongoing impairment in social, occupational, and overall functioning. The exacerbation in his symptoms at the time of admission appeared to be related to his nonadherence to treatment and lack of involvement in any treatment program, his ongoing marijuana and alcohol use, and his strained relations with his family.

Kurt Schneider (1959) could have had someone like Antonio in mind when he described several of the first-rank symptoms that he proposed to distinguish schizophrenia from affective disorders: voices talking with one another, somatic passivity experiences ("being controlled by the people"), loss of a sense of one's own volition and affects, and delusional perceptions (experiencing bodily sensations as signs of other people's presence), among others. Although these first-rank symptoms have been shown not to be pathognomonic of schizophrenia (Pope and Lipinski 1978), as they can be present in other psychiatric disorders, they are nonetheless more common in schizophrenia.

In addition, we considered the diagnosis of a comorbid major depressive disorder, given his depressed mood, weight loss, loss of energy, hopelessness, and suicidal ideation. However, these symptoms did not last for 2 weeks at a time, and some were directly directly related to his psychotic symptoms. Nonetheless, suicide is a significant risk for individuals with schizophrenia, especially in the first few years of illness. A recent meta-analysis revised the lifetime risk of suicide in schizophrenia from the widely quoted 10% to 5.6%, still a significant burden of the illness (Palmer et al. 2005).

Antonio met criteria for alcohol and cannabis dependence, without physiological dependence, given his maladaptive pattern of use, unsuccessful efforts to maintain sobriety or consistently limit the quantity used and his continued use despite the contribution to recurrent exacerbations of his psychiatric condition. Cannabis has attracted much attention recently as an independent risk factor not only for brief psychotic disorder but also for schizophrenia. Arsenault et al. (2004) reviewed five major studies that indicated an approximately twofold increase in relative risk for schizophrenia in heavy cannabis users and noted a dose-response relation. In a longitudinal study that studied gene-environment interactions from childhood to adulthood, Caspi et al. (2005) found that individuals who carry two copies of the valine allele of the COMT (catechol *O*-methyltransferase) gene have a greatly increased risk of psychosis if they used marijuana during adolescence. Although Antonio's psychosis was likely exacerbated by substances, it also clearly persisted at times when he was abstinent, indicating the presence of a primary psychotic disorder.

Given the course of Antonio's illness and the lack of findings, other than weight loss, on a review of systems, physical examination, laboratory tests, MRI, and electroencephalogram, the likelihood that Antonio had a psychotic disorder due to a general medical condition was small. Antonio's weight loss was likely attributable to the effects of his psychosis; medical etiologies such as tuberculosis, gastrointestinal disease, and cancer were subsequently ruled out. His history of self-induced vomiting was brief and clearly linked to psychotic content rather than bulimia. Once he was back on medication and given regular meals, he quickly returned to his previous weight and was not preoccupied with losing weight.

A family psychiatric history was not obtainable beyond the information about his biological mother's likely alcohol dependence and subsequent neglect and abandonment of her child. Adoption and twin studies have firmly established that genetic factors play a strong role in the etiology of schizophrenia, although environmental factors, such as influenza during pregnancy, head trauma, and marijuana use, confer increased risk as well.

Although Antonio's English was not as fluent as might be expected for a person living in the United States since age 10 years, he was bilingual and quite well acculturated. He identified as being Catholic and did not frame his symptoms as a form of spirit possession. His adoptive family treated him as their own son and did not display any ambivalence about continuing to care for him. However, the family's avoidance of discussing his adoption may have led Antonio to develop deep-seated anxieties about his sense of belonging, painful questions about why his biological family abandoned him, and fears about losing his adoptive family (e.g., if he moved to a residence). As Antonio privately struggled with distressing symptoms, he worked hard to be a "good patient" so he could win our acceptance and respect.

TREATMENT

Treatment on an inpatient unit should be collaborative, with input from and good communication among all the disciplines: psychiatry, psychology, nursing, social work, and occupational/recreational therapy. In our team meeting after Antonio's admission, we discussed his case, agreed on a provisional diagnosis, and established a treatment plan. We based our plan largely on principles elaborated in established practice guidelines (Lehman et al. 2004). Our initial goals were to reduce the severity of his psychosis, gather information about his history, and establish a treatment alliance. We chose to treat him with aripiprazole initially because we had the impression from him and his family that his previous medications had not been helpful and had caused significant side effects. Aripiprazole, a partial dopamine agonist, has been shown in randomized controlled studies to be effective for symptoms of schizophrenia and to have a lower risk of extrapyramidal side effects and fewer metabolic side effects (such as weight gain, hyperglycemia, diabetes, and hyperlipidemia) than some other second-generation antipsychotics (El-Sayeh and Morganti 2004). We thought that if this medication were tolerable and helpful to Antonio, then perhaps he would agree to continue taking it after leaving the hospital, although we were well aware that his nonadherence was probably more affected by his lack of insight into his illness. We also temporarily prescribed the benzodiazepine lorazepam, which helped Antonio's intermittent periods of anxiety associated with psychotic symptoms.

While we proceeded with the medical and psychiatric assessments, we worked to establish a supportive therapeutic alliance so that Antonio would trust us and we could thereby gain more credibility in engaging him to become an active member in his treatment. There is evidence that treatment adherence and longer-term outcomes are related to the therapeutic alliance (Frank and Gunderson 1990). We appealed to his desire for scientific explanations, showing him the results of his laboratory tests and MRI to demonstrate our consideration of other possible causes of his experiences, and explained that we felt that these were actually symptoms of schizophrenia and that they were treatable. We tried to help him distinguish normal bodily sensations and common medication side effects from delusional perceptions. The medical student working with him asked him to draw a picture of the people in his body. Antonio proceeded to draw a picture of a train with six cars, each labeled with a different month corresponding to the time when particular people entered him. He explained that he was at the back of the train, while his former boss and others were up front and controlling its movement. Antonio said that the only time he could reach the front of the train was when he smoked marijuana or drank alcohol. We worked with this image to help him regain a sense of control without using marijuana or alcohol, encouraging him to be in the driver's seat and direct the train. He agreed, perhaps genuinely, that these two substances actually made the train feel out of control and likely exacerbated his condition.

Despite our best efforts, we were discouraged by Antonio's seemingly impenetrable lack of insight into his illness and the role of treatment, a common experience in the treatment of schizophrenia. The treatment course was all the more difficult because of the significant side effects he had experienced from his past medications. We agreed that too high a dose of haloperidol may indeed have made him "weak" via its effects on his movements, facial expression, mood, and motivation. Secondary negative symptoms due to dopamine blockade may lead to flattened affect and loss of motivation that need to be distinguished from primary symptoms of schizophrenia. Akinesia, characterized by a sense of lifelessness and lack of spontaneity, along with extrapyramidal side effects such as akathisia (restlessness) and a parkinsonian tremor, contribute significantly to medication nonadherence and rejection of treatment (Perkins 2002; Rosenheck 2005). We explained that we would try to limit the side effects of the medications that had made him feel weak and capitalize on the medication's capacity to strengthen him.

Over the first several weeks of his hospitalization, Antonio still complained of people being inside his body, was heard by nursing staff to make loud snorting and spitting noises in his room, and continued to deny he had a mental illness, but he experienced a decrease in the voices and the intensity of his distress, had resolution of his suicidal ideation, demonstrated a brighter affect, participated in groups on the unit, and stated he felt "calmer" and had "more energy." He proudly noted that he was no longer carrying around a cup to spit into or a string in his mouth, and he talked about wanting to return to work as a forklift operator with his father and finish his GED. His mother said, "He is the best I've seen in years." He participated in research testing, including symptom measures and neuropsychological testing. The latter demonstrated deficits in working memory, processing speed, and verbal memory, all phenomena common in schizophrenia and even more closely linked to functional outcome than the presence of active psychotic symptoms (Green 1996).

The team started to discuss discharging Antonio. As a test, we cautiously sent him home for an overnight stay to assess his readiness for discharge and help him make the transition. However, upon his return, a nurse smelled alcohol on his breath and Antonio was discovered to have a blood alcohol concentration of 0.21%. He had not taken any medication at home, had argued with his family, and had yelled at neighbors on the street to stop getting inside him; he then drank to calm himself down. We realized that his improved functioning in the structured setting of the hospital did not necessarily translate into a readiness for discharge and the challenge of dealing with the stresses of daily life and the impulse to drink. On the unit, he became more agitated again, spitting more, shouting, pacing, and crying at times. He said, "My feelings are like a glass on the edge of this chair." He felt tired of the intense effort he had to exert to contain himself and "be a good patient."

We decided to revise his treatment plan and give him another trial of a long-acting injectable antipsychotic as well as urge him to consider a residential dual-diagnosis program. Because injectable risperidone was not covered under Medicaid, we chose fluphenazine decanoate. We were wary of trying a medication similar to haloperidol, which had caused such significant side effects previously. However, we were encouraged to pursue this course by evidence from the Department of Veterans Affair's cooperative study (Rosenheck et al. 2003), a large randomized clinical trial, which found haloperidol to be equivalent to olanzapine in level of adherence, overall symptom reduction, parkinsonian side effects, and quality of life, but without the weight gain. The use of prophylactic anticholinergic medication with haloperidol (to prevent extrapyramidal side effects) differentiated this study from others that had found advantages for olanzapine and other second-generation antipsychotic medications.

Antonio was started on oral fluphenazine and benztropine and then transitioned to fluphenazine decanoate, eventually settling on a dosage of 18.75 mg injected intramuscularly every 2 weeks with benztropine 3 mg/day. Because of his intermittent anxiety, which likely played a role in his drinking and overall distress, clonazepam 1.5 mg/day was added. With this combination, he was again able to make progress and he worked hard to follow the unit rules and engage in treatment to increase his privileges and be discharged. One of the few times he demonstrated some insight into his illness was during a structured therapy group that I ran, along with medical students, in which he had to respond to the question, "What do you hope people will notice about you?" He became tearful and said quietly, "That I don't have schizophrenia." We discussed how hard he tried to appear well, both to himself and to others, and how he actually became much less fragile when in treatment. I hoped that this would signal a turning point in his treatment, but he continued to struggle against accepting his illness.

Meanwhile, the treatment team continued to work with Antonio and his family to educate them further about the risks of relapse if Antonio discontinued his medication or used alcohol and marijuana and about the benefits of a structured outpatient program. Antonio was strongly opposed to a residential program and insisted on returning to work after being discharged. Despite his history, his parents were reluctant to send him away from home. We worked together to establish a discharge plan that we could all agree on, which would take into consideration Antonio's desire to work and his family's and our concerns about the risk of relapse of both his schizophrenia and his substance dependence. We wanted to encourage Antonio and his family and maintain hope for Antonio's good prognosis, a key ingredient to successful outcomes and reduced suicide risk, while recognizing the seriousness of his illness. We eventually referred Antonio to an outpatient, dual-diagnosis day treatment program in which he was assigned an intensive case manager, and sent him on more visits home, which took place without incident. He contracted with his parents to continue his treatment and abstain from using substances, with the consequence of noncompliance being that they would not allow him to continue living at home. On his eventual discharge, he was appreciative of the care he had received, was quite pleased with his condition and how well he was tolerating the medication, and appeared motivated to continue treatment.

I contacted Antonio 3 months after his discharge. He was excited to report to me that he was not spitting and was working with his father as a forklift operator again, as he had planned, but that he was going to move to Florida to live near his brother and regretted that he would not be able to make it to our annual patient reunion. He said he had continued his medication and visits to the clinic for nearly 2 months but was now feeling well enough to manage without treatment. I felt disappointed and quite powerless to change his decision, but I still encouraged him to keep taking his medication, seek treatment in Florida, and avoid yet another relapse.

DISCUSSION

In summary, this case illustrates the types of severe symptoms and distress that individuals with schizophrenia can experience, the exacerbation of symptoms and overall course caused by comorbid substance dependence, the detrimental impact of a lack of insight into illness, and some of the obstacles to maintaining treatment. In the hospital we were able to develop a therapeutic alliance with Antonio to understand his experiences in depth and try to engage him in treatment. He worked hard to be a good patient but ultimately could not integrate our explanations and recommendations, especially once he left the hospital. It is likely that he will again feel "like a glass on the edge," and we can only hope that he will be able to find more solid ground in the future.

REFERENCES

Arsenault L, Cannon M, Witton J, et al: Causal association between cannabis and psychosis: examination of the evidence. Br J Psychiatry 184:110–117, 2004

Caspi A, Moffitt TE, Cannon M, et al: Moderation of the effect of adolescent-onset cannabis use on adult psychosis by a functional polymorphism in the COMT gene: longitudinal evidence of a gene X environment interaction. Biol Psychiatry 57:1117–1127, 2005

El-Sayeh HG, Morganti C: Aripiprazole for schizophrenia. Cochrane Database Syst Rev CD004578, 2004

Frank AF, Gunderson JG: The role of the therapeutic alliance in the treatment of schizophrenia: relationship to course and outcome. Arch Gen Psychiatry 47:228–236, 1990

Green MF: What are the functional consequences of neurocognitive deficits in schizophrenia? Am J Psychiatry 153:321–330, 1996

Lehman AF, Lieberman JA, Dixon LB, et al: Practice guideline for the treatment of patients with schizophrenia, second edition. Am J Psychiatry 161(suppl):1–56, 2004

Palmer BA, Pankrantz VS, Bostwick JM: The lifetime risk of suicide in schizophrenia: a reexamination. Arch Gen Psychiatry 62:247–253, 2005

Perkins DO: Predictors of noncompliance in patients with schizophrenia. J Clin Psychiatry 63:1121–1128, 2002

Pope HG Jr, Lipinski JF Jr: Diagnosis in schizophrenia and manic-depressive illness: a reassessment of the specificity of 'schizophrenic' symptoms in the light of current research. Arch Gen Psychiatry 35:811–828, 1978

Rosenheck R: Open forum: effectiveness versus efficacy of second-generation antipsychotics: haloperidol without anticholinergics as a comparator. Psychiatr Serv 56:85–92, 2005

Rosenheck R, Perlick D, Bingham S, et al: Effectiveness and cost of olanzapine and haloperidol in the treatment of schizophrenia: a randomized controlled trial. JAMA 290:2693–2702, 2003

Schneider K: Clinical Psychopathology. New York, Grune & Stratton, 1959

CHAPTER 11

On a Mission From God

An Integrative Psychoeducational Treatment Approach to Schizophrenia

Helle Thorning, Ph.D., L.C.S.W.

Helle Thorning, Ph.D., L.C.S.W., is the Director of Social Work at New York State Psychiatric Institute and Co-Director of the Center for Family Education and Resilience (CFER). She is also an Assistant Professor of Clinical Psychiatric Social Work Columbia University and Adjunct Professor at Columbia University School of Social Work. Dr. Thorning has a long-standing interest in understanding the impact of severe mental illness on all members of the family and has worked as both a clinical social worker and a researcher in this area for many years. With her colleagues at CFER, Drs. Ellen Lukens, Dan Herman, and Peggy O'Neill, she has conducted research on Multiple family group intervention, psychoeducation groups for persons with severe mental illness, the experience of having a brother or sister develop severe mental illness, and theory and practice of psychoeducation.

WHEN I FIRST SAW MICHELLE 8 years ago, she was about to be discharged from the hospital. As she sobbed uncontrollably, this 32-year-old woman newly diagnosed with schizophrenia said that no one had ever been able to understand her. She recounted the number of hospitalizations and clinicians, psychics, healers, and family members who over the years had failed her. This was Michelle's ninth hospitalization, and although she had improved much since her admission, she still had persistent frightening hallucinations, delusions, and nightmares. Although, she did not believe I could help her, she judged me harmless and nice enough to "give it a try"; I saw her intelligence and resilience as a basis for hope. We have met twice a week since then.

HISTORY

Michelle was a Caucasion, single, unemployed college graduate from a middle-class background who is the oldest of three siblings. Michelle reported having a normal childhood with close friends and having been fully engaged in after school activities. However, she always felt different from her parents and siblings to the point where she experienced herself as if she were from another planet. In high school, she was driven by a strong desire to excel academically and studied exceptionally hard. This resulted in withdrawal from friends and social engagement. In college she continued to perform at a very high academic level and received multiple awards and honors. Nonetheless, she also continued to be isolated from peers and to feel apart from the college culture. All through college she aspired to become a professor of history.

Michelle's parents divorced when Michelle was in her mid-teens. Her mother has remained in close contact with her over the years whereas her father, unable to face Michelle's illness, sees her only occasionally. For most of her adult life, Michelle has been estranged from her two younger siblings

Michelle's psychiatric history began when she first graduated from college. Faced with decisions about finding a job and a place to live, she had her first psychotic break. In an effort to make decisions about her life she made numerous and repeated phone calls to her family and family friends during which she oscillated between tearful requests for help and enraged outburst for them not understanding her. However, more alarming was the fact that she began acting bizarrely: she approached strangers at all hours of day and night and demonstrated little insight into the unusual nature of her behavior. Later, Michelle reported that during this period she discovered that she had been chosen by God to carry out a special mission. Michelle related that she felt a force that guided all of her behavior. She would receive messages from God through many sources in the environment that told her how to act and who to interact with. To date, the nature of the mission is elusive, but in preparation for carrying out this mission, God's voice commanded her to perform unique tasks, and she felt obliged to carry them out.

DIAGNOSIS

Since this initial onset, Michelle's psychiatric history has been characterized by multiple hospitalizations, participation in many day programs, and work with numerous clinicians. Her illness has been marked by symptoms such as hallucinations, delusions, thought disorder, ideas of reference, an initial decline in cognitive abilities that now seems to be improving, and a loss of motivation.

Although Michelle had had symptoms consistent with the diagnosis of schizophrenia for some years, this was the first hospitalization in which schizophrenia was the primary diagnosis. Prior to this hospitalization, Michelle's presentation of profound difficulties in her interpersonal relationships and the volatile nature of her interactions with others had been identified as borderline personality disorder. Her special relationship with God (i.e., hearing the voice of God, the delusion of being on a mission from God) had not previously been detected. Hence, at the point when I met her, her new diagnoses of schizophrenia allowed her to be treated with a new atypical neuroleptic medication, clozapine. On the new medication, her weight rapidly increased, a common and troubling side effect of this and similar medications, but her symptoms became more manageable. Michelle left the hospital with a treatment plan composed of individual therapy sessions twice a week and meetings with her psychiatrist for medication management once a month. Although Michelle had tried and rejected a number of treatment programs, the hospital social worker had been able to find her a new day program at which she could participate in various group activities. This is where I met Michelle.

TREATMENT

Central Treatment Issues

In treating individuals with schizophrenia, mental health providers tend to focus on the management of the symptoms, often through a pharmacological treatment approach, and on the basic needs for health and social care at the expense of understanding the personal and subjective meaning of the illness for the individual (Wagner and King 2005). In this discussion, I will not address the medications that Michelle was treated with but rather will focus on the constructions of ideas that influenced her everyday life. The meaning she attributed to her symptoms had significant influence on how she conducted her life. Hence, her meaning-making process, albeit severely disturbed due to her psychotic thinking, was important in helping her adapt to living with a chronic illness and therefore needed to be a focus of therapy.

The central treatment issue presented in the individual sessions was Michelle's profound disappointment in herself—a feeling that left her with a persistent preoccupation with things she wanted to accomplish but felt incapable of doing. As Michelle became better able to articulate her thinking, it became evident that her preoccupation her profound disappointment in herself needed to be understood in the context of the persistent delusional idea that she had been singled out by God to save the world. She received special messages from God to perform certain acts or "tests" to demonstrate that she was worthy of this mission. Although Michelle was never quite sure of the scope of the mission, she knew that it would be grand and require extraordinary strengths from her. According to Michelle, she would not be able to perform this mission until she was well and happy—not just ordinarily happy, but filled with an overwhelming sense of bliss that would put her in a position to save the world. She was terrified of not being able to complete God's mission.

Despite the intense psychopharmacological interventions prescribed for Michelle over the past 8 years, this central idea has always remained. Therefore, my work with Michelle centered around facilitating her adaptation to being an "ordinary person," accepting her vulnerabilities as a result of her illness, and letting go of destructive and hateful feelings toward herself—in all, not so different from psychotherapy with many nonpsychotic patients.

Integrative Psychoeducation

Integrative psychoeducation is a strength-based treatment approach that combines education and psychotherapy. Psychoeducation is defined as the synergy of education and the therapeutic process that together integrates information regarding illness in ways that promote an individual meaning-making process (Lukens and Thorning 1998; Lukens et al. 2004). The intervention is designed to instill self-awareness;

suggest options for growth and change; identify resources within the individual, family, and community; and assist the individual in developing an understanding of the recovery process. Integrative psychoeducation draws on a rich range of complementary theories and models related to education and clinical practice, such as social learning theory, cognitive-behavioral theories, systems theories, models of resiliency, and stress and coping models (Andersen et al. 1986; Lukens et al. 1999). The intervention follows stages of healing similar to those of people recovering from trauma: 1) safety, 2) care for self, 3) hope, and 4) anticipatory planning (Lukens et al. 2004). The emphasis of this approach is on understanding the human experience of living with the trauma of schizophrenia and enhancing the quality of life for the individual whose sense of self has been devastatingly impacted by the illness (Thorning and Lukens 1996). Psychoeducation has been established by expert panels as an evidence-based practice for patients with schizophrenia and their families and is supported by persuasive evidence of positive outcome for patients (American Psychiatric Association 1997; Coursey et al. 2000; Lukens and McFarland, in press).

Course of Treatment

As noted above, Michelle had worked with numerous clinicians during the years of her illness. Because she was exceptionally well read in the issues of psychology and therapy, *being* in therapy was a real challenge for her. She had unrealistic expectations and fantasies of what therapy could do, what the role of a clinician should be, and what she should be able to accomplish as a patient. Michelle wanted to get to the roots of her problem so that she could understand why she was not able to do what she wanted to do. She expected therapy to provide a great emotional catharsis at each session and thus free her to do great things. However, slowly over time, she was able to talk about her daily cotidian concerns and the psychotic experiences that clearly interfered with her day-to-day, moment-to-moment functioning. Although she experienced this type of discussion as pedestrian and ordinary, it also was a great relief for her to share these mundane details with me.

More troubling to Michelle was her feeling of being compelled to do bizarre things to satisfy the commands or tests from God, such as stand in the street in the middle of the night screaming at the top of her lungs, approach and talk to strangers in the street, stand for long periods of time in certain stores waiting for signs, or be unable to disengage from conversations with family members. Together Michelle and I embarked on a long journey of reviewing step by step how her experiences and behaviors were motivated by distortions in perception and cognition. Hence we moved away from pathologizing her experiences ("What is the problem?") to asking "What happened?", with her telling the story of the critical situations in which she would find herself. Over time she has become less and less compelled to act on these demands and has since moved toward critically examining the messages from God and making decisions about whether or not to act on them. This has been a delicate, sensitive process that has involved introducing information about psychosis and the symptoms of schizophrenia in a way that does not threaten Michelle's sense of self and her adaptation to being an ordinary person.

Viewing television was always a source of stress for Michelle because of the noise and visual overstimulation, and she preferred not to watch. However, not watching television made her feel "out of the loop" culturally and politically. Michelle watched television often and found herself at times watching from the other room in an attempt to use distance as a buffer between herself and the noise and visual stimulation. With regard to this issue, Michelle was able to reframe her behavior from "being weird" to being an attempt to take care of herself by identifying her vulnerabilities and finding new ways to manage them.

These detailed discussions of Michelle's home situation allowed us to explore her environment and the possible areas of overstimulation that triggered her vulnerability to psychosis.

An avid reader when she was not ill, Michelle began to read again during the course of my work with her and has allowed herself to read nonfiction books. Consequently, she has been able to achieve a sense of accomplishment about her increased ability to concentrate.

Over time, her increased understanding of the severity of her illness made her more forgiving of herself for not having accomplished the dreams of her adolescence. This in turn allowed her to pursue other avenues for finding meaning in her life. Although Michelle's delusion of her mission from God has not gone away, she has been more accepting of her ability to accomplish goals in an ordinary manner, which has allowed her to explore the idea of volunteering at political and environmentally conscious advocacy groups that are consistent with her idea of saving the world. Several organizations have offered her regular volunteer positions, but she has so far been able to only occasionally participate in them.

DISCUSSION

Michelle called me the other day in between sessions to let me know that she had been unable to sleep the night before because she could not stop thinking about how "weird" she had behaved as a younger person. She recounted that, although she felt her behavior had been strange, she also felt sad for her younger self and stated, "I really was not myself. I was out of sorts. My brain was just not acting well." In this phone call, Michelle for the first time experienced empathy for herself rather than self-hatred, and she demonstrated that she is better able to integrate the nature of her illness into her story—a story that is beginning to make sense to her. The integrative psychoeducational approach thus has facilitated Michelle in developing a better understanding of her vulnerabilities stemming from to the symptoms of schizophrenia. This is an enormous accomplishment that has provided her and me with optimism and hope for her future capacity to adapt to living with schizophrenia.

REFERENCES

Andersen C, Reiss DJ, Hogarty GE: Schizophrenia and the Family: A Practititioner's Guide to Psychoeducation and Management. New York, Guilford, 1986

American Psychiatric Association: Practice guidelines for the treatment of patients with schizophrenia. Am J Psychiatry 154:1–63, 1997

Coursey R, Curtis L, Marsh DT: Competencies for direct service workers who work with adults with severe mental illness: specific knowledge, attitudes, skills and biography. Psychiatr Rehabil J 23:370–392, 2000

Lukens EP, Thorning H: Psychoeducation and severe mental illness: implications for social work practice and research, in Mental Health Research: Implications for Practice. Edited by Williams JBW, Ell K. Washington, DC, NASW Press, 1998, pp 343–364

Lukens E, McFarlane W: Psychoeducation as evidence-based practice: considerations for practice, research, and policy, in Foundations of Evidence-Based Social Work Practice. Edited by Roberts AR, Yeager KR. New York, Oxford University Press (in press)

Lukens EP, Thorning H, Herman DB: Family psychoeducation in schizophrenia: emerging themes and challenges. Journal of Practical Psychiatry and Behavioral Health 5(6):314–325 1999

Lukens E, O'Neill P, Thorning H, et al: Building resilience and cultural collaborations post September 11th: a group model of brief integrative psychoeducation for diverse communities. Traumatology 10:103–123, 2004

Thorning H, Lukens E: Schizophrenia and the self, in Schizophrenia: New Directions for Clinical Research and Treatment, Vol. 1. Edited by Kaufman CA, Gorman, JM. Larchmont, NY, Mary Ann Liebert, 1996, pp 177- 188

Wagner L, King M: Existential needs of people with psychotic disorders in Porto Alegre, Brazil. Br J Psychiatry 186:141–145, 2005

PART VI

Mood Disorders

CHAPTER 12

The Suffering Suburban Soprano

Interpersonal Psychotherapy for Major Depressive Disorder

Kathryn L. Bleiberg, Ph.D.
John C. Markowitz, M.D.

Kathryn L. Bleiberg, Ph.D., is an Assistant Professor of Psychology in Psychiatry at Weill Medical College, Cornell University, where she investigates psychotherapy and pharmacological treatments of mood disorders and has a private practice. In addition to providing interpersonal psychotherapy for depression in several clinical trials, she has worked on and published papers relating to adaptations of interpersonal psychotherapy for posttraumatic stress disorder, borderline personality disorder, and depression after a pregnancy loss.

John C. Markowitz, M.D., is a research psychiatrist at the New York State Psychiatric Institute, Clinical Professor of Psychiatry at Weill Medical College of Cornell University, and Adjunct Professor of Clinical Psychiatry at Columbia University College of Physicians and Surgeons in New York City. He has conducted research on interpersonal psychotherapy, other psychotherapies, and the use of medications in the treatment of mood and other psychiatric disorders. He is the author of *Interpersonal Psychotherapy for Dysthymic Disorder* (1998), coauthor with Drs. Gerald L. Klerman and Myrna M. Weissman of the *Comprehensive Guide to Interpersonal Psychotherapy* (2000), and author of more than 150 peer-reviewed articles and chapters.

LAUREL, A 35-YEAR-OLD married mother of a 10-month-old daughter, was referred to us for interpersonal psychotherapy (IPT). The referring colleague said Laurel had been experiencing depression and was interested in time-limited, structured psychotherapy because previous, open-ended therapies had been unfocused and unhelpful. Her chief complaint was, "I need to change my life. I'm disappointed in my career. I've had a huge loss of identity."

Laurel reported at least 3 months of feeling unhappy most days and being unable to enjoy things she used to enjoy, such as cooking, exercising, and socializing. She felt tired and had difficulty falling and staying asleep nearly every night. She overate, cried easily, and felt bad about herself. She felt like a failure for having given up her career as an opera singer when she became pregnant and felt guilty for missing her job when she was blessed with a healthy, beautiful child. She also feared her depression would impair her daughter's development. She reported experiencing several previous episodes of mild depression that lasted no more than a week, which were usually precipitated by the end of a romantic relationship. She felt worse, however, since aborting her career to become a full-time mother and moving from New York City to suburban Connecticut a few months before the birth of her daughter, Emma.

An attractive woman of average height and weight, Laurel appeared her stated age. She was casually dressed in sweatpants and a sweatshirt. Her movements were slightly slowed, although her speech was fluent. Her mood was depressed with a congruent, minimally labile affect. She denied current or past suicidal ideation, any history of substance abuse, and psychotic symptoms. Although she did not appear to have a full-blown personality disorder, her speech was excessively impressionistic and lacking in detail, and her affect and gestures were somewhat histrionic. She denied current or past medical conditions, including thyroid dysfunction.

Laurel reported having received individual weekly psychotherapy from a college counselor in her freshman year and again in her late 20s with a therapist who described herself as following a psychodynamic approach. Each therapy lasted no more than a few months and focused on Laurel's relationship and career issues. Laurel found neither treatment helpful. At her initial evaluation, she reported taking a sleep medication prescribed by her internist but said she had never tried antidepressant medication.

TREATMENT

Principles of Interpersonal Psychotherapy

IPT is a time-limited (12–16 session), symptom-focused, empirically tested treatment that examines current interpersonal difficulties and symptoms (Weissman et al. 2000). Initially developed to treat major depressive disorder, IPT's success with depression has led to its adaptation for various subpopulations of patients with a mood disorder, including dysthymic disorder, atypical depression, and "double depression" (major depressive disorder superimposed on dysthymic disorder); as well as for patients with eating disorders, anxiety disorders, and other syndromes. It has been shown to improve social skills (Weissman et al. 2000).

IPT is based on principles derived from psychosocial and life events research on depression, which has demonstrated a relation between depression and complicated bereavement, role disputes (e.g., bad marriages), role transitions and meaningful life changes, and interpersonal deficits. These stressful life events can trigger depressive episodes in vulnerable individuals; conversely, depressive episodes often impair psychosocial functioning, thereby provoking negative life events. Based on the presumption that the etiology of depressive episodes is multifactorial, IPT focuses on the connection between current life events and the onset of depressive symptoms as a practical strategy to help patients understand and combat their illness.

Treatment With Interpersonal Psychotherapy

IPT treatment focuses on an interpersonal crisis in the patient's life, a focal problem area connected to the patient's episode of illness. By solving an interpersonal problem (e.g., complicated bereavement), the IPT patient improves his or her life situation and simultaneously relieves the symptoms of the depressive episode.

IPT uses the medical model and includes psychoeducation about depression. By emphasizing that depression is a medical illness and giving the patient the "sick role" (Parsons 1951), the therapist helps the patient recognize that he or she is experiencing a common mood disorder with a predictable set of symptoms, and not the personal failure, weakness, or character flaw the depressed patient often believes to be the problem. Temporarily casting the patient in the sick role allows the patient to be relieved of his or her self-blame and permits the clinician to focus the patient on the medical diagnosis of depression.

Laurel was a good candidate for IPT: her symptoms met criteria for major depression and her life was replete with recent events that could be easily linked to the onset or exacerbation of her symptoms. She was also a potential candidate for cognitive-behavioral therapy, pharmacotherapy, or IPT or cognitive-behavioral therapy combined with medication, all of which have been shown to have efficacy in clinical trials. However, after a discussion of the various treatment options, Laurel indicated that she did not want medication or written homework and was interested in working on the interpersonal problems associated with the onset of her symptoms.

Laurel's Treatment Course

The first 16 sessions followed the IPT format for acute treatment (Weissman et al. 2000). In the first three sessions, I (K.L.B.) obtained a thorough psychiatric history for Laurel and set the treatment framework. I explained IPT to Laurel as a time-limited, diagnosis-targeted treatment focused on how recent life events affect one's mood and how mood symptoms complicate the handling of current life events, particularly interpersonal interactions. I said I would take time to gather information about her history, but that sessions would focus on her current relationships and difficulties, not on the past. I explained that IPT has demonstrated efficacy in research studies and that acute treatment often comprises 16 weekly sessions. If indicated, acute treatment may be followed by continuation sessions (often of lesser frequency) to continue work on issues and maintain progress already achieved.

After taking a thorough psychiatric history and administering the Hamilton Rating Scale for Depression (Ham-D) (Hamilton 1960), I determined that Laurel's symptoms met DSM-IV-TR criteria for major depressive disorder, single episode, of moderate severity (American Psychiatric Association 1994). I gave her this diagnosis and the sick role: "You have an illness called major depression, which is treatable and is not your fault." I explained that her Ham-D score of 24 indicated moderately severe depression and that I would readminister the Ham-D every 4 weeks to monitor her progress. I provided psychoeducation about the constellation of symptoms that define major depression in the context of Laurel's specific symptoms. Given the moderate nature of her symptoms and her reluctance to take medication, I did not think medication was needed. I referred her to a psychiatrist to confirm this judgment and evaluate her sleep medications.

After the first session, Laurel felt more hopeful, but she was still skeptical about the prospect of symptom relief in 16 sessions. Although she could appreciate the link between her mood and recent life events, she still felt her symptoms represented character flaws rather than an illness. I was unsurprised by her initial skepticism and recognized it could take time for her to accept the medical model. We agreed to work for 16 weeks and then at that point decide whether further sessions were needed.

In obtaining Laurel's psychiatric history, I conducted an interpersonal inventory, a careful review of her past and current social functioning and close relationships. The goal of the interpersonal inventory is to help the therapist and patient understand how the patient interacts with others, what social supports may be available to him or her, and how relationships may have contributed to or been affected by the depressive episode. The inventory also provides a framework for understanding the social and interpersonal context in which the depressive syndrome arises and should lead to a treatment focus.

Laurel reported having mixed feelings about her family. She complained that her parents, who lived in her hometown of Chicago, were always overly critical of her. She had an older sister in California with whom she did not get along. She suspected that her mother and sister had been depressed in the past but was uncertain whether either had received treatment.

She reported having a few close girlfriends, all of whom lived in other states. She spoke to each friend every couple of weeks, but saw them only a few times a year. Although Laurel was shy in social situations, she could open up once she felt comfortable. Her relationships, once formed, usually lasted a long time. Laurel reported rarely arguing with friends. Because she "hate[d] creating conflict," she avoided confronting friends and coworkers when she disagreed or felt angry with them. She said her friends would describe her as cheerful and having a great sense of humor and probably did not know how badly she felt. She admitted that she tried to appear normal no matter how bad she was feeling. As her depression worsened, she spoke to friends less frequently and often did not return their calls; she explained her reluctance stemmed from her not wanting to burden them with her problems. I responded that depressed people tend to minimize their own needs and avoid seeking help from their friends lest they burden them, yet it is appropriate and can be helpful for them to seek support from others, particularly when they are depressed. Social supports protect against depression.

Since stopping work and moving to the suburbs, Laurel had felt isolated and had difficulty forming relationships. She befriended an older neighbor, but they shared little in common. Laurel and her husband,

Bob, often attended church on Sundays, but she avoided speaking with other members of the congregation. She occasionally took Emma to a local park, but rarely initiated conversations with the other mothers.

Before meeting her husband, Laurel had dated men who were "very passionate" yet had "commitment issues." At age 29 she met Bob, several years her senior, whom she found charming and kind. Unlike previous boyfriends, he had a stable career as an investment banker and was interested in marriage and having a family. Bob was very attentive to her and admired her singing and artistic career, since he and his peers were involved in corporate jobs. After 5 years of marriage, they agreed to start a family and a child was quickly conceived. Laurel enjoyed pregnancy, was excited about motherhood, and looked forward to staying home with her baby. Her delivery was uncomplicated and she breast-fed Emma without difficulty. Although Laurel was able to care for and enjoy Emma when she was born, she felt she was never doing enough for her and felt inadequate because she no longer had a career.

Since the family's move and Emma's birth, Laurel began to feel distant from Bob, and they began to argue frequently. Earlier she had enjoyed dating and living with him in Manhattan. They enjoyed going to movies, restaurants, and theater together. Since moving to Connecticut, they occasionally had dinner with couples he knew through work but rarely went out by themselves. Laurel saw her husband less and less because he had a lengthy commute to his Manhattan office.

Laurel missed being pregnant, when Bob had shown concern for her and helped around the house based on his wish that she not exert herself. Since Emma's birth, she found him no longer attentive but instead unappreciative of how hard she worked in caring for their child and home. Although interested in having sex with her, he was less affectionate toward her than during her pregnancy. When she felt frustrated with Bob, she would keep her feelings to herself for several hours, then end up bickering with him. I explained that depressed patients frequently have difficulty in asserting their needs, confronting others, or becoming angry effectively and taking social risks. These were things to work on: if Laurel could communicate with her husband more effectively, she might improve their relationship and, with it, her mood.

By the end of the first phase of treatment, I had connected Laurel's depressive syndrome to her interpersonal situation in a formulation centered on an IPT focal problem area (Markowitz and Swartz 1997). The formulation simplifies and organizes the patient's story by highlighting one (or at most two) salient interpersonal problem(s) related to the depressive episode. Laurel's chief complaint involved feeling depressed and as though she were a failure by ending her career to become a full-time mother and moving from the city to the suburbs, all role transitions. My formulation underscored that she was in the midst of a role transition—giving up her opera career for motherhood—and that this transition precipitated her depression. Although she was happy about becoming a mother, she simultaneously had experienced a loss in relinquishing her career. This role transition and depression affected her relationship with her husband (a role dispute, although not our chosen focus), and she had difficulty expressing these feelings. Laurel said she felt validated by the formulation and agreed that managing this role transition should be the focus of treatment. With this agreement, we began the middle phase of the treatment.

During the middle phase (sessions 4–12), we worked on resolving Laurel's interpersonal problem area. I continued providing psychoeducation about how depression affects social functioning and repeatedly linked her depression to the identified problem areas. I began each session by asking, "How have things been since we last met?" to elicit an interval history of mood and events between sessions. This opening question elicited affect and kept Laurel focused on her current mood and life events. Trying to elicit affect was sometimes challenging and frustrating for both of us, given her propensity toward somewhat histrionic speech. At times I found it difficult to empathize with her when she spoke in an overly dramatic way. For example, when describing her relationship with her sister, she stated, speaking intensely, "My sister was the evil stepsister and I was Cinderella being made to scrub the floors." When I asked further questions, I learned that her sister was somewhat bossy and critical but not quite so evil. She acknowledged that she had difficulty identifying specific emotions and often used dramatic words in describing her feelings to ensure she was taken seriously. As she analyzed specific interactions with others in treatment, she realized that this could be off-putting and inhibit effective communication.

Our sessions focused on external events, not transference in the office. I assigned no formal homework but encouraged Laurel to work toward resolving the focal problem area by the end of treatment. The strategy for role transitions was to help Laurel mourn the loss of her old role, in which she generally saw herself as happier than now, and to recognize and adjust to possibilities in the newer role. I took a friendly, supportive, optimistic, encouraging therapist stance.

Given that Laurel was in the midst of the transition from being a Metropolitan Opera singer to a stay-at-home suburban mom, I first helped her mourn her old singing role. I encouraged her to describe her experience and what she missed about singing. She tearfully described missing the music, being on stage, and receiving attention and recognition from the audience and colleagues. She missed collaborating with the rest of the cast, recalling that she was never alone when she worked in opera companies. She had enjoyed going out late with other singers after performing and traveling around the country and abroad to perform. She regretted not trying harder to succeed in her field. Having allowed her to experience these emotions, I asked whether there was anything she did not miss—was there anything good about not being an opera singer? She said she did not miss the fierce competition, long work hours, auditioning, or the periods of unemployment between productions. Although she enjoyed traveling, the time demands of opera made it difficult to see her husband and friends who had day jobs.

I empathized with Laurel's sense of loss and linked her experience of loss and life change to her depression. I encouraged her to consider what she could retain from her old role. Did she still have opportunities to sing? She had, in fact, considered joining her church choir, but was scared that she would feel depressed about not performing professionally. She feared that the choirmaster would ask why she had not been singing for over a year and consider her a failure. We role-played her answering questions about her career and expressing interest in the choir. Role-playing helped Laurel to feel prepared and less hesitant in approaching the choir director. She did audition with him, and he was so impressed that he asked her to be a soloist. Pleasantly surprised by the director's enthusiasm, she quickly began rehearsing and singing with the choir. She felt great about singing again and enjoyed the compliments from members of her congregation. She also made friends with other choir members. One month into treatment, Laurel's mood had somewhat improved and her Ham-D score had fallen to 17. She felt more hopeful and less self-critical.

I encouraged Laurel to reconnect with old friends and consider opportunities to form new relationships. I explained that depression tends to isolate people and deny them previously pleasurable activities, both of which can perpetuate depression. She reported that talking to other mothers made her feel anxious, that she feared she had nothing to say and that others would see she was depressed and find her uninteresting. I was struck by her self-deprecation, as I found her witty and engaging in sessions. I explained that depression tends to make people feel down on themselves and assume that others share their depressed self-view. I reassured her that everyone is self-conscious when meeting new people and that she need not convey that she was depressed. I empathized with her feeling that she had to push herself to be social but encouraged her to take social risks to improve her situation.

We explored options for meeting other mothers and role-played introductions and potential conversations. Laurel joined a music class for mothers and toddlers where she socialized and enjoyed seeing her daughter with other children. She also began attending a local gym that had day care facilities. Resuming exercise helped her mood and provided another opportunity to meet other stay-at-home mothers. She felt more comfortable with these women than she had anticipated and felt validated to discover that they, too, felt overwhelmed at home and missed working. She also learned that their husbands shared child care responsibilities, which helped her gauge her expectations of her husband as reasonable. By mid-treatment, her Ham-D score was 11, consistent with mild depression.

Laurel suddenly noticed that I was wearing an engagement ring and asked when I was to be married. I felt uncomfortable, caught off guard, because she had never asked personal questions until now. IPT focuses on the patient's outside life, not on the transference. I answered that I was to be married in a few months. She appeared sad. I asked what she was feeling. She said she feared her experience with her husband would dissuade me from marriage. I said I appreciated her concern, then used the opportunity to express hope about her improving her relationship. Although Laurel seemed concerned about the negative impact she might have on me, I wondered whether she was also feeling envious. This in turn made me feel bad that I might have caused her distress.

Using communication analysis (the reconstruction and evaluation of recent, affectively charged life circumstances), I asked Laurel to recount arguments or unpleasant interactions with Bob: what she was feeling during the interaction, what she said or did, and what he said or did. She described a recent incident. She had asked Bob if he could care for their daughter and let her sleep later on Saturday mornings. He agreed, but did not follow through; he stayed in bed, made lots of noise once he did arise from bed, and woke her to ask questions. She felt that Bob did not appreciate how hard she worked taking care of Emma or cared about her needing sleep. We explored what she wished Bob would do and what options she had for asking him to do these things. We role-played her telling her husband how she felt and asking him to do specific things that would allow her to sleep.

Laurel felt good about being able to assert herself with Bob but resented having to ask him for assistance with Emma and found him only somewhat responsive to her requests. Laurel found a babysitter and made plans with her husband to go out alone on dates. She enjoyed this, but wished he would also initiate plans. She was able to express these feelings to Bob. I was concerned that the conflicts between them would persist.

In the final sessions (14–16), Laurel reported her mood was much improved. Her affect was brighter and her grooming was better than in our initial sessions. Her sleep had improved. Her Ham-D score was now 5, consistent with euthymic remission. She had taken trazodone under psychiatric supervision for the first 6 weeks of treatment then was slowly tapered off the medication. During these final sessions, we reviewed the progress she had made. Laurel reported, "I am more accepting of my role as a mother." She felt happy about how Emma was developing and looked forward to having a second child. She felt good about asserting herself more effectively and achieving more satisfying social interactions. Her improved self-assertion with peers and her husband generalized to her other relationships, to confronting her parents and the contractor who was working on her house. She had begun relationships with other mothers in her neighborhood and was socializing with them and their children. She felt better about continuing to sing, even if she was not singing professionally.

Laurel felt her relationship with her husband still needed improvement. In the course of treatment, we both realized that their conflicts had begun before she left her career and had had Emma. I offered to continue working with her to maintain her progress and continue working on this role dispute. We continued therapy weekly for several months and ultimately tapered to monthly sessions.

DISCUSSION

Although each patient is unique, Laurel's therapy resembled other IPT treatments of major depressive disorder. Laurel felt comfortable performing in front of large audiences yet very anxious in more intimate social situations. Many people with major depressive disorder who experience social anxiety also have performance anxiety. The time limit and brief duration of IPT and my frequent encouragement helped keep Laurel motivated and protected against regression and passivity. She said she felt understood when I linked her mood symptoms and interpersonal difficulties to depression. Defining depression as a medical illness ultimately relieved her of some of her guilt about her difficulty functioning, especially about feeling depressed around her child. Furthermore, her seeing depression as a set of discrete symptoms made them seem manageable and less overwhelming. This performer found role-playing very helpful and said it gave her confidence when initiating plans with other mothers and expressing her thoughts and feelings to her husband.

REFERENCES

American Psychiatric Association: Diagnostic and Statistical Manual of Mental Disorders, 4th Edition. Washington, DC, American Psychiatric Association, 1994

Hamilton M: A rating scale for depression. J Neurol Neurosurg Psychiatry 25:56–62, 1960

Markowitz JC, Swartz HA: Case formulation in interpersonal psychotherapy of depression, in Handbook of Psychotherapy: Case Formulation. Edited by Eells TD. New York, Guilford, 1997, pp 192–222

Parsons T: Illness and the role of the physician: a sociological perspective. Am J Orthopsychiatry 21:452–460, 1951

Weissman MM, Markowitz JC, Klerman GL: Comprehensive Guide to Interpersonal Psychotherapy. New York, Basic Books, 2000

CHAPTER 13

Gay and Depressed

Combined Pharmacotherapy and Long-Term Psychodynamic Psychotherapy With A Depressed Gay Man

Jack Drescher, M.D.

Jack Drescher, M.D., is a Distinguished Fellow of the American Psychiatric Association (APA); Past Chair of the APA's Committee on Gay, Lesbian, and Bisexual Issues; and a Past President of APA's New York County District Branch. He is a Training and Supervising Analyst at the William Alanson White Institute in New York City and a Clinical Assistant Professor of Psychiatry at the State University of New York's Downstate Medical Center. Dr. Drescher is a Fellow and former trustee of the American Academy of Psychoanalysis and Dynamic Psychiatry.

Dr. Drescher is Editor-in-Chief of the *Journal of Gay and Lesbian Psychotherapy*. He has coedited numerous books from the Haworth Press, including *Sexual Conversion Therapy* (2001), *Transgender Subjectivities* (2004), *Handbook of LGBT Issues in Community Mental Health* (2005), and *Barebacking: Psychosocial and Public Health Approaches* (2005). Dr. Drescher is the author of *Psychoanalytic Therapy and The Gay Man* (1998) and edits the *Bending Psychoanalysis* series from The Analytic Press. He is in full-time private practice in New York City.

JOSEPH, AN ARCHITECT IN his early 50s, had recently moved to New York City from the southern United States, having left a long-term heterosexual marriage with the intention of living as an openly gay man. At the time of the initial consultation, his chief complaints were feeling depressed and having difficulty adjusting to recent life changes.

A friend of Joseph's, a therapist himself, had made the referral based on the patient's stated wish for an openly gay psychiatrist. Joseph told me at our first meeting, however, that I was not the first New York therapist to whom his friend had referred him. He had briefly seen another gay therapist but found the experience unsettling. At their first session, after telling the therapist how isolated he felt, the therapist encouraged Joseph to socialize more actively. He suggested some gay social activities that Joseph might attend. At their next session, the therapist "grilled" Joseph about his week's activities and seemed "annoyed" that Joseph had not followed through on the therapist's suggestions. Joseph, feeling coerced and judged by the therapist, left after the third session. Although Joseph said he wanted to be gay, he gave me the immediate impression that he was ambivalent about it. I filed that thought away for future reference as I chose instead to address what I felt to be Joseph's more immediate clinical concerns.

HISTORY

Joseph had a 30-year history of depressive episodes. His first occurred in his early 20s and was treated with cognitive-behavioral therapy. A second episode in his late 30s was treated with tricyclic antidepressants (TCAs), which he took intermittently as his depressive episodes came and went. In his 40s, with the advent of selective serotonin reuptake inhibitors, Joseph was treated with fluoxetine; it ameliorated his depression but caused erectile dysfunction that exacerbated his marital difficulties. His last episode of depression, which occurred 2 years before our first meeting, had responded to bupropion 300 mg/day. At the time of the consultation, Joseph was not taking any psychotropic medications.

At our initial consultation, Joseph reported experiencing the following symptoms: a month-long, unremitting, depressed mood that was worst in the morning (diurnal variation); an inability to find pleasure in anything; a diminished sex drive and, although Joseph was not in a relationship, a loss of interest in masturbating; an increased appetite, but no weight gain; early morning awakening; psychomotor retardation; daytime fatigue; an inability to focus; and intense feelings of hopelessness but no suicidal ideation or thoughts of death. Joseph had had suicidal feelings in the past but had no history of suicide attempts.

Joseph had a significant family history of mood disorder: his father, who had bipolar disorder, underwent repeated courses of electroconvulsive therapy; he eventually committed suicide when Joseph was in his 30s. Joseph had no history of manic episodes. There was no significant history of alcohol or other substance abuse and no significant medical history. Joseph's DSM-IV-TR diagnosis was major depressive disorder, recurrent.

Development of Joseph's Sexual Identity

Many gay adults recall being attracted to members of their own sex since early childhood. However, the adoption of a gay identity is a developmental process that occurs over time. Models of gay identity development (Cass 1979) usually portray a series of linear progressive stages involving tasks such as coming out (the process of recognizing one's homosexual attraction and acknowledging it to oneself and others), becoming involved in gay communities, establishing same-sex relationships, and integrating one's sexual identity into other aspects of the self. However, not all individuals who experience homoerotic desire or participate in homosexual behavior follow such a linear path, nor do they necessarily develop a stable lesbian, gay, or bisexual identity. In other words, a sexual identity is not always equivalent to a sexual orientation (Drescher 1998; Drescher et al. 2004).

The history of Joseph's sexual identity development is a case in point. He had lived most of his life "in the closet"; that is, he had denied his homosexuality to himself and hid it from others. Although he recalls being attracted to men since childhood, Joseph struggled against those feelings, experiencing them as deeply shameful. He was raised in a conservative Christian tradition, was deeply religious, and believed that homosexuality in general was a sin and that his own homoerotic attractions were a punishment for which he had to atone. He never told anyone about his sexual feelings and, throughout adolescence, tried to suppress them through prayer, bible study, and fellowship in his church.

Joseph's efforts to suppress his homosexuality continued into college. He had his first same-sex experience at a religious retreat when he and a fellow student had sex in a shared bed. However, their subsequent sexual relations, which occurred intermittently over the next 2 years, were never talked about openly. In fact, their sexual activity—which included mutual masturbation, oral sex, and intracrural frottage (rubbing one's genitals between the other's legs)—usually took place in a dissociated state (Drescher 1998) while one of them acted as if he were asleep. They never kissed.

Joseph's sexual partner married after college graduation and moved to another state. Neither of them tried to stay in contact. This is when Joseph, now in his early 20s, had his first depressive episode. He sought out a Christian therapist, who identified Joseph's homosexual behavior as the source of his depression. With the help of the therapist, who used a cognitive-behavioral approach, Joseph was able to block out both his depressed cognitions and his homosexual thoughts. His depression eventually resolved.

In the course of their work, the therapist suggested that Joseph could prevent future episodes of depression by solidifying his heterosexual identity. He encouraged Joseph to date; Joseph subsequently became engaged to a woman he had met in college. It was Joseph's fervent hope that the love of a caring Christian woman would make his homosexual feelings go away. His therapist, who encouraged this belief, advised Joseph not to tell his fiancée about his feelings or his past homosexual experiences.

Things did not work out the way Joseph had hoped. Although he and his wife became loving friends, Joseph was never sexually attracted to her. Although they did have physical relations, during vaginal intercourse he was able to maintain his erection and reach orgasm only by fantasizing about sex with men. Joseph and his wife had three children. The psychotherapeutic relationship that began before he married ended amicably after the birth of the first child, with the therapist reassuring Joseph that his homosexuality was now "cured."

Throughout the rest of his marriage, Joseph struggled against strong wishes to engage in homosexual contacts. He remained physically faithful to his wife until after their children were born, 5 years into the marriage. Then he began to have occasional, anonymous sexual encounters in public spaces. He never exchanged names with his sexual partners. He never kissed anyone. If he were out of town, he would go to a pornographic video store catering to gay clients. Again, he always maintained anonymity with sexual partners, being fearful that someone might identify him, reveal his secret to his wife or religious community, or blackmail him.

In one incident about 15 years into his marriage, Joseph narrowly avoided being arrested for public lewdness at a highway rest stop. This event precipitated a second and more severe depressive episode for which he sought treatment with a self-identified "Christian psychiatrist." In addition to medicating Joseph's depression with TCAs, the psychiatrist suggested twice weekly psychotherapy to rid Joseph of his homosexual feelings and impulses. The psychiatrist believed Joseph's homosexual behavior arose from a distant childhood relationship with his depressed father. The psychiatrist also said he disagreed with the American Psychiatric Association's decision in 1973 to delete homosexuality from DSM-III (Bayer 1981) and told Joseph he believed homosexuality was both a mental and a spiritual illness.

Although TCAs reduced his depressive symptoms, Joseph's homosexual attractions and fantasies did not abate. He intermittently continued to have anonymous sexual contacts. After 5 years of twice weekly psychotherapy, the psychiatrist told Joseph he was "just not trying hard enough" and encouraged him to work harder. Joseph decided to end the treatment because he felt he was not receiving the help he needed. He also felt blamed and criticized by the psychiatrist's remarks; they made him feel responsible for the failure of the treatment. This feeling of failure made him even more depressed and hopeless and Joseph began to contemplate suicide.

Joseph's "Coming Out"

Joseph then found another psychiatrist who, in addition to continuing to medicate Joseph's depression, offered a different psychotherapeutic approach. The psychiatrist neither condemned nor praised homosexuality nor did he offer any psychodynamic formulations regarding its causes (Drescher 2002a). Instead, he focused on the lifelong conflict between Joseph's wish to have a heterosexual identity and his strong homosexual desires. It was the first time Joseph had ever spoken to anyone about his homosexuality without that person judging his same-sex attractions (and by extension, him) as unacceptable. Just being able to talk about his feelings in this manner significantly reduced his shame. Although Joseph continued to have anonymous sexual encounters, he found himself wanting more intimacy; during one clandestine episode, he kissed another man on the mouth for the first time. He decided, on his own initiative, to tell his wife about his homosexuality, timing his revelation shortly after their last son left for college. As his individual therapy proceeded and he continued to speak more openly with his wife, Joseph came to the conclusion, "I am gay."

Although having had no inkling of his homosexual struggles before he told her and now being sympathetic to Joseph's struggle, Joseph's wife did not wish to remain married to him if he were gay. The couple divorced amicably and Joseph moved to New York City in the hopes of living, for the first time, as an openly gay man. However, 1 year after the move, he had a recurrence of his depressive symptoms that led to our initial consultation.

TREATMENT

Early Treatment

Given Joseph's history of recurrent depression, one immediate goal was to restart antidepressant medication. Because bupropion had been effective in the past with a minimum of troubling side effects, he was started with a low dosage and his dosage was tapered upward to 400 mg/day over the next few weeks. Many of his depressive symptoms began to gradually remit although his insomnia persisted. Trazodone was added, both to aid his sleeping and as an augmenting agent. This combination proved effective and, after 4 months, Joseph's depressive symptoms were significantly reduced and no longer interfered with his functioning.

In addition to taking medication, Joseph agreed to begin a course of psychodynamic psychotherapy with me. Given his clinical depression and his degree of identity confusion, I suggested he would benefit from intensive treatment, perhaps two or three times a week. However, Joseph could only afford to come once a week. He was not open to a referral to a low-fee clinic where he could receive affordable, intensive treatment and insisted that he wanted to work with a more experienced clinician. I reluctantly agreed, not entirely certain if once a week treatment would be sufficient.

What struck me in the early weeks of therapy was the rather offhanded manner in which Joseph spoke of his transition from being a married Southern gentleman to an aspiring New York gay single. He seemed to have the impression that changing identities was like changing clothes. It was also my impression that his recent three-session therapy had not challenged this implicit assumption, given how the therapist immediately had made directive efforts to socialize Joseph. Determined not to repeat that error, my more immediate psychotherapeutic goal was to help Joseph understand how moving to a new environment, far from family and long-time friends, had exacerbated his depressive diathesis. In his excited focus on the prospect of coming out as gay, Joseph had not given much thought to what sacrifices doing so would entail. I listed his losses for him: 1) dissolution of his marriage to a woman he loved and who loved him, 2) the breakup of a family he had worked for years to keep together, 3) the loss of a carefully cultivated image of himself as a heterosexual man, 4) a painful separation from his children's day-to-day lives, 5) the abandonment of a long-held wish that he might one day rid himself of his homosexual feelings, and 6) his disillusionment with the religious beliefs that had shaped most of his life. As he gradually came to realize the severity of his losses, Joseph wept openly—not because he was clinically depressed, but because he was grieving the loss of his previous life and the person he had been trying so hard to become.

The remission in Joseph's depressive symptoms coincided with adjustments in his medication and our psychotherapeutic focus on his losses. After 6 months, with the resolution of his depressive symptoms and a reduction in the intensity of his grief, the therapeutic focus shifted. No longer in a depressive crisis, Joseph was now in a better position to deal with the "life issues" he faced as an openly gay man. He agreed to embark on open-ended psychotherapy to address several ongoing issues that I had delineated for him during the first months of treatment. For example, I pointed out to Joseph that he had lived for years as a heterosexual married man who engaged in only furtive homosexual activities. As a consequence, he had little experience socializing as an openly gay man; he did not know how to date or how to make gay friends. Furthermore, although he now thought of himself as gay, in my opinion, Joseph remained deeply ambivalent about openly expressing his homosexuality. Complicating matters further, he had a tendency to talk about his homosexuality in clinically disparaging terms. For example, in discussing his feelings, he would say things like, "This is so pathological" or "I know this behavior is regressive." This led me to see Joseph's current efforts to accept himself as gay as having been adversely affected by his earlier efforts to change his sexual identity.

Long-Term Treatment

Most cultures offer socially sanctioned, albeit sublimated, outlets for children that serve the purpose of modeling their roles as future heterosexual adults. For example, teenage dating and supervised coeducational activities such as high school dances are useful in developing the interpersonal skills required for later life and relationships. In these interactions, an adolescent develops confidence by learning conventional gender roles and expectations. However, although the rituals of adolescence teach children lessons about future adult heterosexual behavior, those same rituals generate confusion, shame, and anxiety in adolescents who grow up to be gay. Gay adults can sometimes become anxious, superficial, or detached at a time when their heterosexual peers are learning social skills they will need for adulthood (Drescher 2002c; Kooden 1994).

Joseph's interpersonal style had been shaped by years of hiding in the closet. His first homosexual relationship had occurred in a dissociated state, with either Joseph or his partner feigning sleep. In the decades that followed, he had met other men furtively at rest stops and in adult video stores where he engaged in anonymous sexual encounters. He had no idea where and how—and by what rules—gay people made contact with each other when they did not have to hide their sexual identities. This led to some contradictory presentations of himself in our relationship. On the one hand, Joseph was extremely competent: educated, professionally successful, and a caring and thoughtful father. Yet, when it came to his conduct as a professional, gay man, I repeatedly (and sometimes surprisingly) experienced him as oddly naïve and ingenuous.

One such example occurred during the first year of therapy. Joseph began a session talking about a group of coworkers who had gone out to dinner to celebrate the completion of a project. In the course of the evening, one gay man who directly reported to Joseph confided in him about his personal problems, which included the recent breakup of a long-term relationship. Joseph's initial efforts to comfort his subordinate ultimately led to their going home together and having sex.

I was surprised to hear this because, up to that moment, my sense was that Joseph had reasonably firm professional boundaries. I wondered aloud what his company's policies were regarding sexual relations between employees in general and between managers and their subordinates in particular. Joseph said he knew heterosexual relations were prohibited, but he never thought that these restrictions applied to homosexual activities. As he put it, "I don't think there are any rules when it comes to being gay."

Although startled by Joseph's response, I found it not altogether surprising. Like many gay men who come from conservative, religious backgrounds, Joseph experienced acceptance of his homosexuality as confirming that he had crossed a line and entered a world where none of the "normal" rules applied. After all, if he were willing to defy his strong religious prohibitions against homosexuality, what moral and ethical guidelines could possibly guide him in this new and forbidden arena?

In response, I offered a practical and readily available example—our therapeutic relationship—to suggest that it was possible for gay people to engage in social behaviors with boundaries akin to those adopted by heterosexuals. After all, I told Joseph, he had come into treatment seeking a gay psychiatrist; the fact that we were both gay did not mean that we could not or should not maintain professional boundaries. Furthermore, there are many places in the world where ethical and moral behavior are not guided by literal readings of the bible. There were other socially acceptable codes of conduct governing human relationships. For example, my behavior toward him was guided by my professional code of ethics (American Psychiatric Association 2001; Drescher 2002b).

As we further explored Joseph's encounter with his subordinate and similar lapses in judgment, I came to understand that Joseph was trying to resolve his internal conflicts about being gay by acting as if he had successfully rid himself of his long-standing antihomosexual identifications and beliefs and that this psychological splitting was a lifelong defensive maneuver. Before he came out, Joseph had idealized heterosexuality and lived his homosexuality in a dissociated manner. After he came out, being gay became idealized while Joseph's disapproving feelings were pushed out of direct awareness. In our sessions, I encouraged Joseph to express aloud all of his unarticulated doubts about being gay. By bringing his conflictual feelings to the surface, he began the long and slow process of integrating his wish to be gay with his own antihomosexual attitudes.

As he did so, Joseph, of his own accord, began putting himself into new environments where he could socially interact with other gay men. Because he did not drink, he was extremely anxious about the prospect of going to a gay bar. Instead, he tried to find some other social settings that would help him define and practice his new gay identity. He discovered the Lesbian, Gay, Bisexual and Transgender Community Center of New York City (http://www.gaycenter.org), which offered a wide range of social activities, including bingo and dance nights. Again, I was struck by the way Joseph serially tried out different gay identities as if he were trying on new clothing. In his efforts to separate his needs for nonsexual relationships from his sexual desires, he found gay reading groups, a gay fathers' group, and even gay Alcoholics Anonymous (after one of his sons developed a drinking problem). One social difficulty immediately emerged in this process: as Joseph met new people in these settings, he was anxiously confused by his difficulty in distinguishing gestures of friendship from sexual advances or romantic overtures. After learning that it was possible and necessary for gay men to make such distinctions, he used his sessions to try and sort out the differences.

Joseph also began attending welcoming and affirming churches of Christian denominations that accept openly gay worshippers. He believed his capacity to relate to others was connected to his deep religious faith. Without his faith, Joseph felt incapable of forming relationships. Such feelings and attitudes are not uncommon among individuals who grow up in religious communities where social and religious activities are closely intertwined (Haldeman 2001). However, Joseph's internalized, conservative belief was that he could not maintain his religious convictions and be a gay man at the same time. He inwardly was suspicious of religious denominations and institutions that provided him opportunities to do so. He spoke openly in our sessions of his belief that religion and heterosexuality represented his potential for goodness and that being gay meant he was sinful. He also spoke at length about how his first two experiences with Christian therapists had reinforced these beliefs. Both of those therapists were openly disapproving of homosexuality and spoke disparagingly of all same-sex relationships. For Joseph, the concept of being a gay Christian was an anxiety-producing oxymoron (White 1994). However, his being able to speak in a nonjudgmental manner about his long-standing contradictory wishes and beliefs provided him with a new and anxiety-reducing perspective.

Throughout the next 6 years of his weekly treatment, Joseph gradually came to see that gay relationships did not have to be forbidden, furtive, or sexual. As he gained a broader perspective on his initial sources of anxiety about being gay, he was able to openly interact with other gay men in a range of social settings and activities. In the process, he was able to establish several new and enduring friendships. He also struggled with anxieties associated with dating men and had ongoing concerns about being rejected and rejecting others. As he had done during his marriage, when he became frustrated, Joseph turned to pornography and masturbation for relief and critically judged himself for doing so. I repeatedly pointed out that he had spent a lifetime expressing his sexuality in solitude and that masturbation provided relief from his anxieties. I told him he knew how to masturbate, but that he did not know—and he was uncertain if he would ever know—how to be a gay man openly relating to others. Although he said he wanted a gay relationship, when he became frustrated in his dealings with others, he reflexively chose the path of least (sexual) resistance and would treat his anxieties by masturbating. Over the years, through our repeated reframing of his masturbatory activities as defensive rather than as evil and sinful, Joseph found a way out of the cycle of disappointment and shame in which his social withdrawal would lead to further disappointment and shame.

During our the seventh year of treatment, Joseph met Richard. Despite his misgivings about their differences (education, economic status, ethnicity, and religion), Joseph pursued the relationship. Richard was receptive to his advances and for the first time since we began working together, Joseph seemed truly happy. Nevertheless, he was anxious about his ability to sustain the relationship, fearing that he might withdraw or that it might not work out. Joseph had erectile dysfunction at times, but Richard seemed patient and understanding. The two of them continued to grow closer and eventually moved in together. About 6 months into his new relationship, Joseph decided to end his therapy. Although I expected future difficulties might arise in his new relationship and told him I thought so, I respected his wish to go it alone. We spent 2 months discussing the termination of our psychotherapy relationship.

DISCUSSION

In looking back at our psychotherapeutic work together, I had a range of personal, inner responses to Joseph. First and foremost, I was deeply affected by the intensity of his painful lack of self-acceptance. From our first session, I experienced him as a man who had hated himself for a long time. In addition, as mentioned earlier, surprise was a recurrent feeling over the years for me, usually evoked by the sharp disparity between Joseph's surface presentation as a seemingly mature, professional man and his naïveté in the realm of intimate, interpersonal relationships. His outer, social self—created after many years of closeted life—was not well integrated with what Winnicott (1965) termed the "true self," the individual's authentic feelings and desires. As it became possible for him to explore his hidden wishes and desires, Joseph began a process of social and sexual experimentation. This left me, at times, feeling like a parent watching his adolescent child painfully make his way through the wider world. Racker (1968) refers to this normal countertransferential response as a complementary identification with the patient's objects. I consequently felt sad for Joseph if he was hurt and disappointed if a date did not work out, pleased for him if he made a new friend, and at times annoyed when he repeatedly made overtures to someone who seemed obviously (to me) wrong for him.

Finally, given the strong antihomosexual elements of Joseph's personal developmental history, I was challenged to engage with religious views that were foreign to me and that I did not share. I found Joseph's internalized antihomosexual attitudes to be permeated with rigid moral absolutes characterized by an intense disdain for anything that he experienced as relativism. Exploring these attitudes required both tact and ongoing efforts to avoid any defensive confrontations with his beliefs. Even if I did not like what he had to say, I was not there to prove he was wrong. In fact, Joseph's internalized religious beliefs were not limited to the condemnation of homosexuality; they also included moral and ethical beliefs that were integral to his adult self. I found the psychotherapeutic challenge was to integrate his adult feelings and understanding of sexuality, ethics, and morality with his internalized antihomosexual beliefs. In other words, I always tried to keep in mind that Joseph did not need me to preach my own beliefs to him, although I felt free to tell him what they were. Instead, I chose the role of a sounding board who, despite my own gay identifications, could be respectful of Joseph's most hateful, antihomosexual thoughts.

Because efforts to lower Joseph's antidepressant had always led to an increase in his depressive symptoms or an episodic recurrence, he had decided during our time together to take medication prophylactically. Even though we had terminated our psychotherapeutic relationship, Joseph still required periodic follow-up. We agreed to meet for a medication checkup every 3 months. During the course of those visits, Joseph would fill me in on developments in his relationship. He still had anxieties but wished to work them out on his own. After 2 years, he decided to resume psychotherapy; however, he wanted a therapist who would focus more on his religious beliefs and spiritual needs. I referred him to such a therapist and at the time of this writing, Joseph continues to see him for therapy and to see me for quarterly medication visits. Joseph and Richard are still together—not a perfect couple, but a gay one.

REFERENCES

American Psychiatric Association: The Principles of Medical Ethics, With Annotations Especially Applicable to Psychiatry. Washington, DC, American Psychiatric Publishing, 2001

Bayer R: Homosexuality and American Psychiatry: The Politics of Diagnosis. New York, Basic Books, 1981

Cass VC: Homosexual identity formation: a theoretical model. J Homosex 4:219–235, 1979

Drescher J: Psychoanalytic Therapy and the Gay Man. Hillsdale, NJ, Analytic Press, 1998

Drescher J: Causes and becauses: on etiological theories of homosexuality, in Rethinking Psychoanalysis and the Homosexualities (The Annual of Psychoanalysis, Vol. 30). Edited by Winer JA, Anderson JW. Hillsdale, NJ, Analytic Press, 2002a, pp 57–68

Drescher J: Ethical issues in treating gay and lesbian patients. Psychiatr Clin North Am 25:605–621, 2002b

Drescher J: Invisible gay adolescents: the developmental narratives of gay men. Adolesc Psychiatry 26:73–94, 2002c

Drescher J, Stein TS, Byne W: Homosexuality, gay and lesbian identities, and homosexual behavior, in Kaplan and Sadock's Comprehensive Textbook of Psychiatry, 8th Edition. Edited by Sadock B, Sadock V. Baltimore, MD, Williams & Wilkins, 2004, pp 1936–1965

Haldeman DC: Therapeutic antidotes: helping gay and bisexual men recover from conversion therapies, in Sexual Conversion Therapy: Ethical, Clinical and Research Perspectives. Edited by Shidlo A, Schroeder M, Drescher J. New York, Haworth Press, 2001, pp 117–130

Kooden H: The gay male therapist as an agent of socialization. Journal of Gay and Lesbian Psychotherapy 2:39–64, 1994

Racker H: Transference and Countertransference. Madison, CT, International Universities Press, 1968

White M: Stranger at the Gate: To Be Gay and Christian in America. New York, Simon & Schuster, 1994

Winnicott DW: Ego distortion in terms of true and false self, in The Maturational Processes and the Facilitating Environment: Studies in the Theory of Emotional Development. Edited by Winnicott DW. New York, International Universities Press, 1965, pp 140–152

CHAPTER 14

Stabilizing Sarah

Interpersonal and Social Rhythms Therapy of Bipolar Disorder

Andrea Fagiolini, M.D.
Ellen Frank, Ph. D.

Andrea Fagiolini, M.D., is Associate Professor of Psychiatry at the University of Pittsburgh and Medical Director of both the Bipolar Disorder Center for Pennsylvanians and the Depression and Manic Depression Prevention Program at the Western Psychiatric Institute and Clinic. He specializes in the treatment of bipolar, depressive, and anxiety disorders. He is the attending psychiatrist for patients participating in a number of research studies and has published numerous papers on mood and anxiety disorders and their treatment.

Ellen Frank, Ph.D., is Professor of Psychiatry at the University of Pittsburgh and Director of the Depression and Manic Depression Prevention Program at the Western Psychiatric Institute and Clinic in Pittsburgh. An expert on mood disorders and their treatment, Dr. Frank has conducted a series of controlled maintenance treatment trials in recurrent unipolar and bipolar disorder using pharmacotherapy and psychotherapy that have received international recognition. She served on the Mood Disorder Work Group and the Task Force for DSM-IV. Dr. Frank is the developer of Interpersonal and Social Rhythm Therapy, which has been shown to reduce the risk of recurrence in patients with bipolar I disorder.

SARAH WAS A 30-YEAR-OLD woman who was referred to me (A.F.) for psychotherapy by a colleague, who was seeing her for medication management. The referral letter ended with a statement about the colleague feeling "sure she would be an easy and quickly successful case." No doubt the statement was intended to encourage me; however, it resulted in the opposite effect. First, the words "easy and quick" immediately brought to my mind the memories of all the cases that seemed easy and quick at the beginning then turned out to be very difficult once the patient and I had moved beyond the initial encounter. Second, the information that was provided in the referral letter seemed to contradict the optimistic conclusion. Third, the conclusion was followed by a post-script: "Make sure you read and remember all the details above. She hates going through them over and over again and will test you on how well you have studied her case." When I finished reading the referral letter, I could not help noticing that although I had not seen the patient yet, I was already feeling uncomfortable. Not a very encouraging start.

HISTORY

The referral letter reported, among other things, that Sarah had grown up in a large and chaotic family. Her mother and father raised her until they divorced when Sarah was age 16. When Sarah was a child, her father, who abused alcohol, was often physically abusive. Sarah has three siblings, all now reported by her to have mood disorders and alcohol abuse problems. She began using cocaine and alcohol while still in high school. At age 19, Sarah married Mark, her physically abusive, drug-addicted, and alcoholic boyfriend and increased her cocaine and alcohol abuse. Sarah continued to using substances until about age 23, when she became pregnant. At that time, she stopped her substance use.

Shortly after her son was born, Sarah experienced a period of time when she went without sleeping for days, feeling unusually good, cheerful, and overly excited. During this time, Sarah spoke loudly and rapidly and bought many things she could not afford, including a new car and new furniture for her house. She eventually was hospitalized after she assaulted a bank teller who refused her a $5 million loan, which she wanted to open the largest kindergarten in the state.

Sarah was discharged about 2 weeks later, felt relatively well for about 10 days, and then experienced a depressive episode, which lasted almost 2 years. She described the episode as entirely related to the domestic violence that she endured during that time from her abusive husband, who continued to use drugs and alcohol. Sarah also endorsed posttraumatic stress disorder (PTSD) symptoms related to the domestic violence that she endured during the marriage. Those symptoms included distressing recollections of the events and a feeling of detachment or estrangement from others. The depressive episode and the PTSD symptoms resolved when she was age 26, at which time she divorced her husband, found a new boyfriend, and, with her son, moved in with her mother.

Things continued to go relatively well until about 1 year before she came to see me when she began experiencing new depressive symptoms. At that time, she experienced several social stressors, including relationship problems that culminated in her discovery that her boyfriend was actually engaged to be married to someone else. She was also very dissatisfied with her employment as a housecleaner. In addition, her mother, with whom she and her 6-year-old son were still living, died unexpectedly after having recurrent episodes of untreated chest pains. Sarah, who had been largely dependent on her mother's support, reported that the death of her mother strained her already troubled relationship with her father and siblings and caused her severe financial problems. The house where Sarah lived belonged to her mother, and her father and siblings wanted to sell it immediately.

DIAGNOSIS

On her first visit, Sarah appeared as a slightly overweight young woman of her stated age. Based on the referral letter, I was prepared to meet a relatively hostile woman. I did not feel anxious or threatened in anticipation of the upcoming "test," but I found myself going through each detail of the referral letter again and again before I went to meet her in the waiting room. To my surprise she looked very different from the way I had pictured her. Sarah's dress was clean, neat, and appropriate. When we walked to my office, she was pleasant and cooperative. She started the conversation commenting on some pictures in my office, but then quickly moved to the reason why she decided to visit me. "I am going to tell you how I am feeling now. I am sure you have already read the [referring clincian's] report." I felt relieved because she had obviously waived the test. Sarah started to relate her feelings. Although she was crying, she was able to maintain good eye contact. She described herself as being very depressed, often irritable, and full of guilt because of her inability to offer her son the future that she would like him to have. She also described her inability to enjoy any food and her lack of interest in the things that she used to enjoy in the past. She reported long periods of intense fatigue, which were occasionally (about once a week) followed by very brief (lasting only minutes) periods when she experienced racing thoughts, bursts of energy, and agitation. She also reported that she was having difficulty sleeping and as a result was going to bed at very irregular times. She admitted that she often hoped to fall asleep and not wake up the following day; however, she adamantly denied any suicidal intention or plan and was able to establish a contract for safety with me. Sarah also endorsed experiencing limited symptom panic attacks approximately twice a day and relatively frequent and severe headaches. She stated that a recent magnetic resonance imaging test did not find evidence of any macroscopic brain abnormality. She denied current symptoms of psychosis or alcohol or other substance abuse.

Sarah's symptoms met the DSM-IV-TR criteria for bipolar I disorder, with her currently experiencing a major depressive episode. Although she had manic symptoms concurrent with her depressive episode, those symptoms were present less than nearly every day and were numerically insufficient to permit a DSM-IV-TR diagnosis of a mixed episode (American Psychiatric Association 2000).

TREATMENT

Sarah and I discussed the possible relation between her symptoms and both her interpersonal relationships and the disruption of her biological and social rhythms. I presented her with the possibility of and rationale for a treatment based on interpersonal and social rhythm therapy (IPSRT). I explained the structure and goals of IPSRT (Frank 2005; Frank et al. 2000). We discussed the possibility that psychosocial stressors mainly related to interpersonal relationships and changes in her biological rhythms had led to and sustained the current affective episodes. Sarah had several questions about IPSRT and doubts about her ability to "stick to any homework." Despite her doubts, she seemed to like the IPSRT approach to her symptoms and problems, which she found "kind of practical," and agreed to begin therapy.

Initial Phase of Treatment

The initial phase of treatment focused on my taking Sarah's history, completing an interpersonal inventory, identifying a problem area, initiating the social rhythm metric, and educating Sarah about her bipolar disorder. The therapy began with a review of Sarah's experience of the illness. She was reluctant to review her personal history. She said that she had already seen five psychiatrists and two therapists and was tired of going over her past and saying the same things each time. Although I understood her frustration, I tried to explain to her that this review was very important for her therapy. She became more cooperative once she understood that reviewing the symptomatic and interpersonal aspects of her earlier episodes could give us very important indications as to the best way to treat her current and future symptoms.

Sarah was relatively surprised to gradually discover the relation between her symptoms and the alterations and disruptions in her daily life and interpersonal interactions that preceded their development. For example, she described having a very unhealthy relationship with her ex-husband and recalled that her first depressive episode followed a period when this relationship was particularly difficult. At that time, she started using drugs, sleeping during the day, partying at night, and eating irregularly. She described her social routines at that time as completely disrupted. Although she loved her husband, she frequently had sex with other men, sometimes in the presence of her husband. At the time, she was experiencing frequent periods of excessive happiness and racing thoughts but, as best as she could recall, those periods never lasted more than 1–2 days.

Sarah clearly recalled her first full-blown manic episode, which occurred after the birth of her child and lasted at least a couple of weeks; during the episode she was not using alcohol or other substances. At that time she experienced intense worry about the impact of this birth on her life and about her ability to be a mother. Her sleep-wake cycle and eating habits were again completely disrupted by the baby's schedule. In an interesting development, in describing her present episode, she was able to link her first symptoms of being unable to sleep regularly to the discovery that her boyfriend was engaged to another woman. After she broke up with her boyfriend, Sarah started going to bars to look for a "replacement" and stopped going to work at the appropriate times. About that time her mother died and Sarah's daily routine became even more disrupted. She began skipping most of her meals and then eating large amounts of food every 2–3 days at very irregular times: one day at 3:00 P.M., one day at 8:00 A.M., and another day at 2:00 A.M. While collecting the information above, I completed the interpersonal inventory (Klerman et al. 1984) and found that the most significant individuals in Sarah's life were her son, Eric, and her friend, Susan, who was helping her by paying her utilities and buying food for her son.

Throughout the initial phase of treatment, I attempted to educate Sarah about bipolar disorder and the ways in which her interpersonal problems and disruptions in her daily routines could be related to the onset and continuation of her manic and depressive episodes. By the fourth session, Sarah was knowledgeable about the relation of her bipolar symptoms and interpersonal problems with the social and biological rhythm disruption that had preceded and been present during all of her acute episodes. I was pleased with her progress. At that point, Sarah was highly motivated to change.

During the first three to four sessions, Sarah completed the Social Rhythm Metric (SRM) (Frank, in press; Frank et al. 1994) on a daily basis. While doing so, she was instructed not to alter her routine until she and her therapist had had a chance to review the first few weeks of SRM recordings.

After the interpersonal inventory and SRM were completed, Sarah and I identified what the primary problem area was among the four possible choices: grief (including grief for the lost healthy self), interpersonal dispute, role transition, and interpersonal deficit (Frank, in press). At first, Sarah attributed all her symptoms to the loss of her mother. As the discussion proceeded, however, she acknowledged that the feelings related to this loss were more one of sadness and "normal" grief than depression and that most of her depressive symptoms were instead related to the severe financial difficulties that her mother's death had caused her. In fact, she spent most of the session describing how difficult it was for her to deal with her failure to achieve financial stability and ensure a safe future for her son. Sarah did not seem too worried about the interpersonal difficulties with her father and siblings. After fully discussing Sarah's complex interpersonal problems, Sarah and I agreed to focus on role transition; that is, we focused on the problems related to the change in her duties and responsibilities after her mother's death.

Intermediate and Later Phases of Treatment

The intermediate phase of therapy focused on 1) the search for triggers of rhythm disruption, 2) finding and maintaining the right balance with respect to activity and stimulation and adapting to changes in Sarah's routine, and 3) the resolution of the identified interpersonal problem.

After Sarah completed 3 weeks of SRMs, we reviewed them together looking for those rhythms that seemed to be particularly unstable. Sarah was going to bed at 11:00 P.M. one night, 5:00 A.M. the next night, and 8:00 P.M. the third night. She alternated days when she went without eating and days when she ate very large quantities of food. She did not distinguish breakfast from lunch or dinner; some days she had dinner when she woke up and breakfast when she went to bed. She alternated between periods when she avoided any social interaction and periods when she left her son with her friend, Susan, and spent 3–4 nights in a row in bars and clubs, hoping to find a new boyfriend. Sarah and I discussed the risks of such unstable rhythms, reviewed the implications of such instability for her symptoms, and agreed to work toward stabilizing them. Sarah gradually became convinced that social rhythm stabilization could have a therapeutic effect on the symptoms that she was experiencing and a prophylactic effect once those symptoms resolved, thus helping to prolong her intervals of being well and improve her functioning during them. I felt that Sarah had reached a turning point.

We then devised an initial, tentative plan for regularizing her routines and managing her symptoms in the Social Rhythm Stabilization Schedule for the forthcoming week. She also completed the Future Stabilization Goals Chart. This gave Sarah a sense of what the most immediate and more distant goals were as well as some confidence that her goals were attainable. Sarah could then focus on the relatively modest goals of getting out of bed by 9:00 A.M. for the next 7 days and having a regular breakfast.

In the next sessions, we started the process of finding the right balance of activity and stimulation and adapting to changes. Using the SRM to review activities and social interactions, we searched for the amounts of social interaction, sleep, and interpersonal stimulation that were associated with the most balanced mood state. We reviewed the SRM data and other recent historical information, trying to determine what in Sarah's life led to increased or decreased sleep, increased or decreased social stimulation, and so on. In addition, we evaluated the inputs from the outside (physical and social *zeitgebers*) that might affect her biological rhythms. To this end, I tried to help her identify situations (e.g., going to bars) that might be overstimulating and eventually develop strategies for modulating the frequency and intensity of overstimulation. Although the development of the initial plan and the search for triggers of disruption were accomplished in a relatively short amount of time, finding a balance in her activities and adapting to these changes took more experimentation. In fact, this aspect of social rhythm stabilization took many weeks of effort, along a "two steps ahead, one step back" trajectory.

Interpersonal Intervention

In the intermediate phase of treatment, we focused on the problem area formulated during the initial phase of IPSRT. The focus that Sarah and

I had chosen was role transition. Role transitions become the focus of treatment when events in the patient's life have caused major changes in the patient's roles and/or lifestyle and seem to be linked to the most recent illness episode. Role transitions can precede or follow a manic or depressive episode. In fact, all of Sarah's bipolar episodes appear to be related to a role transition. The multiple role transitions that Sarah experienced before and during the present depressive episode (from being 'partnered' to single and from being daughter to head of household, with the related loss of financial stability and increased responsibilities), clearly affected her mood stability, altered her self-esteem, and led to unstable social rhythms. Thus we agreed to focus our attention on role transitions.

My goal was to help Sarah structure her life during these role transitions, grieve over the roles that had been lost, and cope with the new roles she involuntarily had to assume. We gradually worked toward stabilizing her relationships while still working on stabilizing her social, and indirectly, her biological rhythms. A first success was achieved when Sarah realized and accepted that the loss of her boyfriend could be managed without desperately seeking a new boyfriend in each and every bar.

As a second step, once her social rhythms had achieved an acceptable level of stabilization, we started focusing on Sarah's dissatisfaction with her financial situation and the related distress of feeling unable to provide for her son. Sarah was clearly dissatisfied with her job of cleaning houses. She found it unrewarding from economic and psychological standpoints. She described it as mentally humiliating. Sarah talked of her ideal job as one in which she would interact with people instead of "cleaning germs," one in which she would feel important and be appropriately compensated. The reality was that she did not have either a qualifying degree or a set of skills that could be translated into her ideal job. In an attempt to address those issues, I helped her to gradually reset her job expectations to more reasonable goals. After one failed attempt to work as a waitress, which ended with her pouring a pound of salt over the head of a customer who had been "rude and excessively complaining," she accepted a job involving the home care of an 80-year-old woman. Although she found this job difficult at first, she accepted my encouragement not to give up. As time passed, she gradually established a good relationship with the elderly woman and started liking her and the job she was doing for her. At this point, Sarah started spending many more hours at her employer's house than she was being compensated for and, whenever possible, brought her son with her. Sarah's son established a good relationship with his new "grandmother," and Sarah started to think of her the woman not only as an employer but also as a friend. Sarah had been working for her client for about 9 months when the court issued an order for Sarah to immediately vacate her mother's house, which her father and siblings had sold. Sarah accepted her client's offer for her and her son to move in and share her home.

Termination

During the termination sessions, we reviewed the progress Sarah had made, focusing on the stabilization of her symptoms and social routine and her interpersonal problem areas. We talked a lot about the importance of continued vigilance for maintaining regular social routines and sleep patterns. We reviewed Sarah's typical prodromal signs of both depressive and manic episodes and developed a plan for how she might minimize and/or prevent future episodes. I tried to help Sarah develop coping strategies for stressors that may arise in the future. In particular, we discussed the possibility of her elderly client becoming too ill to remain at home or dying. Sarah said she would be sad when either of these occurred but appeared well prepared for the events. She had started saving money and Sarah's client had provided for her and her son in her will. Sarah seemed determined to continue her present kind of work even after the death of her employer and friend. I raised a question about the similarities between the new situation and the situation in which she was living before her mother's death. Sarah pointed out that the situations were in reality very different: "This time I am the one in charge. This time I am the one who is helping and providing the care for another person." At this point, I determined that she was ready to start decreasing the number of sessions and possibly complete her IPSRT course.

DISCUSSION

Interpersonal and social rhythm therapy is a modification of interpersonal psychotherapy based on our social zeitgeber hypothesis (Ehlers et al. 1988, 1993), which assumes that unstable or disrupted daily routines lead to circadian rhythm instability and, in vulnerable individuals, to affective episodes (Frank 2005; Frank et al. 2005). In the case that we have presented, a disruption in the patient's routine coupled with her interpersonal difficulties could easily be identified as the trigger for her depressive episode. Thus, we decided to intervene early and aggressively, seeking to enhance circadian integrity and focusing on the regular scheduling of daily activities and the avoidance of the activities that were disrupting the patient's rhythms. We also attempted to address the interpersonally based stressors the patient was experiencing, with the ultimate goal of reducing the patient's depressive symptoms, which we felt were at least partially related to her interpersonal difficulties.

Increasing the regularity in Sarah's life clearly contributed to the resolution of her symptoms and at the same time provided her with tools and knowledge that might be helpful in preventing future episodes. The ability of IPSRT, provided as adjunctive treatment to pharmacotherapy, to reduce the risk of future acute episodes of bipolar disorder represents one of the major strengths of this psychotherapy. In fact, we recently demonstrated that IPSRT is effective in reducing the risk of new episodes once the acute episode has resolved (Frank et al. 2005). We have also demonstrated that the ability of IPSRT to prevent new episodes is directly related to the extent to which patients are able to increase the regularity of their daily routines.

IPSRT can be a very helpful adjunctive treatment to pharmacotherapy during the acute treatment of the bipolar depressive episodes in cases like the one that we have described. We chose to present the Sarah's case because of the clear relationships among the patient's symptoms of bipolar disorder, her interpersonal problems, and the disruption of her biological and social rhythms. It is true that such a relationship may not be evident at this level of clarity in all patients with bipolar disorder; however, it is rare to be unable to identify any role of interpersonally based stressors or any destabilization of the circadian integrity during an acute bipolar episode, whether it is depressive, manic or mixed. In cases when the relationship between the acute bipolar episode and the presence of interpersonal difficulties and biological rhythm disruption is not as strong as in the case we have presented, a more general psychosocial intervention based on an intensive clinical management and psychoeduacational approach may produce results similar to those observed with IPSRT (Frank et al. 2005). However, even those cases can benefit from the development of a clear knowledge of the importance of maintaining regular social rhythms, adequate sleep, and appropriate levels of stimulation during the acute phases of bipolar disorder, as well as from the evaluation of the interpersonal stressors that may contribute to a patient's symptoms. In summary, IPSRT is an established adjunctive treatment for the prevention of new bipolar episodes (Frank et al. 2005) but can also be a very useful adjunctive treatment for the acute bipolar episodes, particularly depressive episodes and those depressive episodes in which a disruption of the biological rhythms and the level of interpersonal distress play a clear role, as in the case of Sarah.

REFERENCES

American Psychiatric Association: Diagnostic and Statistical Manual of Mental Disorders, 4th Edition, Text Revision. Washington, DC, American Psychiatric Association, 2000

Ehlers CL, Frank E, Kupfer DJ: Social zeitgebers and biological rhythms. A unified approach to understanding the etiology of depression. Arch Gen Psychiatry 45:948–952, 1988

Ehlers CL, Kupfer DJ, Frank E, et al: Biological rhythms and depression: the role of zeitgebers and zeitstorers. Depression 1:285–293, 1993

Frank E: Interpersonal and Social Rhythm Therapy for Bipolar Disorder: A Manual for Clinicians. New York, Guilford Press, 2005

Frank E, Kupfer DJ, Ehlers CL, et al: Interpersonal and social rhythm therapy for bipolar disorder: integrating interpersonal and behavioral approaches. Behav Ther 17:143–149, 1994

Frank E, Swartz HA, Kupfer DJ: Interpersonal and social rhythm therapy: managing the chaos of bipolar disorder. Biol Psychiatry 48:593–604, 2000

Frank E, Kupfer DJ, Thase ME, et al: Two-year outcomes for interpersonal and social rhythm therapy in individuals with bipolar I disorder. Arch Gen Psychiatry 62:996–1004, 2005

Klerman GL, Weissman MM, Rounsaville BJ, et al: Interpersonal Psychotherapy of Depression. New York, Basic Books, 1984

CHAPTER 15

Baby Got the Blues

Treating Depressed Pregnant and Postpartum Teens

Heather B. Howell, M.S.W.
Kimberly Ann Yonkers, M.D.

Heather B. Howell, M.S.W., is a Clinical Social Worker working in Yale University's PMS, Perinatal, and Postpartum Research Program under Dr. Kimberly Ann Yonkers. She provides mental health counseling to pregnant and postpartum women with mood and anxiety disorders and substance abuse issues. She earned a master's degree in Social Work with a specialized concentration in mental health and substance abuse. She has coauthored publications on perinatal mental health, anxiety disorders in women, and premenstrual dysphoric disorder.

Kimberly Ann Yonkers, M.D., is an Associate Professor of Psychiatry and an Instructor of Epidemiology at Yale University. She directs the PMS, Perinatal, and Postpartum Research Program, with research interests centering on the detection and treatment of depression in pregnant and postpartum women as well as treatments for premenstrual dysphoric disorder. She is widely published in the area of women's mental health.

HISTORY

The typical patient seen in our practice is a pregnant or postpartum woman referred by our affiliated maternal health obstetric clinic. The referral issue usually centers psychological problems requiring further evaluation and/or treatment. Such centers care for the city's residents, providing not only basic prenatal and postnatal care but also education about self-care, personal safety, community resources, mental health, and substance abuse, as appropriate. Overall rates of prenatal depressive symptoms in this clinic are 23%; rates among African-American patients are 31% (Smith et al. 2004).

Kayla was an African-American teenager who presented in her third trimester of an unplanned first pregnancy; she was referred by her obstetrician for evaluation of a possible mood disorder. She volunteered that she felt frequently anxious and worried and reported a low mood and lack of interest. She denied using alcohol or drugs, but the referring obstetrician revealed that her clinic urine toxicology screen tested positive for marijuana. She had received prior grief counseling as a younger adolescent after the death of her mother, which she ended on her own after only a few sessions. She stated that she did not like the treatment and did not find it helpful.

Kayla expressed a diffident attitude toward her pregnancy. Many elements of her life seemed in disarray: her housing was unstable and of questionable safety, she was neither employed nor attending school, and the pregnancy was neither planned nor entirely welcomed. However, as seemed to be a pattern in her life, she felt stuck dealing with what came her way, neither able to accept responsibility for nor determine to take control over the outcome.

Although Kayla described her symptoms as uncomfortable, she outrightly declined my offer of outpatient individual and group supportive services, clearly stating that she was not ready for psychotherapy. She believed she was able to handle current life problems on her own, that therapy was not important to her at this time, and that she would not be inclined to attend. To push her seemed disrespectful and confrontational; however, her obstetrician continued to express concern about her emotional well-being, apparent marijuana use, and the possible influence of these factors on her fetus.

Therefore, after completing the preliminary evaluation in a conversational manner, I elected to employ motivational interviewing, a systematic assessment approach designed to encourage internally motivated change (Miller et al. 2002). The purpose of this technique at this time was to shore up her internal motivation to attend counseling, as well as to clarify her own self-assessment of her symptoms and her life stressors. It was my thought that, once she made a commitment to attend outpatient mental health care, a broader range of treatment techniques could relieve depressive and anxious symptoms.

DIAGNOSIS

My initial goals were to introduce her to the benefits of psychotherapy and encourage her to decrease her drug use. We discussed ways in which her symptoms of depression and anxiety were interfering with her daily functioning, and we also touched on her ongoing use of marijuana. She was initially wary of speaking with me but warmed up to our conversations surprisingly easily. I was aware that she lacked a maternal figure in her life and recognized that she responded easily to my nurturing, supportive interpersonal contact. She was given educational information about fetal development and offered brief advice to reduce or cease drug use. She was also encouraged to discuss her use openly with her obstetrician to facilitate the best possible prenatal care. Finally, she was referred to a community mentoring program that offered specialized education and support for first-time mothers. Until her delivery, I heard nothing more from Kayla.

Kayla was re-referred to me after she delivered her baby. I hoped that she would now be able to engage in treatment. I imagined that the transition into motherhood might challenge her determination to go it alone. She had delivered a full-term baby girl who was rehospitalized at age 3 weeks with respiratory complications, for which she was treated and released. This stressor seemed to impress on Kayla the value and fragility of her maternal role. She continued to work with her volunteer support mentor and spoke quite positively of that service.

My therapeutic aims at this point were to reassess her mental state and connect with her in such a way that she would accept outpatient counseling. Now at 5 weeks postpartum, her depression had worsened. She had thoughts that life was empty and not worth living and that she would be better off dead; she had considered harming herself by taking pills. Her sadness and irritability were persistent, and she felt dismal about the future. She was overeating and gaining weight; she overslept during the day and was unable to sleep at night. The anxiety of which she had complained during our prior sessions could clearly be delineated into episodic attacks of shortness of breath, heart racing, and overwhelming fear that something awful was imminent, all consistent with panic attacks.

She was more isolative and was feeling the effects of her dwindling social network; she also had difficulty accepting what minimal support was available from family and friends. Her friends did not have children and were appropriately focused on high school sports and the upcoming class prom. She felt sad that she could not relate to her peers and struggled to balance the fulfillment and emptiness of motherhood.

Kayla denied using marijuana, stating that she had stopped late in the pregnancy. However, given her history of using marijuana to cope with emotional and interpersonal strain coupled with her living environment where others used the drug, her potential to use remained an ongoing concern.

Her relationship with her boyfriend (the father of her child) had been problematic since she conceived, and he was emotionally unavailable to her. He enjoyed seeing his daughter but did not feel compelled to offer financial support. The memories of the loss of her own mother at an early age recurred during the postpartum period; Kayla felt that her mother would have been able to help her, both emotionally and physically, during this time of early motherhood.

TREATMENT

After discussing her treatment options, I offered her psychopharmacology coupled with cognitive-behavioral therapy. I prescribed a serotonin reuptake inhibitor that would alleviate symptoms of depression and panic. Kayla had elected not to breast-feed, so medication was a logical component of her psychiatric care. I felt that the psychotherapy would help control her panic attacks, encourage medication adherence, and teach Kayla skills that could help her manage and overcome her depressive symptoms as well as negotiate her interpersonal relationships.

My therapeutic goal in helping her transition into motherhood was complex. This young woman was developmentally appropriate for her age, but the responsibility of motherhood demanded from her a new and unfamiliar set of skills. She struggled to find a balance in her attitude toward her daughter, which fluctuated between adoration and panic. She cherished her daughter, was pleased with the unconditional love that she felt from her, and even stated that her daughter loved her "the most." She felt good about herself in the moments when she was able to sooth her daughter's crying but overwhelmed during the times when her daughter was uncontrollably fussy or when she could not understand how to meet her infant's needs. She worried aloud about her daughter's basic needs but was proud when she was able to show her off to others, especially if she was wearing new clothes or a cute bonnet. Kayla hesitated to let others hold or touch the baby, however, even resisting such a connection with the baby's father. It seemed clear that he also supported this distance, as he was spending little time with her and was chronically unable to baby-sit, even when Kayla attended appointments or sought personal time.

Kayla struggled with the contrast between the joy she felt being a mother and performing the role well and her initial desire not to be pregnant and to live a single life. She reminisced about the times when she had attended school, worked, and had friends independent of her boyfriend. She felt she had lost those aspects of her life when her daughter was born. Although she struggled to verbalize her feelings, I sensed that she harbored some resentment toward her daughter, as her mere existence meant that she was "stuck" with her boyfriend in a deteriorating relationship and that she was often literally stuck at home with few resources to expand her day-to-day experiences.

This ambivalence about motherhood became a focus of our talk therapy. At times, I verbalized this observation for her, suggesting that many new mothers feel such a conflict. I suggested that it was normal to feel a pull toward the previous luxury of teenage irresponsibility. She would respond with a thoughtful "Hmmmm," suggesting to me that she was considering her own scenario internally but was unwilling to outwardly admit any negative feelings toward motherhood or her daughter in particular.

Treatment with this patient did not progress smoothly. She was reasonably adherent with her medication, at times taking an extra dose to cope with a tough day. Her boyfriend belittled her for being in therapy, saying she was crazy and incapable of being a good mother if she were depressed. She took these words very seriously and would call in crisis, tearful, and overwhelmed. At these times she would say that motherhood was too hard, she never wanted to have a baby, and she wanted her old life back. After one of these conversations, she would miss one or several therapy sessions and then regain her balance and seem stable again. My sense was that after she opened this window of honesty, she felt guilty and exposed. Afterwards, she strongly resisted further such conversations, brushing off any of her controversial words by saying she was "all better now."

The medication offered substantial relief to Kayla. Over the course of the next month, her antidepressant dose was increased to a normal therapeutic dose. She was simultaneously making therapeutic gains by setting limits with her partner, encouraging family time, and supporting him as a father. She applied and was hired for a part-time job; although the work was uninspiring and unchallenging, she considered it a step toward moving back into the job market and gaining financial strength. She enjoyed having some money for personal spending, contributing to household expenses, and buying the baby something special. She continued to feel validated by the adoration that her baby offered her and struggled with hard decisions about the future of her relationship with her partner.

When she ended therapy after eight sessions, it appeared to me that she had been patient with the process for as long as possible and had reached her limit. Her primary care physician in the clinic agreed to continue psychopharmacology under my guidance. I had wished that Kayla would remain in therapy for a longer period of time, but I also understood that the changes that she enaceted were dramatic, given her life circumstances and limited ability to effect change. I also recognized that a few months of therapy was quite a long-term commitment for her. In the midst of chaos, she had struggled to develop a relationship with me as her therapist, and it was my hope that she would be able to generalize these skills to relationships with other people in her life.

DISCUSSION

Women often do not receive the support and validation they may need to acknowledge some of the difficulties inherent in new motherhood. Social systems continually reinforce the joy and gift of motherhood, supporting the idea that it should be a happy, blissful time. The reality is that there are many challenges to being a new mother and that even mothers who are not depressed may need support around a variety of issues; these difficulties include raising a child, starting a new family, negotiating the changing roles among existing household members, and adjusting to dramatically altered future goals and plans.

My experiences working with these young mothers, thanks to our affiliation with a primary care clinic, are eye opening and career affirming. I have sampled various therapeutic approaches, trying to fashion the right fit to meet each patient's needs. These young women struggle with every impoverishment imaginable and demonstrate amazing resilience. Their community-based resources are limited. Surrounded by drugs and violence, they try to balance family responsibilities with creating an opportunity for themselves.

I generally find that women flourish when they feel good in their relationships, which sways my clinical orientation toward interpersonal psychotherapy. However, the usefulness of cognitive-behavioral skills training is undeniable in helping patients solve problems and promoting their self-worth. The common lack of health insurance among the population seen in the primary care clinic creates a problem when clinicians try to prescribe antidepressants or antianxiety medications for these patients. The occasional use of drugs and alcohol is an unfortunate fact in these patients and only furthers my allegiance to motivational enhancement and cognitive-behavioral therapy, as these approaches are known to be effective with substance use disorders.

Pregnancy and motherhood are not guaranteed times of happiness or mental wellness. A clinician or provider should not assume the positive status of a mother's emotional health. It is a time when a mother may feel unable to discuss her struggles, in part influenced by external pressure to present a happy and optimistic front. Her silence about the pain only further contributes to her feelings of isolation, loneliness, and possible depression. She is likely to feel grateful and relieved if her provider can offer her an opportunity to speak truthfully about her emotional experiences.

In reflecting back on this case and others similar in profile, I leave the reader with some key summary points.

There is a trend in health care to integrate the treatment of depression and anxiety with primary care services. This move, which has been influenced by managed health care insurance companies as well as patient preferences, has the possible benefit of increasing patient adherence, as individuals complaining of depression or anxiety symptoms are likely to contact their primary care physician, someone with whom they already have a professional relationship, before seeking services with a mental health specialist (Regier et al. 1993). For practical reasons, I have paired my clinic, which specializes in perinatal mental health, with a prominent obstetric clinic.

Depressed and anxious people face many barriers to receiving quality mental health care, not the least of which is their own ambivalence regarding seeking treatment. The stigma attached to talking with a "shrink" is not trivial, and part of a mental health provider's task is to help individuals overcome such struggles. I have standardized the use of one to three sessions of motivational enhancement therapy for every patient I see. The focus of these sessions is to address a patient's readiness for receiving care and her existing fears and concerns that might contribute to her decision not to return to my office. I find that having this discussion at the beginning of therapy gives a patient the option to decline services and still feel supported by the clinic. It also increases the chance that she might change her attitude toward mental health care in the future. (For a review of the foundations of motivational interviewing, see Miller et al. 2002.)

The rate of drug and alcohol abuse generally found in our clinic's prenatal population is 9%, a percentage that is consistent with that found at other sites (Ebrahim and Gfroerer 2003; Substance Abuse and Mental Health Services Administration 2003). Current standards of care are to offer brief advice about the detrimental effects of substance use to the mother and her fetus and a referral for recovery care in the community.

Untreated depressive symptoms during pregnancy often continue and may worsen during the postpartum period (Altshuler et al. 1998; Hobfall et al. 1995; Yonkers et al. 2001). It is my aim to offer prenatal mental health care, as it is not only pertinent and effective but can also prevent potential serious postpartum illnesses; for example, rates of postpartum depression in our area clinics range from 10% to 30%, with especially high rates for adolescents. At a time when a woman has the additional stress of a newborn infant and her changing role as a woman, partner, and mother, it seems only prudent to offer her some skills and services ahead of time. An obstetric practice that does not address this health concern is missing a key component of providing health care to mothers, babies, and families.

REFERENCES

Altshuler LL, Hendrick V, Cohen LS: Course of mood and anxiety disorders during pregnancy and the postpartum period. J Clin Psychiatry 59 (suppl 2):29–33, 1998

Ebrahim SH, Gfroerer J: Pregnancy-related substance use in the United States during 1996–1998. Obstet Gynecol 101:374–379, 2003

Hobfoll SE, Ritter C, Lavin J, et al: Depression prevalence and incidence among inner-city pregnant and postpartum women. J Consult Clin Psychol 63:445–453, 1995

Miller WR, Rollnick S, Conforti K (eds): Motivational Interviewing, 2nd Edition: Preparing People for Change. New York, Guilford Press, 2002

Regier DA, Narrow WE, Rae DS, et al: The de facto US mental and addictive disorders service system: epidemiologic catchment area prospective 1-year prevalence rates of disorders and services. Arch Gen Psychiatry 50:85–94, 1993

Smith MV, Rosenheck RA, Cavaleri MA, et al: Screening for and detection of depression, panic disorder and PTSD in public-sector obstetrics clinics. Psychiatr Serv 55:407–414, 2004

Substance Abuse and Mental Health Services Administration: Results From the 2002 National Survey on Drug Use and Health: National Findings. Rockville, MD, Office of Applied Studies, 2003

Yonkers KA, Ramin SM, Rush AJ, et al: Onset and persistence of postpartum depression in an inner-city maternal health clinic system. Am J Psychiatry 158:1856–1863, 2001

CHAPTER 16

Depressed Electrician

Cognitive-Behavioral Therapy of Major Depression

Cory F. Newman, Ph.D.

Cory F. Newman, Ph.D., is Associate Professor of Psychology in Psychiatry at the University of Pennsylvania School of Medicine. He graduated summa cum laude and Phi Beta Kappa from the University of Pennsylvania in 1981, and earned his Ph.D. in clinical psychology from the State University of New York at Stony Brook in 1987. Dr. Newman completed a postdoctoral Fellowship under the mentorship of Aaron T. Beck in 1988, and became the Director of the Center for Cognitive Therapy in 1994, a post he currently maintains. Dr. Newman is a Diplomate of the American Board of Professional Psychology and a Founding Fellow of the Academy of Cognitive Therapy. He has coauthored four books and is primary author of dozens of chapters and articles on topics related to cognitive therapy. An international lecturer, Dr. Newman has presented seminars and workshops across the United States and Canada as well as in 12 countries in Europe and South America. He has been a protocol cognitive therapist and supervisor on a number of randomized, controlled trials, including the National Institute on Drug Abuse Multisite Collaborative Study on Psychosocial Treatments for Cocaine Abuse, and the Penn-Vanderbilt-Rush multisite studies on the pharmacotherapy and cognitive therapy of severe depression.

Dr. Newman was listed by Philadelphia Magazine as one of the Best

Therapists in the Philadelphia Area, and he was the recipient of the Earl Bond award for outstanding supervision and mentoring of Fellows and Psychiatry Residents in 2004. When he is not actively engaged in his role as a clinical psychologist, Dr. Newman plays amateur-league ice hockey with the Philadelphia Roadrunners, and is a serious classical pianist who gives annual recitals at the University of Pennsylvania.

KENDALL, A 53-YEAR-OLD electrician and divorced father of two, was advised by his college-age son to seek therapy for his clinical depression. Kendall's son had taken a course in abnormal psychology, recognized that his father had most of the symptoms characteristic of a major depressive episode, learned that cognitive-behavioral therapy was efficacious in treating this disorder (Gloaguen et al. 1998), and thus recommended that his father go for treatment. At first, Kendall felt very little motivation to pursue therapy other than to please his son. However, within 2 months, Kendall had changed his mind after a woman with whom he was in love made it clear to him that the most she could ever give him was friendship. Heartbroken, Kendall called the Center for Cognitive Therapy, a university-affiliated outpatient center specializing in cognitive-behavioral therapy, to commence treatment.

DIAGNOSIS

The first appointment involved a complete diagnostic work-up, including a structured diagnostic interview (the Structured Clinical Interview for DSM-IV-TR, Clinician Version; First et al. 2000); open-ended questioning about Kendall's reasons for seeking therapy; assessment of his high risk factors (e.g., Kendall's past and present thoughts about suicide); self-report scales such as the Beck Depression Inventory (A.T. Beck et al. 1961), Beck Anxiety Inventory (A.T. Beck et al. 1988), and Beck Hopelessness Scale (A.T. Beck et al. 1974); and take-home questionnaires in which Kendall wrote about his current life situation, personal history, and goals for therapy. Kendall was struck by what an extensive and rigorous process this intake evaluation was. It was explained to him that proper therapy required a thorough assessment of his symptoms and overall functioning and that this process would continue throughout therapy as new information came to light. Kendall said that the initial interview fatigued him, but he was appreciative of the professionalism that was brought to bear on his case, and he expressed some hope that therapy could be a positive experience.

As a result of the diagnostic evaluation, Kendall was given the following provisional multiaxial DSM-IV diagnosis:

Axis I: Major depressive disorder, recurrent, moderate severity; social phobia (mild); and nicotine dependence

Axis II: None (some avoidant features)

Axis III: Early signs of chronic obstructive pulmonary disease

Axis IV: Moderate life stressors, including chronic overwork and stress in his job as an electrician, never-ending monetary difficulties with his financially irresponsible ex-wife, college expenses for his son, social loneliness

Axis V: Score on Current Global Adaptive Functioning of 65, indicative of symptoms that are prominent enough to have a moderately adverse impact on everyday functioning and quality of life, but not sufficient enough to require intensive intervention (e.g., hospitalization, vigilant assessment of suicidality, immediate commencement of psychotropic medications). The patient's best score in the past year was 70, indicating that the patient's levels of symptomatology and functioning were fairly consistent throughout the past year.

Kendall's most prominent current symptoms included sad mood, anhedonia (diminished ability to enjoy things), low energy, self-reproach (feelings of guilt, sense of worthlessness), hopelessness about the future, loneliness, and early morning awakening. Kendall also noted that he was generally uncomfortable in social situations and therefore spent most of his free time alone. Aside from interacting with his son and daughter, he did not have socially meaningful contacts with anyone other than a supervisor at work, whose praises for Kendall's skills as an electrician Kendall did not entirely believe. Kendall was more than humble; he was self-deprecating. I felt that his low self-esteem would be a target for intervention, as this factor impacted both his clinical depression and his social avoidance problems.

Kendall did not report suicidal ideation or intent at the time he commenced cognitive therapy, although he acknowledged that there had been two times in his life when he thought about ending his life: once when he was in college and the object of his affections announced her engagement to someone else and again years later when he learned that his wife had been having affairs with both a neighbor and a tennis instructor. However, Kendall stated that he had never taken any concrete steps to harm himself, that he had not felt suicidal for more than 5 years, and that he was interested in improving his life, not ending it. As Kendall's therapist, I was relieved to hear him state his commitment to life, but when dealing with a patient with major depression it is always important to be alert to signs of suicidality. Thus I knew that I would keep a watchful eye on Kendall's condition, paying special attention to his responses on the three Beck inventories mentioned above, because exacerbations in symptom clusters such as hopelessness and dysphoria might signal a renewed risk for suicide.

Almost as an aside, Kendall offered that his chronic smoking habit might represent a "sort of slow suicide." On hearing this, I asked if he would like to put "quitting smoking" on the list of goals for therapy. Kendall's raised eyebrow indicated that he was intrigued by this suggestion, but he did not exactly jump at it. He noted that his primary care physician and pulmonologist had been adamant that he needed to quit smoking to prevent the progression of his chronic obstructive pulmonary disease. Perhaps, Kendall reasoned, this entry into cognitive therapy might be his best shot at pursuing this most important goal for his general health. Kendall was quick to add that he was "making no promises"; I responded by saying that Kendall's willingness to even consider working on his smoking problem was a welcome development.

HISTORY

An examination of Kendall's personal history was revealing, although he wrote about it (and discussed it in session) in a characteristic low-key tone. He was raised in a household where the father ruled with an iron fist. Kendall's two older brothers were "just like Dad," following in his footsteps to play football in high school and college. By contrast, Kendall said that he was seen as a "momma's boy," and indeed he shared more of her characteristics, such as a love of reading, poetry, and painting. Kendall was ostracized by his father (as well as his male schoolmates) on a regular basis for these interests, and so Kendall retreated into a silent world in which he rarely if ever discussed anything of emotional significance with anyone. In the meantime, Kendall honed his crafts and excelled as a student.

By the time he reached college, Kendall still had never gone on a date, but he came to idealize a young woman named Sylvia who he met during his freshman year. Being shy, he never openly declared his love for Sylvia, but he came to assume that somehow they would always be together; indeed they spent a great deal of time together as friends. However, in their senior year, Sylvia announced to Kendall that she had become engaged. This stunned and crushed the naïve young man who had envisioned a lifetime together with his heretofore platonic love object. Kendall's chief reactions were to be mercilessly self-reproachful (e.g., "How could I have been so innocent and so stupid?"), to become unable to eat or go to class, and to pour out his grief in dark poetry and painting. His mother became alarmed about his reactions to Sylvia's engagement and hand-walked Kendall to the student counseling center, whereupon a finding of "vegetative depression and suicidal ideation" led to his hospitalization just before and during final exams, all of which he missed.

When he was discharged a month later, Kendall made two fateful decisions that would continue to haunt him until the present. First, he assumed that he had now flunked out of college and that he had no recourse. In actuality, there is every reason to believe that he could have gone back to school and completed his degree by finishing some incomplete course requirements and enrolling for an additional semester. Second, rather than take his prescribed antidepressants, Kendall took up smoking ("Just like Dad; isn't that ironic?"), and nicotine became his chief form of self-medication.

Kendall rebounded by going to a trade school to become an electrician, where he excelled. He continued to paint and write poetry in private and even set up his own art studio in the apartment he rented. Kendall's mood improved, although he continued to isolate himself socially. He entered his first romantic relationship when he was age 30 in which the woman (Giselle, who was later to become his wife) was the aggressor. Years later, well after they were married, he learned the painful truth of his wife's propensity for infidelity, yet he stayed with her to keep the family intact for the sake of his two young children. Kendall tried to focus his attention on his job and on raising his kids, silently enduring the indignities of his marital situation, until things came to a head when he discovered his wife's affairs with both a neighbor and a tennis coach. At this point, Kendall opted to end his marriage, although in keeping with his mild-mannered, nonassertive approach to life, he pursued a "no-fault" divorce. Although he shared custody of the children with his ex-wife, the kids gradually chose to spend more time with Kendall, resulting in a de facto full-custody situation that the ex-wife never contested.

For the next few years (leading up to the present), Kendall continued to function reasonably well, being a competent and loving father to his children and earning a living as a master electrician. Nevertheless, his existence was fairly lonely and melancholy, with his only outside interests being art and poetry (he had compiled quite an impressive portfolio that nobody ever saw). Kendall probably would have gone on this way indefinitely, feeling a general, pervasive sadness in life but seeking no treatment, except for the following situation. Kendall fell in love with a woman named Laura whom he met at a book-reading event, although (reminiscent of his college experience with Sylvia) he never openly expressed his romantic interest to her. Although Kendall asked Laura to attend other cultural events with him and to meet for conversations over coffee, he never so much as tried to hold her hand or kiss her. Nevertheless, Laura surmised that his romantic interest was much greater than her own and thus she made herself less available. When Kendall continued to call, Laura acknowledged that she could only be his friend and that their relationship would never be anything more. Just as with Sylvia in college, Kendall felt despondent and self-reproachful, declaring to himself that he must be undeserving of a real, mutual relationship with a woman. Kendall's depressive symptoms worsened, and he decided to follow his son's advice to seek therapy.

TREATMENT

As is customary for all patients at the Center for Cognitive Therapy, Kendall came to his sessions 10 minutes early to fill out three Beck inventories prior to each meeting with me. These data allowed me to track Kendall's functioning and progress on a week-by-week basis in addition to providing me with an early warning system in case his condition should suddenly decline. At the time of his initial intake evaluation, his scores were as follows: Beck Depression Inventory, 24 (moderate level of depression); Beck Anxiety Inventory, 7 (mild level of anxiety); Beck Hopelessness Scale, 14 (moderate to severe hopelessness).

Kendall's scores were nearly identical at the time of his first therapy session 1 week after intake. Kendall talked about having some difficulty "facing the day" in the aftermath of Laura's declaration that "nothing would ever happen" between them, but otherwise presented his mood and life situation in an understated fashion.

The two main objectives for the first session were to establish a positive, collaborative working relationship with Kendall and to set some goals for therapy as a whole. To build rapport with Kendall, I offered him a sympathetic conceptualization of his life issues, then asked him for feedback on the accuracy of what I had just said. I noted that Kendall had experienced repeated, significant interpersonal rejections in his life, including those by his father, Sylvia (in college), his wife (who had shunned him but had sex with others), and Laura, and that these experiences contributed to his being chronically low in self-esteem and lonely. I added that it was remarkable that Kendall did not seem to be bitter and angry and that he still exhibited a pleasant and polite demeanor. I applauded him for raising his children well in spite of the adverse situations of his marriage and divorce and for achieving a high level of proficiency in his profession. At the same time, I acknowledged that Kendall was significantly depressed and offered to collaborate with him on a clinical plan that would have the best chance of improving his quality of life.

As a psychologist, I was not in a position to prescribe antidepressant medication for Kendall. However, I explained to Kendall that talk therapy (in this case, cognitive therapy) and pharmacotherapy sometimes go well together (Hollon et al. 1992; Pampallona et al. 2004) and that it might be useful to consider this sort of combined treatment approach. Given that Kendall had stated previously that he was interested in smoking cessation, I reminded him that there was a medication (bupropion [Wellbutrin]) that doubled as both an antidepressant and an inhibitor of nicotine cravings (Lief 1996). Kendall seemed intrigued by this medication but was not ready to commit to pharmacotherapy, saying, "Let me think about it." My response was, "That's okay. You can think about it, but in the meantime would it be fair for me to assume that you and I are still going to try to help you with your depression and smoking via cognitive therapy?" My message was clear: I would respect Kendall's opinion about his own treatment directions, but I would still be assertive and eager in helping him pursue sensible, attainable goals.

Kendall was a man with many admirable qualities. He was humble, pleasant, intelligent, a good father, a stable provider, a talented poet and artist, and a resilient individual who had suffered but survived a number of significant interpersonal injuries in his life. My sense was that Kendall's strengths would serve him well in treatment. It was unfortunate (and perhaps predictable) that Kendall did not share this positive view of himself. He described himself as awkward, passive, and, much worse still, as unlovable and a failure. This was certainly the self-image of a depressed person. His subjective sense of himself was much worse than how others would view him, including myself. As therapy started, I had much more respect for Kendall than he had for himself.

To engage in sophisticated cognitive therapy, I had to avoid simply contradicting Kendall about his self-image by merely imploring him to think more highly of himself and rid himself of the "negative, dysfunctional beliefs" he held about himself. Instead, it was crucial for me to show genuine empathy for Kendall by treating him with kindness and compassion but also trying to understand how it was that he came to view himself the way he did. Kendall, insightful fellow that he was, made it easy for me. He noted that he felt like a failure in that he had never earned his college degree and therefore, he reasoned, the high regard his colleagues had for him was really bogus because they (as full-fledged electrical engineers) were more highly educated and successful than he was. Kendall seemed unmoved by the fact that his nickname at work was "mild-mannered Clark Kent," a tribute to the quiet heroism he displayed in preventing a number of catastrophes owing to his quick thinking and diligence on the job. Kendall simply focused on his lack of a college degree, which haunted him to this day.

In describing why he felt unlovable, Kendall said, "I can explain that in three words: Sylvia, Giselle, Laura." I understood entirely, and I did not even bother to add that he probably did not get much affirmation or love from his father either. So it made sense that Kendall would undervalue himself. On the other hand, there was compelling evidence that he was extremely lovable as a father, and I made certain to ask about his ongoing interactions with his son and daughter to play up this point. In fact, Kendall told me quite a few heartwarming anecdotes about meaningful times he had spent with his kids and the affection they had showered on each other over the years. When Kendall mentioned that his daughter had said to him, "Dad, we really need to find you a girlfriend," I seized the opportunity and said that his daughter was quite wise in making this suggestion. Before long, we were brainstorming ways for Kendall to meet new people in social situations.

As we began to generate a list of ambitious goals for therapy, I expected that Kendall would have doubts about his ability (or perhaps even his "worthiness") to attain such goals. I often asked him for feedback to make sure that I had his consent to pursue the lines of inquiry and interventions that would have him face things that were arguably beneficial to his life but that might trigger a sense of helplessness and hopelessness in a depressed, socially anxious individual such as Kendall. Part of our work involved monitoring and documenting (both in and between sessions as homework) Kendall's automatic thoughts that, if left unaddressed, might lead him to avoid taking active steps to help himself. For example, whenever he had the inclination to give up on a homework assignment (e.g., giving a reading of his poetry at a promotional event at a nearby bookstore), he was instructed to write down the thoughts that were discouraging him and then to counter them with new ways of thinking that would give him the impetus to follow through on his initial plan. This sort of self-help requires much instruction and practice in session, something we did together on a regular basis. One of the most prominent of Kendall's pessimistic thoughts that we addressed was his concern that he would fail in therapy. Aside from giving him a lot of genuine moral support, I helped Kendall conceptualize everything he did in therapy as an experiment in improving his life and not as a task that would be judged in terms of pass or fail. Kendall acknowledged after some time that he was finally getting the message that every step he took to help himself was part of a collective triumph in the long run, regardless of the immediate outcome of the exercise.

Another way in which we worked to boost Kendall's self-esteem was to focus on his relationship with his son and daughter. He noticed that his mood was consistently at its best when he was most involved in his kids' lives, including helping them with homework, attending their extracurricular activities, and (ironically) giving them pep talks whenever they felt discouraged. I pointed out that Kendall's parenting style seemed to have transcended his own parents' skills by a healthy margin, in that he did everything he could to make his son and daughter feel valued and validated. Kendall's own children became a constant reminder that he was not a failure and certainly not unlovable. Still, he had additional goals to pursue, and pursue them we did!

Throughout our sessions, Kendall made reference to his poetry and artwork, pursuits I strongly encouraged (in light of the fact that his father had discouraged them, which had pained Kendall so deeply). I asked him to bring in samples of his work, and some of our sessions turned into mini-lessons, with Kendall as the teacher and me as the student. I was amazed when Kendall stated that he had never shared his work so extensively with anyone, not even with the women he had loved, and certainly never with his family of origin. I looked at Kendall as if he were sitting idly on a treasure and implored him to continue this work and make it more public. For example, over the course of a number of months of treatment, Kendall wrote editorials to local newspapers, submitted short stories for publication in magazines, volunteered to paint murals for public facilities, and so on. By now Kendall was adept at noticing his own depressed and anxious cognitive-emotional reactions, and he quickly responded therapeutically to thoughts that his work would be rejected and judged harshly and that this would "prove" he was a failure. Kendall reasoned that rejection was the norm for submissions of literary and artistic works and that it was the acceptances he should focus on, enthusiastically taking full advantage of them. He documented these "point-counterpoint" thought processes in his daily thought records, standard forms that are often used in cognitive therapy as part of the technique called "rational responding" (J. S. Beck 1995). As a nice, individualized twist to the technique, Kendall wrote his rational responses on his daily thought records in poetic fashion.

A quantum leap in Kendall's recovery from depression and social anxiety occurred when he enrolled in a painting and sculpting course at a local school of fine arts. Here he encountered a peer group that shared his interests and appreciated his work. As an added bonus, Kendall began dating a fellow classmate named Lanie, a woman who not only gave Kendall affection and affirmation but also served as his greatest motivator to stop smoking. Lanie apparently told Kendall that she could be more amorous toward him if she did not smell smoke on his breath and shirt and if she didn't have to worry that he would have a coronary sometime soon. At last, Kendall had a compelling reason to deal with the difficulties of nicotine withdrawal. He explained this development to me in session, stating wryly, "No offense, Doc, but Lanie can give me motivation to stop smoking in a way that none of your techniques can touch!" Kendall proceeded to contact his family physician, whereupon he commenced using a nicotine patch to curb his cravings while he quit smoking cold turkey. Ultimately, Kendall succeeded in becoming smoke free, a significant accomplishment that further increased his self-esteem.

After approximately a year in weekly therapy sessions, Kendall's mood scores on the three Beck inventories were much improved, being consistently in the "normal" range (e.g., below 8 on the depression and anxiety inventories and averaging less than 5 on the hopelessness scale). I offered my opinion that he was doing well enough that we could aim for one more goal—perhaps the biggest and most daunting—namely, it was high time that Kendall investigated what he had to do to finish up the bachelor's degree program he had fatefully abandoned more than 30 years earlier. This was the one remaining piece of unfinished business in Kendall's emotional life that he could still resolve, and his improved life situation and mood state seemed to indicate that he was ready. Kendall contacted the university and learned that he could still complete his degree by taking courses over the next two semesters. Whenever Kendall noticed that he was talking himself out of following through on this plan, he would create a mental image of his framed diploma. As a further incentive, Kendall's son remarked how it would be "so cool" if they graduated college at the same time, which would mean that they could "party twice as hearty."

Kendall tapered the frequency of his sessions with me. He continued to touch base just so we could make sure he was doing well, that his Beck inventory scores were still low, that he was still abstinent from smoking, and that depressive relapses were nowhere in sight. When Kendall received his college diploma, he proudly brought it to a session and announced that he was also going to graduate from therapy that day. We shared a back-slapping hug and a joyous laugh and said our goodbyes.

DISCUSSION

Kendall's recovery from depression (primarily) and anxiety (secondarily) was not just the result of cognitive therapy. There were many variables, including the salubrious effects of a meaningful romantic relationship with Lanie. However, cognitive therapy helped him notice the strengths and gifts he already possessed (his children, his artistic skills, his successes as an electrician) and helped him overcome his doubts about pursuing goals that would improve his lot further still (e.g., make his writings and artwork more public, take courses, meet new people, stop smoking, finish his bachelor's degree). Kendall learned to be his own best supporter, and in the process he was able to more fully and legitimately internalize the care and support of others in his life, including his kids, his supervisor at work, his new girlfriend, and yes even his sentimental therapist who shed a tear on saying goodbye on "graduation day."

Although Kendall's depressive syndrome was chronic—a condition that usually would make it more difficult to achieve success in treatment than if he had been experiencing acute depressive episodes—he had a number of personal strengths that helped him respond well to cognitive therapy. First, he was successful in the major life areas of work and child rearing, having been gainfully employed in the same profession for nearly 30 years and successfully raising two well-functioning adolescents as a single parent. Second, Kendall was intelligent and talented, although he did not appreciate these qualities until they were recognized and validated by a new peer group and by his therapist. Third, he was a genuinely friendly person who had the ability to bond with others. I never experienced a conflict with Kendall, and we always respected each other's opinions. He was very appreciative of and responsive to my interest in his poetry and artwork, and trusted me when I nudged him in the direction of activities that tested his resolve (e.g., submitting articles for publication, asking Lanie to go out with him for the first time, reapplying to college). Although Kendall was an appropriate candidate for a combined treatment of cognitive therapy and pharmacotherapy, he wound up responding favorably to cognitive therapy alone, and his therapeutic gains were maintained for the entire period of booster sessions that lasted over a year. Seeing Kendall change from a chronically depressed, lonely, self-deprecating, smoking individual to a happier, funnier, healthier (smoke-free), more confident man who had a new girlfriend and a college diploma was extremely rewarding for me. Accompanying people such as Kendall on their journey to a better life is a joyful reminder of the reasons I entered the profession of mental health care.

REFERENCES

Beck AT, Ward C, Mendelson M, et al: An inventory for measuring depression. Arch Gen Psychiatry 4:561–571, 1961

Beck AT, Weissman A, Lester D, et al: The measurement of pessimism: the hopelessness scale. J Consult Clin Psychol 42:861–865, 1974

Beck AT, Epstein N, Brown G, et al: An inventory for measuring clinical anxiety: psychometric properties. J Consult Clin Psychol 56: 893–897, 1988

Beck JS: Cognitive Therapy: Basics and Beyond. New York, Guilford Press, 1995

First MB, Spitzer RL, Williams JW, et al: The Structured Clinical Interview for DSM-IV-TR Axis I Disorders, Clinician Version (SCID-CV). Washington, DC, American Psychiatric Association, 2000

Gloaguen V, Cottraux J, Cucherat M, et al: A meta-analysis of the effects of cognitive therapy in depressed patients. J Affect Disord 49:59–72, 1998

Hollon SD, DeRubeis RJ, Evans MD: Cognitive therapy and pharmacotherapy for depression singly and in combination. Arch Gen Psychiatry 49:774–781, 1992

Lief HI: Bupropion treatment of depression to assist smoking cessation. Am J Psychiatry 153:442, 1996

Pampallona S, Bollini P, Tibalbi G, et al: Combined pharmacotherapy and psychological treatment for depression: a systematic review. Arch Gen Psychiatry 61:714–719, 2004

CHAPTER 17

An Actress With More Going on Than Meets the MRI

An Unusual Case of Bipolar Affective Disorder

Benjamin R. Nordstrom, M.D.
Philip R. Muskin, M.D.

Benjamin R. Nordstrom, M.D., is currently a Fellow in Addiction Psychiatry in the Division on Substance Abuse at the New York State Psychiatric Institute. Dr. Nordstrom received his medical degree from Dartmouth Medical School. He completed a residency in adult psychiatry at the New York State Psychiatric Institute/New York-Presbyterian Hospital–Columbia University Medical Center program where he served as Chief Resident.

Phillip R. Muskin, M.D., is the Chief of Consultation-Liaison Psychiatry at the Columbia University Medical Center of the New York-Presbyterian Hospital; Professor of Clinical Psychiatry at Columbia University College of Physicians and Surgeons; and a faculty member of the Columbia University Psychoanalytic Center for Training and Research. He received his medical degree from New York Medical College and completed his psychiatric residency at the New York State Psychiatric Institute.

Dr. Muskin's research and publications have examined mood disorders and AIDS, the psychodynamics of the failure of empathy toward AIDS patients, panic disorder, medical presentations of psychiatric disorders, treatment of anxiety and depression in medically ill patients, maladaptive denial of physical illness, personality disorders in the primary care setting, the role of religiosity in patients' decisions regarding do-not-resuscitate status, the psychodynamics of physician-assisted suicide, and the impact of intercessory prayer on medical outcomes.

Dr. Muskin was the editor of *Complementary and Alternative Medicine and Psychiatry* (2000). He was Past President of the Association for Academic Psychiatry and the Society for Liaison Psychiatry. He has been a member of the Scientific Program Committee of the American Psychiatric Association (APA) since 1990, serving as the Committee Chair for the 2001 and 2002 annual meetings. He is currently the head of the APA Council on Psychosomatic Medicine.

JEANETTE, A 23-YEAR-OLD, unemployed, Caucasion actress, was brought to the emergency room by her father who was seeking an explanation for her recent change in behavior. She described several weeks of experiencing a persistently euphoric mood, greatly increased productivity and energy, and a decreased need for sleep. She denied having racing thoughts, irritability, subjective pressure to keep talking, or impulsive behavior. Her mood and thinking had changed several weeks prior to the emergency department visit, after she read an evangelical Christian novel about the rapture and the "end times." Her concerns about the rapture turned into a preoccupation with the concept of rape, with preoccupations about being raped, "being horny," and child molestation. She was concerned that people thought she was "staring at their crotches" and concluding that she was "some kind of pervert." She endorsed some ideas of reference about people she passed on the street saying "rape" regarding her, but denied other delusions or hallucinations. She denied having used any drugs in the past month, but she reported a history of daily marijuana use and experimenting with lysergic acid diethylamide (LSD), psilocybin-containing mushrooms, and cocaine in college. She denied drinking alcohol. She also gave a vague history of having had her first mood disturbance, an episode of depression, during her first year of college.

On examination, Jeanette was a thin young woman with a close-cropped hairstyle and wire-rimmed glasses. She was gregarious, congenial, pleasant, and engaging and seemed delighted to have the opportunity to discuss her recent experiences. She displayed mild psychomotor agitation in that she repeatedly wrung her hands and took her glasses on and off. On a number of occasions, she appeared to be responding to internal stimuli in that she laughed inappropriately to herself and muttered under her breath, "Oh, for sure, dude." She was markedly distractible and craned her neck to try to locate the source of any trivial sounds that emanated from outside of the interview room. She described her mood as good; her affect was elated and expansive, and she remained giddy even when discussing topics she claimed were distressing to her. Her speech was fluent and pressured. Her thought processes were tangential with some flight of ideas. Her thought content was notable for paranoid ideation about being assaulted and for ideas of reference. She denied experiencing auditory or visual hallucinations and having any suicidal or homicidal ideation. She was oriented to person, place, and time and had no trouble with naming, repetition, and simple calculation tests. She struggled with serial sevens (i.e., counting backward from 100 by 7) and listed the months of the year in reverse with one error.

HISTORY

Jeanette's father, a polite and appropriately anxious man with a heavy Eastern European accent, provided an account of Jeanette's history. He reported a 2–3 month change in his daughter's "thinking." He said that her ideas did not "line up and make sense" and that she could "speak very fast when she was excited about something." He denied that she had had any prior psychiatric illness, but did note that she seemed depressed after a play in which she appeared ended its run some months ago. When asked about this, Jeanette said she was bothered by hearing other actors say critical things about her while onstage during performances. Her father, who attended every performance, was perplexed and said he never heard anything of the kind. Her father explained that the family's cultural background prohibits a free and open discourse about mental illness, and he reluctantly reported that Jeanette had a maternal aunt who had bipolar disorder.

DIAGNOSIS

The results of the laboratory studies, including an HIV test and a urine toxicology screen as well as comprehensive physical and neurological examinations, were unremarkable. The emergency department psychiatrist insisted that she undergo brain imaging because this was her first episode of psychosis. A computed axial tomographic scan, a computerized X ray that rapidly produces cross-sectional images with intermediate resolution, revealed large ventricles, suggesting that cerebrospinal fluid (CSF) flow out of the brain was obstructed. A magnetic resonance imaging scan, a more lengthy and complicated procedure that uses strong magnetic fields to produce more highly detailed cross-sectional images, showed a cystic mass on the left side of her posterior midbrain. This mass was pinching off the narrow aqueduct through which CSF flows out of the brain. Jeanette and her family denied that Jeanette showed any signs typical of hydrocephalus (cognitive blunting, psychomotor slowing, gait disturbance, or incontinence). She was admitted to the neurosurgery service where she underwent a ventriculotomy, a procedure in which the outflow tract is opened for CSF draining and sampling. The lesion was located too deep within the brain for a safe biopsy or excision.

Jeanette presented with several weeks of abnormally and persistently elevated mood, a decreased need for sleep, and an increase in goal-directed activity, distractibility, and flight of ideas. Her symptoms met DSM-IV-TR criteria for a manic episode. In light of her paranoid and referential delusions, her episode was severe, with psychotic features.

Jeanette also had a brain lesion, thought to be a cyst, which raised the question, Was this mood episode best understood as an episode of bipolar I disorder (bipolar II disorder was ruled out by the presence of frank mania with psychosis) or as being due to a general medical condition (hydrocephalus or midbrain mass)? In support of the former, Jeanette had a history, albeit vague, of one or two prior episodes of self-described depressions and had a family history of bipolarity. In support of the latter was the curious timing in the onset of her manic symptoms relative to the discovery of her hydrocephalus.

There is an extensive literature about ventricular enlargement (as was present in Jeanette's imaging studies) in bipolar disorder (Nsarallah et al. 1982; Pearlson et al. 1985; Rieder et al. 1983; Swaze et al. 1990). There have also been reports of hydrocephalus presenting with mania (Bhanji et al. 1983; Dewan and Bick 1985; Kwentus and Hart 1987; Max et al. 1995; Schneider et al. 1996; Thienhaus and Khosla 1984) and of brain lesions located in the general vicinity as Jeanette's, apparently provoking a bipolar-like syndrome (Benke et al. 2002; Kulisevsky et al. 1993; McGilchrist et al. 1993; Vuilleumier et al. 1998). Therefore, we considered the possibility that the lesion itself could be responsible for the manic-like symptoms.

A third possibility was that Jeanette's manic episode was substance induced. She had a history of heavy cannabis use as well as frequent use of other hallucinogens. However, her negative urine toxicology and the prolonged, persistent elevation in her mood state argued against this diagnosis. Some authors have put forth the controversial idea that bipolar patients frequently self-medicate with cannabis, so perhaps her use of this drug lent indirect support for a bipolar diathesis as the etiology of her mood disturbance (Grinspoon and Bakalar 1998).

Considering all of the above, our working diagnosis was as follows:

1. Bipolar I disorder, current episode manic, severe with psychotic features
2. Rule out mood disturbance, manic type, severe with psychotic features, due to a general medical condition (hydrocephalus or secondary to a lesion in the left tectum or thalamus)
3. Rule out substance-induced mood disorder, manic type
4. Cannabis abuse, rule out dependence
5. Hallucinogen abuse

Jeanette had no symptoms of hydrocephalus, suggesting to us that the mass and the resulting increase in CSF pressure must have been gradual. Her mood symptoms had been present for approximately a year, with an abrupt worsening. If the mania was due to the increase in intracerebral pressure, the mood symptoms would resolve after surgical decompression.

TREATMENT

Surgery restored the normal flow of Jeanette's CSF, as evidenced by normalization in the size of her ventricles and confirmed with subsequent brain imaging. There were no postoperative complications. Laboratory studies and cytology of her CSF failed to shed light on the etiology of the cystic lesion. The consensus of the neurologists and neurosurgeons on the case was that the structure was not indicative of parasitic disease or malignancy and that it was most likely slow growing and benign. They recommended serial radiographic monitoring of the structure.

While recovering from the surgery, Jeanette was followed by the consultation-liaison psychiatry service. During her first postoperative day, she reported that her manic symptoms were far less intense and declined the team's offer of psychopharmacological intervention. However, on the second postoperative day she became markedly manic. She consented to take clonazepam (a sedative) and aripiprazole (a second-generation antipsychotic medication) to control her mania. She was hypersexual, inattentive to the fact that she was not appropriately dressed, and pressured in her speech and lacked insight into the fact that she was psychotic. She was also engaging and funny. Our immediate concern related to her family members, who were reluctant to agree to an inpatient psychiatry transfer. Her father and brother were angry that the surgery had not resulted in either a diagnosis or a cure of her symptoms. We were sure that her mania would quickly respond to antipsychotics and mood stabilizers and were concerned her family would sign her out of the neurosurgery or psychiatry ward. Her transfer to the inpatient psychiatry ward for further treatment of her mania and psychosis was eventually arranged.

Our prediction of a rapid therapeutic response turned out to be in correct. On the inpatient psychiatry service, Jeanette remained persistently manic and hypersexual. She perseverated about "penises and nipples" as well as about the words "horny," "rape," and "child molestation." She eventually consented to the addition of divalproex sodium to her medication regimen, and later to the addition of lithium carbonate, both of which are mood stabilizers used to control the affective extremes of bipolar disorder. Clonazepam was discontinued after she complained of persistent sedation. When she failed to respond to the aripiprazole after 2 weeks she was cross-tapered with another second-generation antipsychotic, olanzapine. Blood tests revealed abnormalities of her liver function, which necessitated the discontinuation of both the divalproex sodium and the olanzapine. An expert psychopharmacology consultation was obtained, resulting in the addition of a first-generation antipsychotic (perphenazine) to the lithium carbonate. Her mood and psychotic symptoms slowly improved.

After 6 weeks of inpatient treatment, Jeanette was discharged to a day-treatment program. At a 4-month follow-up after her discharge from the hospital, she was manic and psychotic, although the intensity of her symptoms had diminished. Her family reported that she had been nonadherent with the follow-up plan and was not taking the prescribed medications. Follow-up information obtained 6 months later revealed that her hallucinations and paranoid ideation had stopped. She continued to take lithium and perphenazine; however, her mood remained somewhat elevated and she remained unable to return to work as an actress.

DISCUSSION

We learned several lessons from this case. The first lesson was to not ignore a brain lesion. The persistence of the symptoms in spite of aggressive treatment suggested that this was not bipolar I disorder, but that the brain lesion had a role in the psychosis. The second lesson was that when you have bad luck, you need good luck. This patient unfortunately had and has a serious psychiatric disorder; however, it was her psychotic symptoms that brought her to the attention of a physician. Although she did not have the typical presentation of a patient with hydrocephalus when we treated her, it was only a matter of time before those symptoms developed. She had the good fortune to be seen by an emergency department psychiatrist who pursued a thorough neurological evaluation. Finally, we learned that physicians should be cautious in what they promise to patients and families. The neurosurgeon was heard by the family as promising that the surgery would lead to a definitive diagnosis. This particular family, already suspicious of the medical system, felt betrayed when the surgery resulted in neither a diagnosis nor a change in Jeanette's symptoms. The family members' preexisting distrust was thus magnified, which made working with them more difficult. This situation could have been avoided by the surgeon who might have taken more time to convey the necessity for the surgery along with the possibility that it might not result in a definitive diagnosis.

We learned to be more humble in our predictions as well. Jeanette did not experience the type of benefit we expected from psychiatric treatment. Cautious optimism on our part might have aided her family in understanding the complexity of her medical disorder.

REFERENCES

Benke TH, Kurzthaler I, Schmidauer CH, et al: Mania caused by a diencephalic lesion. Neuropsychologia 40:245–252, 2002

Bhanji S, Gardner-Thorpe C, Rahavard F: Aqueduct stenosis and manic depressive psychosis. J Neurol Neurosurg Psychiatry 46:1158–1159, 1983

Dewan MJ, Bick PA: Normal pressure hydrocephalus and psychiatric patients. Biol Psychiatry 20:1127–1131, 1985

Grinspoon L, Bakalar JB: The use of cannabis as a mood stabilizer in bipolar disorder: anecdotal evidence and the need for clinical research. J J Psychoactive Drugs 30:171–177, 1998

Kulisevsky J, Berthier ML, Pujol J: Hemiballismus and secondary mania following a right thalamic infarct. Neurology 43:1422–1424, 1993

Kwentus JA, Hart RP: Normal pressure hydrocephalus presenting as mania. J Nerv Ment Dis 175:500–502, 1987

Max J, Richards L, Hamdan-Allen G: Case study: antimanic effectiveness of dextroamphetamine in a brain injured adolescent. J Am Acad Child Adolesc Psychiatry 34:472–476, 1995

McGilchrist I, Goldstein LH, Jadresic D, et al: Thalamo-frontal psychosis. Br J Psychiatry 163:113–115, 1993

Pearlson GD, Garbacz DJ, Moberg PJ, et al: Symptomatic, familial, perinatal, and social correlates of computerized axial tomography (CAT) changes in schizophrenics and bipolars. J Nerv Ment Dis 173:42–50, 1985

Rieder RO, Mann LS, Weinberger DR, et al: Computed tomographic scans in patients with schizophrenia, schizoaffective, and bipolar affective disorder. Arch Gen Psychiatry 40:735–739, 1983

Schneider U, Malmadier A, Dengler R, et al: Mood changes associated with normal pressure hydrocephalus. Am J Psychiatry 153:1366–1367, 1996

Swaze VW II, Andreasen NC, Alliger RJ, et al: Structural brain abnormalities in bipolar affective disorder: ventricular enlargement and focal signal hyperintensities. Arch Gen Psychiatry 47:1054–1059, 1990

Thienhaus OJ, Khosla N: Meningeal cryptococcosis misdiagnosed as a manic episode. Am J Psychiatry 141:1459–1460, 1984

Vuilleumier P, Ghika-Schmid R, Bogousslavsky J, et al: Persistent recurrence of hypomania and prosopoaffective agnosia in a patient with right thalamic infarct. Neuropsychiatry Neuropsychol Behav Neurol 11:40–44, 1998

CHAPTER 18

Mr. Opposite

Comprehensive Treatment of Childhood Bipolar Disorder

Kenneth Towbin, M.D.
Ellen Liebenluft, M.D.

Kenneth Towbin, M.D., is Chief of Clinical Child and Adolescent Psychiatry in the Mood and Anxiety Disorders Program in the Intramural Research Program of the National Institute of Mental Health. He is also Professor of Psychiatry and Behavioral Sciences and Pediatrics at the George Washington University School of Medicine. His research interests are in pediatric bipolar disorder, pediatric anxiety disorders, depression in children and adolescents, and pervasive developmental disorders. He also has published on the diagnosis and treatment of autism spectrum disorders, tics, and Tourette's disorder. Dr. Towbin is a Fellow of the American Academy of Child and Adolescent Psychiatry and is on the editorial board of the *Journal of the American Academy of Child and Adolescent Psychiatry*.

Ellen Leibenluft, M.D., is Chief of the Unit on Affective Disorders in the Pediatrics and Developmental Neuropsychiatry Branch, Mood and Anxiety Program, of the National Institute of Mental Health. Her main research interest is bipolar disorder in children and adolescents, with an emphasis on neural mechanisms underlying the illness. She has also conducted research on how to diagnose and conceptualize the psychiatric problems of children with very severe irritability. She has also authored publications on rapid cycling bipolar disorder (a severe form of the illness) in adults, the role of the sleep-wake cycle in bipolar disorder, and gender differences in mood disorders. She has authored approximately 100 professional publications and is a member of the editorial boards of *Biological Psychiatry, Bipolar Disorders,* and the *Journal of Child and Adolescent Psychopharmacology.*

Dr. Leibenluft is a member of the American College of Neuropsychopharmacology, Child and Adolescent Bipolar Foundation Professional Advisory Board, the Scientific Council of the National Alliance for the Mentally Ill, and the Program Committee of the American Academy of Child and Adolescent Psychiatry. She is Co-Chair of the DSM/ICD Conference Steering Committee on Externalizing Disorders of Childhood of the American Psychiatric Institute for Research and Education. Her awards include the Distinguished Psychiatrist Award of the APA, special service awards from the National Institutes of Health, the National Institute of Health's Director's Award for Mentoring, and the Virginia Tarlow Memorial Lectureship at Northwestern University.

FRANK WAS A 12-YEAR-OLD boy with dark eyes that fixed on you forcefully when he spoke. You could tell from the outset that he meant business. "I'm here for the study to help understand kids with bipolar disorder," he announced when I asked him what he knew about why he had come into the hospital. "I want to feel better and, if it helps, I want other kids to feel better, too." It was a forward remark that said a lot about Frank. I was struck that his knowledge and communication skills were advanced for his age. It is not what I expected given his history. Things had not been easy for Frank; his resilience was but one remarkable feature of his life.

HISTORY

Our research group was contacted by Frank's mother after she learned about our studies from a parent support group Web site. Frank's difficulties were always apparent to his mother, particularly his difficulty calming himself and controlling his anger. His first psychiatric evaluation, prompted by severe outbursts, aggression, and intense temper tantrums, occurred when he was just age 4. Although the referral was for Frank, his mother recognized that Frank's behaviors mirrored the aggression and marital tension at home. Frank frequently witnessed his father's physical abuse of his mother and younger brother, although Frank himself was not a target of his father's cruelty.

Over the next 4 years Frank continued to have verbal outbursts, destroyed his toys and furniture when angry, and refused to comply with rules at home. His parents' separation and subsequent divorce when Frank was age 6 did not moderate his behavior. Frank then entered psychotherapy for his outbursts and aggression, and his mother noted improvements in his academic performance and peer relations during kindergarten and first grade.

Over the next year Frank had regular visits with his father, but there were always arguments and tensions surrounding the visits—both Frank and his brother often asked not to go but were required to go under the custody agreement. Later it was learned that Frank frequently witnessed his brother's physical abuse during the visits. Finally, there was a visit after which Frank's father refused to return the boys. Their father forced them to stay with him while he eluded authorities; Frank and his brother were recovered 3 months later.

When Frank was age 7, he was evaluated by another psychiatrist and diagnosed with oppositional defiant disorder, attention-deficit/hyperactivity disorder (ADHD), and posttraumatic stress disorder. He was not prescribed medication because his mother was concerned about the dangers it might pose. He returned to psychotherapy and his behavior improved once again, but more in school than with peers or at home.

The pattern shifted markedly the following year. Frank began having aggressive outbursts at school and was quite sad. There appeared to be no precipitant for these feelings or outbursts. He was prescribed and began taking sertraline (an antidepressant) and methylphenidate (a stimulant used in the treatment of ADHD). He later voiced suicidal ideation, saying he "hated his life" and thought about "killing myself if it is going to be like this." He complained that the medication made him tired all the time. After 9 months, all medication was stopped and Frank's mood appeared to improve. He was given a long-acting form of methylphenidate (Concerta) for the next 9 months, although whether or not it was helpful was in doubt. His mother finally stopped it and Frank had stopped taking all medication by the time he was age 10. Around this time, Frank's mother remarried. Frank got along well with his stepfather and their relationship grew into a mutually close one.

The family moved to a new state, where Frank had to establish a new peer group and attend a new school. The adjustment proved to be difficult for him; after 6 weeks, the police called saying that Frank had been in a fight at school and was disrespectful to an officer who had been called to assist. There were other fights at school, which Frank claimed were all in self-defense. He complained that his classmates teased him about his behavior and appearance. His irritable outbursts returned at home too. Frank was home schooled after being put out of school for fighting and for outrageous, provocative, oppositional behavior.

In the late spring of 6th grade, when he was age 11, there was a 2-week episode during which Frank's mood and behavior were obviously uncharacteristic. He was extremely happy, was quite excited by "everything," and had "thousands of ideas of things to do." Frank was usually self-effacing, but during this time he boasted about how brilliant, talented, and creative he was. His attitude change even led to a fistfight when his younger brother challenged Frank's boasting. Frank was impossible to converse with because he could not be interrupted long enough to have an exchange, and he talked "really fast." He tried to construct a scooter of his own design that "would go 50 miles an hour," and he searched for the right motor. He slept 4 hours a night or less, otherwise wandering the house or cleaning his room. He engaged in uncharacteristic activities, such as dismantling his stereo, the family's computers, and the VCR. He was much more distracted than usual and could not stay with anything long enough to complete it. He talked back to his mother constantly. He decided he was going to remodel the house by himself. One day during this period, he was reported to the police for holding on to passing cars while riding his bike, something he did for "thrills." He had a short fuse and was quite irritable; he seemed much worse than his typical grouchy, overreactive demeanor. On one occassion, his parents discovered he had climbed out his bedroom window onto the roof, where he was sweeping with a broom and running a hose "to get it cleaned off." Because his parents feared for his safety, he was hospitalized. During that hospitalization he was treated with dextroamphetamine (a different type of stimulant) for his ADHD symptoms and he became much more irritable. During this first hospitalization, bipolar disorder was added to his diagnosis.

Frank was rehospitalized with depression 2 months later. For several weeks his attitude had been lackluster, he had no interest in being with friends or riding his bike, he had increased his eating and weight, and his movements were so slowed that he could barely function. Frank also expressed feelings of helplessness, hopelessness, and worthlessness, and he felt guilty about minor everyday events. He voiced suicidal ideation, wrote a suicide note, and subsequently attempted to exit a moving car. He was rehospitalized days after he was found playing with a loaded handgun. In the hospital, he was withdrawn from dextroamphetamine and was given citalopram (an antidepressant) 20 mg/day. A few weeks later, olanzapine (an antipsychotic medication also used to treat mania) was added and later oxcarbazepine, an anticonvulsant used as a mood stabilizer, was added at a dosage of up to 600 mg/day.

On the combination of citalopram, olanzapine, and oxcarbazepine, Frank continued to experience depressive symptoms and suicidal ideation. Citalopram was stopped after 2 months. Eventually Frank was given a new atypical antipsychotic medication, aripiprazole, and a relatively new anticonvulsant, zonisamide, which it was hoped would work as a mood stabilizer; he continued the oxcarbazepine at this time.

In school, Frank had become such a problem in class and with his peers that the school authorities requested that he be removed from the school. He was placed on homebound education and, for several months prior to his hospitalization at our research facility, his mother home-schooled him for want of an appropriate educational program. Frank was fearful of attending school because of his aggression and because he could not tolerate his classmates' teasing and rebuffs.

DIAGNOSIS

Frank was brought to our research facility for evaluation. On admission his affect was flat, but he was conversant, personable, articulate, and highly cooperative. His mother was an excellent source of information and an astute observer. Based on a diagnostic assessment using a research interview, Frank was noted to have current (i.e., within the last 6 months) mania (bipolar I disorder, remitted), major depressive disorder (currently in partial remission), ADHD (predominantly inattentive type, current, ongoing), and oppositional defiant disorder (current, ongoing). He also had lifetime diagnoses of posttraumatic stress disorder and social phobia (social anxiety disorder).

One of our research studies in pediatric bipolar disorder allows us to hospitalize children with the disorder, taper their medication, and then restart treatment after roughly 2 weeks of the patient being medication free. Frank seemed an appropriate candidate for this study insofar as he was not doing well on his current regimen but was not so impaired or dangerous that a medication-free period was contraindicated. From a clinical standpoint, we believed that Frank's current medications were not optimal because he continued to have significant problems at home and school and his mood disorder was only partially remitted. His psychiatrist did not feel that it was safe to reduce Frank's medications as an outpatient and there were no inpatient resources that would allow admission for this purpose unless a patient was dangerous to himself or others.

TREATMENT

Frank and his mother accepted our invitation to enter the inpatient study. Frank's mental status examination at the time of admission revealed a mildly overweight boy who displayed blunted affect and sad mood. He was hypoactive and had moderate psychomotor retardation. He was intelligent and had no impairment in memory, language, insight, or judgment. He showed no symptoms of psychosis or suicidal ideation nor was he clinically depressed. On the first day of the study, he was appropriately anxious, and as the first hospital days unfolded, he was noted to be socially reluctant, somewhat given to isolation, and sad in appearance. He was occasionally irritable but not to the point of displaying aggressive behavior. He could be cheerful for short periods, especially in the gymnasium, but cheerfulness was not sustained. On occasion he would threaten staff. Although he was sometimes irritable for approximately 30 minutes at a time, he became aggressive on only two occasions, usually in response to limits being set or needing to complete school assignments.

As the hospitalization continued, Frank readily engaged staff and patients; he was hungry for social interaction. He was polite and thoughtful and showed a precocious ability to understand others and to anticipate how they might feel. At school, he was slow in completing his work and in picking up on new facts or concepts. The combination of sedation, psychomotor retardation, and inattention had conspired to interfere with his learning and progress.

Our clinical impression was that most of Frank's impairment resulted from his mood disorder and ADHD, and our primary therapeutic targets were Frank's aggressive outbursts, threatening behavior, irritability, and low mood. In addition, we noted Frank had attentional symptoms and learning problems that needed to be addressed pharmacologically and educationally. We wanted to ensure that Frank's medication regimen would treat his current mood disorder effectively while also providing prophylaxis against future episodes but with minimal side effects. Finally, we were concerned about the long-term effects on Frank's self-concept of being diagnosed with bipolar disorder and of his difficulties with family and peers.

Prior to his admission into our study, Frank was having explosive outbursts nearly every day, including attacking others, and he constantly displayed threatening behavior. We did not observe as much aggressive behavior at our center as was reported prior to Frank's admission. Having the consistent presence of nursing staff members and our giving him space and not pressing him to comply immediately with program requirements appeared to help him control his outbursts. The nursing staff taught Frank techniques that he could use to calm himself and helped him practice them when needed. Frank was able to talk about how frightened he was when he became very angry, and gradually the frequency of his angry episodes diminished.

An important question was whether Frank's irritability, blunted affect, and restlessness might be associated with his aripiprazole treatment. Our research protocol called for stopping all medication. However, even if the protocol had not required this, a dosage decrease would have been clinically indicated to ascertain the role of medication side effects in Frank's clinical presentation. As the aripiprazole was tapered and stopped, Frank's outbursts declined and his irritability diminished. By the time he was completely off aripiprazole he was emotionally responsive and had more cheerful periods; his outbursts had ended, although he was still somewhat irritable.

When the medication-free period ended, we faced a decision about what prophylactic treatment would be best for Frank. We did not see mania or hypomania during Frank's hospitalization. Based on his history, his response to oxcarbazepine, the only mood stabilizer he had received since his first episode of mania, was inadequate. He also had gained a substantial amount of weight on olanzapine and his affect was dulled by aripiprazole. We considered atypical neuroleptics, lithium, and divalproex sodium, all of which were potentially effective as mood stabilizers. We chose to prescribe lithium carbonate and gradually increased it to a dosage that achieved a stable blood level of 0.9 mg/L. Frank had no ill effects at this dosage.

Even while on lithium, Frank's problems with inattention and distractibility were a barrier to his schoolwork; he was impulsive, unfocused, and forgetful. Stimulants are usually appropriate for treating these symptoms, although caution must be used when treating a bipolar child with stimulants (typically, the stimulant should be cautiously added after therapeutic levels of a mood stabilizer have been reached). Frank's mother recalled how irritable he had become on methylphenidate and the significant insomnia he had developed when taking the long-acting stimulant form (Concerta). She was concerned that adding a stimulant to Frank's regimen would precipitate his mania, and she had read information on Web sites that counseled against using these medications in children with bipolar disorder. We noted how compromised Frank was by his inattention and distractibility and reassured Frank's mother that he would be watched closely. We then added 5 mg of methylphenidate for Frank to take every morning with his lithium regimen. This low dose was surprisingly effective in improving his attention and concentration at school in the mornings. Given these positive results, we added a second 5-mg dose to be taken at noon. Frank was then able to focus on his work throughout the morning and afternoon and completed assignments with relative ease. He was very proud of his ability to complete his schoolwork. In afternoon non–school-related activities, he was calm and better able to enjoy his leisure time. He also was better able to refrain from becoming angry or frustrated in activities with other patients. This form of methylphenidate did not produce insomnia and we did not see any adverse changes in his mood.

Frank frequently said he felt like a failure. His ADHD symptoms made it impossible for him to function in the classroom and confirmed for him his distorted sense of himself as "retarded" and "stupid." He saw himself as damaged and hopeless. When he made errors or did not perform up to his high standards, he experienced intense, short-lived bursts of anger and refused to participate in the unit program. Sometimes encouraging him only led him to threaten violence. He was eventually able to review these events and was apologetic about his actions once he had cooled down.

In developmental terms, we recognized that Frank's onset of mania in early adolescence was particularly burdensome. The capacity for self-control and increasing competence that are so central to successful adolescent development were threatened by his biological illness. For Frank, the anxiety during his outbursts was related to the fear that at any time he could become as disinhibited and helpless as when he was manic. He doubted his ability to control his behavior to the point where he would not end up in the hospital and apart from his family again.

Drawing on his good intellect and ability to self-reflect, we took a psychoeducational approach with Frank. Unit staff taught him about bipolar disorder and helped him understand his different mood states, how they began for him, and what he could do to help himself control his reactions. We also helped Frank see that he could regain control over his behavior by attending closely to his rising frustration and working with us or other adults in his life. We encouraged him to practice calming strategies and to talk with staff members when he was agitated. When these techniques worked, he felt success and his fear of losing control diminished.

Late in his 9-week hospital stay, Frank decided it was fun now and then to have "opposite day." On an opposite day, Frank would begin morning rounds with a broad smile and a piercing look, saying something like, "I just hate it here. Yesterday, I had a terrible time going out to the movies." He would break into laughter when the response was something akin to, "Well, it makes me so miserable to hear that, Frank."

As his discharge neared, we reported to his school how skilled and able Frank now was. We acknowledged that some accommodations for his problems with attention and distractibility might be needed, but noted that he was performing all of his grade-level schoolwork without difficulty and was eager to return to school with his peers. He continued to worry what the other students would do and say, but we pointed out that he had been a wonderful friend to other patients on our unit and that he had a winning personality that he could now show to others.

On his last day (not surprisingly, an opposite day), I informed Frank that I dreaded having to see him on his return, in about 6 months, for our longitudinal study. He told me, "I hated it here and hope never to return."

DISCUSSION

The field of child psychiatry has moved from considering bipolar disorder as a condition that does not arise in children to the modern view as a disorder that creates significant impairment for roughly 1% of children and adolescents (Costello et al. 1996). As of yet, there is no consensus on how the term is applied to children and adolescents, and the application of the DSM-IV-TR criteria can vary widely between clinicians (Leibenluft et al. 2003; National Institute of Mental Health Roundtable 2001). Consequently, any discussion of prevalence, features, prognosis, and treatment must be considered in light of how the diagnostic criteria are being applied.

This case history for mania based on the episode in the Spring of 6th grade illustrates many distinguishing features of what has been termed *narrow phenotype bipolar disorder* (Leibenluft et al. 2003). The hallmarks of narrow phenotype bipolar disorder are at least one discrete episode of mania that is consonant with strict DSM-IV-TR criteria and includes elevated mood and/or grandiosity. Other cardinal features that are particularly congruent with classic mania, such as a decreased need for sleep, increased goal directed activity, and elevated self-esteem, are also portrayed in Frank's history. The presence of comorbid ADHD is common in children diagnosed with bipolar disorder and can complicate making the diagnosis (Beiderman et al. 1998). Symptoms of distractibility, talkativeness, restlessness, impulsivity, and irritability are common in ADHD and during episodes of mania (Beiderman et al. 1998; Reich et al. 2005). Frank's history underscores how these comorbid symptoms can become much worse during periods of mania. A careful diagnostic approach takes information from the child and parent and considers carefully the concept of a manic episode as distinctly different from the child's usual baseline mood and function. Such a careful approach toward the identification of a distinct episode is essential when the child's baseline is characterized by ADHD and chronic irritability. During that episode, the appearance of cardinal features for duration for at least 4 days is highly suggestive of a disorder that goes on to display the classic features of bipolar disorder in adulthood.

Another point illustrated by this case history is the pivotal role of treating current symptoms and impairment using multiple modalities. This bright young man was able to benefit from psychoeducational and cognitive techniques. We also noted that, once a mood stabilizer had been started, providing stimulant medication for ADHD symptoms was important in order for him to attend to these ideas and use them. The use of agents with known efficacy for his comorbid ADHD and bipolar disorder proved crucial to his overall improvement psychologically, socially, and academically. This improvement was reflected in his increasing competence, control, and self-esteem.

REFERENCES

Biederman J, Klein RG, Pine DS, et al: Resolved: mania is mistaken for ADHD in prepubertal children. J Am Acad Child Adolesc Psychiatry 37(10):1091–1099, 1998

Costello EJ, Angold A, Burns BJ, et al: The Great Smoky Mountains study of youth. Goals, design, methods, and the prevalence of DSM-III-R disorders. Arch Gen Psychiatry 53(12):1129–1136, 1996

Leibenluft E, Charney DS, Towbin KE, et al: Defining clinical phenotypes of juvenile bipolar disorder. Am J Psychiatry 160:430–437, 2003

National Institute of Mental Health research roundtable on prepubertal bipolar disorder. J Am Acad Child Adolesc Psychiatry 40:871–878, 2001

Reich W, Neuman RJ, Volk HE, et al: Comorbidity between ADHD and symptoms of bipolar disorder in a community sample of children and adolescents. Twin Res Hum Genet 8(5):459–466, 2005

SUGGESTED READING

Bhangoo RK, Lowe CH, Myers FS, et al: Medication use in children and adolescents with bipolar disorder. J Child Adolesc Psychopharmacol 13:515–522, 2003

Carlson GA: Mania and ADHD: comorbidity or confusion. J Affect Disord 51:177–187, 1988

Dickstein DP, Treland JE, Snow J, et al: Neuropsychological performance in pediatric bipolar disorder. Biol Psychiatry 55:32–39, 2004

Kowatch RA, Youngstrom EA, Danielyan A, et al: Review and meta-analysis of the phenomenology and clinical characteristics of mania in children and adolescents. Bipolar Disord 7(6):483–496, 2005

Leibenluft E, Blair RJ, Charney DS, et al: Irritability in pediatric mania and other childhood psychopathology. Ann N Y Acad Sci 1008:201–218, 2003

Scheffer RE, Kowatch RA, Carmody T, et al: Randomized, placebo-controlled trial of mixed amphetamine salts for symptoms of comorbid ADHD in pediatric bipolar disorder after mood stabilization with divalproex sodium. Am J Psychiatry 162:58–64, 2005

PART VII

Anxiety Disorders

CHAPTER 19

Moving From Trauma to Triumph

Posttraumatic Stress Disorder With Chronic Pain and Alcohol Use

Sheila A. M. Rauch, Ph.D.
Edna B. Foa, Ph.D.

Sheila A. M. Rauch, Ph.D., is a psychologist in the VA Ann Arbor Health Care System and Assistant Professor in the Trauma, Stress, and Anxiety Research Group in the Department of Psychiatry at the University of Michigan Medical School. She received her doctorate in clinical psychology from the University of North Dakota in 2000 and joined the Center for the Treatment Study of Anxiety at the University of Pennsylvania upon completion of her clinical internship in the Department of Clinical and Health Psychology, University of Florida Health Science Center. Dr. Rauch has published scholarly articles and book chapters in the areas of sexual aggression and posttraumatic stress disorder (PTSD) focusing on factors involved in the development and maintenance of PTSD, psychosocial factors in medical settings, and the relation between physical health and anxiety. She has coordinated several research grants, including the development of a bibliotherapy program for anxiety disorders in primary care settings, a study of paroxetine for children with PTSD, and a treatment study for adults with PTSD. She served as coinvestigator in a National Institutes of Health study examining the use of benzodiazepines in older adults in primary care and in an Advanced Center for Intervention and Services Research study focusing on developing, evaluating, and disseminating interventions for depression and related disorders for older adults in medical settings.

Edna B. Foa, Ph.D., is Professor of Clinical Psychology in Psychiatry at the University of Pennsylvania and Director of the Center for the Treatment and Study of Anxiety. She is an internationally renowned authority on the psychopathology and treatment of anxiety. Her research into delineating etiologic frameworks and targeted treatment has been highly influential. Dr. Foa has received numerous grants from the National Institute of Mental Health for the study of posttraumatic stress disorder (PTSD) and other anxiety disorders. Dr. Foa co-chaired the DSM-IV subcommittee on PTSD, coordinated the Consensus Guidelines Initiative on the Treatment of PTSD, and chaired the Task Force for Treatment Guidelines of PTSD of the International Society for Traumatic Stress Studies. The program she has developed for rape victims is considered to be the most effective therapy for posttrauma sequelae. She has published several books and over 200 articles and book chapters and has lectured extensively around the world.

Dr. Foa is the recipient of numerous awards and honors, including the Distinguished Scientist Award from the scientific section of the American Psychological Association, the First Annual Outstanding Research Contribution Award from the Association for the Advancement of Behavior Therapy, the Distinguished Scientific Contributions to Clinical Psychology Award from the American Psychological Association, and the Lifetime Achievement Award from the International Society for Traumatic Stress Studies.

MARILYN, A 35-YEAR-OLD Caucasion woman, sought therapy because she was depressed 2 years after being hit by a bus. She reported that she had become steadily worse in every way since the accident. Her husband's recent move out of the house because he could not relate to her anymore prompted her to seek help.

HISTORY

During the psychiatric evaluation, Marilyn reported a past history of a depressive episode after being date raped at age 17. At that time she did not seek help and things gradually improved over about a 1-year period. She did seek help shortly after the bus accident 2 years earlier and at that time was given a selective serotonin reuptake inhibitor antidepressant. She felt that this made her sleep problems worse, so she discarded the medication after 4 days and did not seek additional mental health care. When asked to briefly describe what had happened during the accident, Marilyn angrily stated that a bus hit her while she was crossing the street with the light at a crosswalk. She felt that her life just kept getting worse after the accident, and she attributed everything bad in her life to the accident, stating that she would never be the same again.

The injuries to Marilyn's back and legs caused her chronic severe pain. Shortly after the accident, Marilyn attempted to go on a long distance hike with her husband but had to have the ranger pick her up due to her knee pain. She said that the incident was quite embarrassing and marked the point when she lost hope of ever being happy again.

Marilyn often focused on her pain during the interview and needed to be prompted to move on to focus on her other difficulties. She had refused to take pain medication due to the impact the medication had on her thinking and her dislike of taking medications. Although her medical doctor had encouraged her to become involved in light physical activity, she had not followed through with physical therapy and avoided any activity where someone might see her limp. She reported that she had severely restricted her activities since the accident. She no longer went into the city, walked as little as possible, and generally avoided people. Marilyn was fired from her job as a realtor due to her avoidance of the city and angry outbursts at work. At the time of the intake, she had been unemployed for 6 months. She was embarrassed by her disability and felt that her friends no longer valued her because of it. Marilyn stated that she had only one friend, and even this friend was "getting on her nerves."

Marilyn's relationship with her husband began souring after the accident. Although he tried to be supportive at first, he eventually began started suggesting that she quit feeling sorry for herself. He moved out of the house 1 month before Marilyn sought help. He acted as though her pain was not real and that she should be able to just move on as though nothing had happened. On top of this, she was no longer interested in sex. With all of this friction in her marriage, Marilyn felt that she no longer cared if her marriage ended.

Marilyn complained of poor sleep. On further questioning, she reported that despite being extremely tired, she rarely slept more than 4 hours at night; she described having difficulty falling asleep as well as waking up early in the morning and being unable to get back to sleep. Her early morning waking was usually triggered by vivid nightmares in which she was trapped under a bus. She started drinking wine about a year ago to help her fall asleep and typically drank three glasses of wine each night. She had never tried to cut down, but her husband had hinted that her drinking was a problem and they often argued when she drank.

DIAGNOSIS

Marilyn's presentation of nightmares and physical and emotional reactions to reminders of the accident, avoidance of activities and things that reminded her of the accident, her feelings that no one could relate to her, her problems sleeping, and her hypervigilance were consistent with a diagnosis of chronic posttraumatic stress disorder (PTSD). Her score on an interview measure (Posttraumatic Symptoms Scale Interview; Foa et al. 1993) suggested that her symptoms were severe. She also met diagnostic criteria for having a current major depressive episode and pain disorder associated with both psychological factors and a general medical condition.

TREATMENT

Reasons for Choice of Therapy

During the evaluation, Marilyn felt that the symptoms of PTSD were the most intrusive in her life at the present time, although she also saw her pain as a significant problem in need of immediate attention. We discussed how her depression and alcohol use seemed to have been a reaction to the posttraumatic stress symptoms and her chronic pain.

Prolonged exposure (PE) therapy was chosen to address Marilyn's PTSD because PE therapy has been demonstrated to be effective for PTSD (Rothbaum et al. 2000). Indeed, PE therapy has demonstrated reductions in PTSD symptom severity as well as in the associated depression and anger (Cahill et al. 2003; Foa et al. 1999). PE therapy consists of psychoeducation about common reactions to trauma, breathing retraining (i.e., an exercise to help slow down breathing), in vivo exposure to feared and avoided situations, and imaginal exposure to the trauma memory (Foa and Rothbaum 1998). Given that Marilyn's depression had developed after the trauma and that depression is often reduced with PE therapy, we determined that we would monitor her depression and reexamine it at the end of PE therapy to determine whether therapy that focused on the depression was warranted.

Given the high rate of comorbidity of chronic pain and PTSD, it has been postulated that there is a common etiology for both conditions; further, and more important for treatment, a mutual maintenance model of chronic pain and PTSD has been developed that indicates the symptoms of each disorder exacerbate and maintain the symptoms of the other (Asmundson et al. 2002; Sharp and Harvey 2001). As an example, when Marilyn experienced pain while walking up steps, it reinforced her feeling that she could not do anything because of the pain and increased her anxiety about being vulnerable and unable to handle crisis situations because she was "damaged goods." Asmundson et al. (2002) have suggested that effective treatment of each condition may require modification of cognitive-behavioral therapy protocols to address the other disorder. For example, when developing an in vivo exposure hierarchy of avoided situations, the therapist must consider how chronic pain may interfere with what the patient can and cannot do and appropriately construct the exposure episodes. In addition, adding items to the hierarchy that encourage activity pacing (gradual reengagement in desired activities without overexertion) can help survivors feel the triumph of finding out they can do something that is important to them. For example, having Marilyn walk up stairs in a gradual manner (i.e., one flight one day, two flights the next day, and so on) could help reduce her hypervigilance as she saw that she could function and help ameliorate her chronic pain as she saw that she could still do things that were important.

With regard to alcohol use, Marilyn did not believe her drinking was a problem and agreed to reduce the number of drinks by one drink per night. She did not have abstinence as her goal but did think that she was relying on alcohol too much to help her sleep. She was not interested in addressing the alcohol use in therapy but was willing to monitor it while she was in therapy. Although I would have preferred to discuss the alcohol misuse in sessions, Marilyn was so adamantly against this that pursuing the issue any further was likely to drive Marilyn entirely away from therapy.

We planned to follow the 10- to 12-session protocol of PE therapy (Foa and Rothbaum 1998) and then broaden our focus to address chronic pain (Philips and Rachman 1996) and depression for an additional 5 sessions. Marilyn agreed with this plan and was optimistic that things might begin to improve.

Treatment Goals and Progression

Our treatment goals were 1) reduction of posttraumatic stress symptoms, 2) reduction of depressive symptoms, and 3) decreased pain perception.

As per the PE protocol, the first two sessions were largely focused on psychoeducation about PTSD, an overview of PE therapy, and the rationale for PE therapy. These sessions provided the groundwork for Marilyn to begin to understand 1) how PTSD develops and is maintained, 2) that having PTSD symptoms did not mean she was crazy, and 3) that she could do things to reduce her PTSD symptoms.

During these sessions, three specific issues had particular relevance for Marilyn. First, avoidance seemed to have overtaken her life, having led to her losing her job, her friends, and her confidence. Furthermore, interwoven with the standard protocol for PE therapy, we discussed how her pain served as a reminder of the trauma and thus became a motivator for avoidance (Foa and Rothbaum 1998). Marilyn was visibly anxious when we discussed confronting her feared situations and activities with in vivo exposure. She stated that the idea of confronting her fears was scary, but she also understood that doing so made sense. During session two, we constructed her in vivo hierarchy and included items that she avoided due to fear of the trauma as well as fear of pain. The hierarchy was constructed to included those activities, people, and/or situations that Marilyn avoided. She then ranked them by rating how difficult she believed each activity would be.

The second issue of special importance to Marilyn was the focus on challenging unhelpful thoughts and beliefs. Since the accident, Marilyn had felt completely worthless and incompetent. These thoughts contributed to her depression, PTSD symptoms, and alcohol use. Challenging these thoughts would be key to Marilyn's making progress. One step toward her confronting these unhelpful thoughts was her pursuing the items on her hierarchy. As she completed the items, Marilyn found over and over again that she could do what was important to her and that for the most part other people did not even detect her disability. Thus these exercises provided extensive data to Marilyn that contradicted these unhelpful thoughts. In addition, we discussed some of these thoughts during session, including gathering evidence for and against the unhelpful thoughts, evaluating the evidence, and coming up with alternative thoughts.

The third issue of particular relevance to Marilyn was how her hyperarousal and depressive symptoms might be actually contributing to increases in her pain. For example, consistent with the hypervigilance seen with PTSD, Marilyn was in a constant state of muscle tension. This tension in her back pulled on the area where the injury occurred and made the pain more severe. The PE therapy model and the explanation of how her depression, PTSD, and pain interacted truly resonated with her. Marilyn was optimistic about therapy and said she was glad she had finally come for help.

After this initial psychoeducation phase of the treatment, I was optimistic about PE therapy with Marilyn. Marilyn completed eight sessions of imaginal exposure to the memory of the accident. In her first imaginal exposure session, Marilyn reported feeling strongly connected to the trauma image and expressed a lot of anger toward herself and others (the driver of the bus, the police at the accident site, the doctors at the hospital, etc.). In the second imaginal exposure, she focused on her anger and sobbed through much of the exposure. During the processing of her thoughts and emotions in these sessions, we discussed and validated her anger and her loss (loss of functioning due to pain, loss of her relationship with her husband and friends, etc.) and her wish that this had not happened. We then discussed how holding on to the anger and hurt over the loss kept her stuck in the accident and how letting go of the anger and accepting and grieving her loss so that she could move on and accept herself as she was might actually be more helpful. Although this sounds like a straightforward process, as with most cognitive challenges of long-held beliefs, the discussion was difficult for Marilyn and me. As the therapist, I was required to remain flexible and yet diligent in asserting the cost of anger. However, as the discussion continued, she began to truly consider alternatives to holding on to the anger.

Then, prior to the third imaginal exposure session, I asked Marilyn to let the anger and sadness be there but to focus on the fear and anxiety she had experienced at the time of the accident. Marilyn reported experiencing a lower anxiety level during that imaginal exposure. During the week between the third and fourth imaginal exposures, she said that she felt that a weight had been lifted from her shoulders. Not having to carry the anger and sadness made sense to her and she felt happy again for the first time since the accident.

In conjunction with the process of accepting her loss, Marilyn and I began to discuss ways to help her accept her injuries and do the things that were most important to her (gardening, moderate exercise, yoga) as well as finding new interests (photography, taking a class) to fill the gap that was left by activities that were no longer feasible (competitive ballroom dancing, long-distance hiking). This fit well with the in vivo exposures because Marilyn had been avoiding many activities due to her fear of pain and fear that others would discover her disability. An important component of this therapy focus was activity pacing (Philips and Rachman 1996). This entailed helping Marilyn to slowly begin each new activity so that she could evaluate its impact on her pain and work toward her goal of doing the things that were most important to her. In addition, Marilyn began physical therapy. Seeing Marilyn's progress and her return to positive activities as well as her increased confidence was quite rewarding.

Marilyn had several "hot spots" or parts of the trauma memory that continued to elicit significant anxiety after the early imaginal exposure sessions (Foa and Rothbaum 1998). As with many PTSD patients, one hot spot focused on the moment when Marilyn realized that she might be killed. A second hot spot occurred in the emergency room when her knees were being examined and she knew that they would never be the same again. Per the PE protocol, we focused on each of these hot spots in the imaginal exposure session. During the hot spot exposure, I asked Marilyn to slow down these brief moments and tell me everything that she could about just those specific moments (e.g., her thoughts and feelings and the things that she did). We then repeated just the hot spot for the remainder of the imaginal exposure until it was worn out and she reported experiencing very low anxiety.

After eight sessions of imaginal exposure, Marilyn reported having very little anxiety related to the memory. She felt like she was finally over the traumatic experience. She could talk about it and she had accepted its impact on her life while still grieving her loss. I pointed out that even though the accident negatively impacted her life, she could adjust and do those things that were important to her (having a family, being active, being artistic).

The focus of therapy then shifted to in vivo exposures. Marilyn's fear of others' perceptions about her disability had made it difficult for her to follow through on many of her in vivo homework assignments. Her noncompliance with homework was frustrating to me and stalled

Marilyn's progress in therapy. Thus I challenged her specific fears (e.g., that others would think she was faking her symptoms for sympathy or that she was lazy) by examining the likelihood, costs, and consequences of her fears as well as through in-session in vivo exercises. Marilyn and I also discussed the importance her being able to do these things had in her efforts to take back her life. As her specific fears were addressed, Marilyn began to follow through on her in vivo assignments and began to fell more confident.

As a last issue of importance to Marilyn, we focused on her decision to try to repair her relationship with her husband. Marilyn was unsure about whether she wanted to try to work on her marriage, so together we used problem-solving techniques to evaluate what she wanted to do.

In total, Marilyn completed 15 sessions over 24 weeks: 10 PE therapy sessions and 5 sessions focused on continued in vivo exposures, activity pacing, acceptance of disability, and relationship issues. Throughout therapy, Marilyn missed several sessions. My being flexible in rescheduling her sessions to keep her motivated was a key to her staying with the treatment. Early in therapy, Marilyn had a difficult case of bronchitis that led to several missed appointments. She also missed several sessions later in therapy due to her increased involvement in social activities and decreased feeling that she needed more assistance from therapy. Her change was gradual over time, but she reported feeling like a new person at the end of therapy. Her PTSD symptoms had substantially subsided and she reported that the trauma felt like "ancient history" and that she was ready to move on with her life. She felt confident that she could do what she needed and desired to do and had even started working again on a part-time basis. Her depression was much less severe. She said she still had bad days that usually coincided with her experiencing increased pain after overexerting herself; however, those days were rare and were becoming less frequent as she settled into her new life.

Throughout therapy, Marilyn continued to drink alcohol (i.e., one to two drinks per episode about 2 nights per week). However, she felt that she no longer was using the alcohol to deal with her pain and depression, but drank only at social occasions. Her husband concurred that she was no longer misusing alcohol. Although Marilyn and her husband entered relationship counseling, she was not sure what would come of it. At the end of therapy, she had decided to try to reconcile with him, but she was not sure that she could forgive her husband for what she thought was his lack of support after the accident.

A year after completing therapy, Marilyn reported maintenance of and continued improvement in her gains. She was employed full time and very active in the city arts organizations. She had reconciled with her husband and felt that she was doing great.

DISCUSSION

In summary, Marilyn was able to make life-changing improvements in her quality of life over the 24 weeks that we worked together. These changes included improvements in multiple problems that were identified at pretreatment. Several factors contributed to her progress: First, establishing a treatment plan with specific goals and associated effective treatment strategies helped to maintain both motivation and focus. Second, remaining flexible with missed sessions and uncompleted homework when Marilyn's motivation waned allowed us to refocus our motivation upon returning to treatment. Finally, given the interrelation of Marilyn's PTSD, depression, and pain, working in a treatment plan that incorporated all of these issues simultaneously allowed for progress in one area to feed progress in the in other areas. The effectiveness and power of our work together is further supported in the maintenance of her gains and continued improvement in her quality of life a year after ending our sessions.

REFERENCES

Asmundson GJG, Coons MJ, Taylor S, et al: PTSD and the experience of pain: research and clinical implications of shared vulnerability and mutual maintenance models. Can J Psychiatry 47:930–937, 2002

Cahill SP, Rauch SA, Hembree EA, et al: Effect of cognitive-behavioral treatments for PTSD on anger. Journal of Cognitive Psychotherapy 17:113–131, 2003

Foa EB, Rothbaum BO: Treating the Trauma of Rape. New York, Guilford Press, 1998

Foa EB, Riggs DS, Dancu CV, et al: Reliability and validity of a brief instrument for assessing post-traumatic stress disorder. J Trauma Stress 6:459–473, 1993

Foa EB, Dancu CV, Hembree EA, et al: A comparison of exposure therapy, stress inoculation training, and their combination for reducing posttraumatic stress disorder in female assault victims. J Consult Clin Psychol 67:194–200, 1999

Philips HC, Rachman S: The Psychological Management of Chronic Pain: A Treatment Manual. New York, Springer, 1996

Rothbaum BO, Meadows EA, Resick P, et al: Cognitive-behavioral therapy, in Effective Treatments for PTSD. Edited by Foa EB, Keane TM, Friedman MJ. New York, Guilford, 2000, pp 60–83, 320–325

Sharp TJ, Harvey AG: Chronic pain and posttraumatic stress disorder: mutual maintenance? Clin Psychol Rev 21:857–877, 2001

PART VIII

Somatoform Disorders

CHAPTER 20

"Doctor, Are You Sure My Heart is Okay?"

Cognitive-Behavioral Treatment of Hypochondriasis

Arthur Barsky, M.D.

Arthur Barsky, M.D., is Professor of Psychiatry at Harvard Medical School and the Director of Psychiatric Research in the Department of Psychiatry at the Brigham and Women's Hospital in Boston, Massachusetts. His major interests are hypochondriasis and somatization, the psychological factors that affect symptom reporting in medically ill individuals, and the cognitive-behavioral treatment of somatic symptoms. Dr. Barsky has been the principal investigator of nine National Institute of Mental Health and National Institutes of Health research grants in these areas. He has authored over 125 articles, 18 book chapters, and the popular books *Worried Sick: Our Troubled Quest for Wellness* and *Stop Being Your Symptoms and Start Being Yourself.* Dr. Barsky received the President's Research Award from the American Psychosomatic Society. He is a Faculty Fellow of the Mind/Brain/Behavior Interfaculty Initiative of Harvard University and chaired one of its interdisciplinary work groups on the experience of illness. He is a Distinguished Fellow of the American Psychiatric Association and served on the council of the American Psychosomatic Society.

LOUIS WAS A 66-YEAR-OLD retired restaurant owner who was referred for a psychiatric consultation by his cardiologist for anxiety. Louis himself readily acknowledged being worried about his cardiac status but added that his real source of distress was physical: a diffuse feeling of pressure in his chest when he climbed stairs and palpitations that occurred unpredictably. He came to his first appointment with me with copies of his extensive medical records, including reports of his exercise tolerance test, ambulatory electrocardiographic monitoring, and cardiac catherization. Louis was most concerned about his serial blood platelet counts. Although his platelet count was actually within normal limits, it had been trending downward on the last few evaluations, leading him to ask me anxiously, "Is that significant?"

HISTORY

Louis had developed atypical chest pain 5 years earlier. Repeated extensive evaluations had failed to disclose any cardiac or other medical cause for his symptoms, and careful medical and cardiac follow-up since the evaluations had not revealed any demonstrable disease. Louis did not find the negative results of the workups reassuring, however, and instead became more and more convinced that he did indeed have significant heart disease. He consulted numerous cardiologists armed with sophisticated and detailed questions about the possible existence and extent of heart disease. In the course of this peripatetic medical odyssey, he noticed that he was having occasional palpitations and episodes of dizziness. Evaluations of these new symptoms revealed occasional ectopic heartbeats but no evidence of clinically significant arrhythmias.

Over the ensuing 4 years, Louis's symptoms continued unabated. They preoccupied his thoughts, and his "illness" governed much of his daily routine. He retired prematurely from the restaurant business and spent his time visiting physicians, reading about and researching heart disease, monitoring and subtly adjusting his stringent low-fat diet, and carrying out an extraordinarily strenuous exercise regimen. He consulted multiple internists and cardiologists for third, fourth, and fifth opinions and pored over their reports and findings. Alarmed by slight inconsistencies or minor contradictions in the reports of his many physicians, equivocal test results, and incidental laboratory abnormalities, he worried that no one had completely grasped or definitively diagnosed his problem.

At the time when I saw Louis, he was recording his blood pressure four times a day using two different machines whose values he then averaged. He noted in a health diary any symptoms that occurred when he exerted himself, and he regularly counted the number of steps it took to increase his pulse by 15 bpm. He collected and filed magazine articles and medical journal reports dealing with heart disease. He also curtailed his travel (he used to be an inveterate tourist with a great passion for photography) for fear that he would have a "cardiac event" while away from home and his doctors. He also curtailed his sexual activity with his wife, fearing that the excitement could precipitate a "heart attack."

Louis's anxiety was restricted to health issues and he was not clinically depressed. He had had a depressive episode 8 years previously when he was diagnosed with angina. He had no history of panic attacks or typical obsessive-compulsive disorder symptoms but had experienced some agoraphobic symptoms (fears of being alone and of leaving the house or traveling away from home) secondary to his cardiac concerns. He had previously completed a stress reduction/relaxation response training program and had seen a psychiatrist on occasion for anxiety. Over the years he was tried on a number of different anxiolytics. None of these interventions proved to be particularly beneficial.

DIAGNOSIS

Hypochondriacal individuals suffer from the mistaken belief that they have an undiagnosed medical disorder. The DSM-IV-TR defines *hypochondriasis* as a preoccupation with the fear or belief one that has a serious disease that is based on a misinterpretation of benign bodily sensations. This preoccupation must persist despite appropriate medical attention and reassurance, last for at least 6 months, and result in significant impairment or distress. Louis clearly mets these diagnostic criteria.

Hypochondriasis is a psychiatric disorder lying midway along the spectrum of pathological somatizing conditions. At one end of the spectrum lie the somatoform disorders in which the patient complains of a disturbing physical symptom, but is not troubled by his or her thoughts or beliefs about the symptom. Thus patients with chronic idiopathic pain and those with somatization disorder are troubled by a physical symptom but not by the meaning or significance of that symptom; they are not afraid that they have a fatal disorder and are not terribly concerned about a diagnostic explanation for their symptoms. Rather, these patients are primarily concerned with symptom relief. At the other end of the spectrum are individuals troubled solely by their *ideas* about disease—they believe that they are sick and fear their condition will worsen without treatment, but have no physical symptoms or bodily discomfort to support the belief. These patients are often diagnosed with disease phobias or obsessive-compulsive disorder. They seek relief from their thoughts, not from bodily distress. Their disturbance lies in the domain of cognition, not of physical sensation or bodily perception.

Hypochondriacal patients lay midway along this diagnostic spectrum, since they have both a disturbing bodily sensation and disturbing thoughts and ideas about the meaning and significance of the sensation. The hypochondriacal patient seeks symptom relief, but even more so, he or she seeks to know the cause of his symptoms and to learn their medical explanation. The patient knows he or she has an undiagnosed illness and desperately wants to obtain a diagnosis. Our patient Louis fits comfortably into this nosological niche and thus exemplifies hypochondriasis.

The major diagnostic dilemma with hypochondriacal patients is the problem of other Axis I comorbidity and, if it is present, the dilemma of deciding which condition is primary and which is secondary. The most common comorbid conditions with hypochondriasis are anxiety and depressive disorders, and well over half of all hypochondriacal patients have at least one of these other conditions (Barsky et al. 1992). The rates of generalized anxiety disorder, panic disorder, dysthymia, and major depression are all elevated in hypochondriasis (Barsky et al. 1992). It is important to search for these comorbid conditions behind the veil of somatic complaints and concerns because they are often eminently treatable, and their successful treatment generally results in the resolution of the hypochondriacal symptoms as well (Keeley et al. 2000; Noyes et al. 1986). In this case example, Louis is clearly anxious, but his anxiety is restricted to health-related issues and does not extend to involve other common sources of worry (such as finances) nor has he had panic attacks. Although he, understandably, has periods of depressed mood, he has not had a major depression and does not suffer from dysthymia. Thus Louis seems to be a clear case of primary hypochondriasis.

TREATMENT

Louis's therapy with me focused on his cognitive appraisal of his physical symptoms, his worry about their meaning and significance, and the illness and sick role behaviors he had developed in response to his symptoms. Four general domains were explored: 1) the development of a trusting and stable relationship with a single primary care physician; 2) curtailing illness-related behaviors that were initially undertaken to reassure himself but that in actuality ended up heightening his anxiety;

3) developing alternative, more benign etiologic explanations for his symptoms; and 4) acquiring a more psychosocial and less biomedical understanding of health and disease in general.

Before these four goals of treatment could be pursued, however, it was necessary for Louis and me to explicitly agree on a formulation of the problem and a rationale for cognitive-behavioral treatment (CBT). Psychological treatment generally makes little sense to hypochondriacal patients who believe that their problem is solely a medical one. Before proceeding with treatment, patients must begin to think about the nature of their problem in a different way; the formulation offered is that their distress results not only from their somatic symptoms but also from their reactions to these symptoms (their thoughts about, emotional responses to, future expectations about, and actions taken in response to them). These reactions amplify physical symptoms and make them seem more intense, ominous, and serious. I often illustrate this process of symptom amplification with the statement that a headache you believe is due to a brain tumor hurts a lot more than a headache you attribute to eyestrain.

I explained to Louis that most bothersome benign symptoms are self-limiting and gradually subside of their own accord over time. (As Lewis Thomas has written, "The great secret …is that most things get better by themselves. Most things, in fact, really are better by morning." Thomas 1975, p. 100). However, people prevent this natural process of symptom resolution from happening when they react to the symptoms by suspecting the most catastrophic cause possible (no matter how unlikely or how remote it may actually be), developing bodily hypervigilance and intensively monitoring themselves, selectively searching for information that confirms their fears, ignoring disconfirmatory evidence that they are not sick, and becoming excessively alarmed. These reactions amplify the symptoms and perpetuate and maintain them. In essence, they obstruct the natural, self-limiting, transient course that most benign ailments follow over time. In the first two treatment sessions, these ideas were presented to Louis and fully discussed with him. Only when he understood and agreed that his distress stemmed not only from his palpitations and chest pains but also from his thoughts and feelings about them could treatment commence.

The first explicit goal of Louis's therapy was to establish a satisfactory and stable relationship with a single primary care physician who would serve as a gatekeeper for further consultation and referrals and as the sole resource for information about his cardiac status. Louis was encouraged to express his misgivings about his doctors and the reasons he had for not trusting them. When he was finally able to identify one physician whom he felt he could trust, we then discussed how he might negotiate an explicit agreement about the goals of his medical care with that doctor. One of these goals was for Louis to schedule regular visits with the chosen physician during which he could seek answers to all his questions but then agree to make no changes in his self-treatment or medical regimen between these regular appointments (unless, of course, a significant medical event occurred). This had the effect of relieving the pressure Louis felt to monitor his symptoms minute by minute and continually update himself on the latest medical information because these actions would not prompt any changes until he next visited his doctor. Thus Louis could gradually decrease the frequency with which he checked his blood pressure and charted his exercise tolerance, because these data would not prompt any change in his regimen until his next regularly scheduled visit.

The second step in Louis's treatment was to examine and then modify some of his dysfunctional illness behaviors. Many hypochondriacal patients find it easier to change some of their behaviors before they try to change their thinking about symptoms and disease. After some reflection, Louis began to see that his attempts to reassure himself about his health actually heightened rather than reduced his anxiety and ultimately made things worse. For example, he would press a consultant to tell him with absolute certainty that he had no heart disease. When the consultant replied that, no matter how unlikely, occult disease could never be ruled out with absolute certainty, Louis then found himself to be more terrified than before he asked. When surfing the Web in the hopes of learning that the tingling he thought he noticed in his fingertips could not be related to heart disease, he learned of many fearsome diseases he had never even heard of before that can cause paresthesias. He came to realize that researching his symptoms, asking others their opinions about his symptoms, and examining himself for evidence of disease were all having the paradoxical and unintended result of actually heightening his anxiety and alarm. Recognizing this enabled him to gradually curtail, limit, and then eventually abandon these behaviors. As a start, Louis agreed to stop his customary habit of reading the obituary column in the daily newspaper, seeking to learn the causes of death of those his own age. He then found he could begin curtailing the amount of time he allowed himself to surf the Web about health-related topics. In the most significant change, Louis decided on his own that it would be helpful to discard the extensive clippings file he had accumulated on various aspects of cardiovascular disease.

As he discovered that behavioral changes could diminish his anxiety and the time he spent worrying about his health, Louis became more willing to entertain new ways of thinking about his symptoms. We focused on the process of symptom attribution and amplification. I illustrated for him how powerful our thoughts, ideas, and opinions about a symptom could be and how they could influence how a symptom feels and actually amplify the symptom itself. We reviewed selected research findings and clinical examples of this (e.g., although the pain of an osteosarcoma of the foot and wearing a tight shoe might be similar, the experience is totally different. From this discussion, it became apparent to Louis that if certain ways of thinking about a symptom can make it worse, then other ways of thinking about it can make it better.

These discussions opened the door to an examination of Louis's disease attributions—his tendency to catastrophize uncomfortable body sensations and attribute them to serious diseases rather than to normalize them. (Normalization is the process whereby people attribute symptoms to nonpathological causes such as dietary indiscretion, aging, lack of proper exercise, daily wear and tear, stress, and so on.) Louis and I examined his symptom attributions, and I encouraged him to consider other possible alternative, nonpathological causes for his symptoms. We discussed the fact that palpitations are common in everyday life but are generally ignored, dismissed, or never even consciously noted. It became clear to him that in most instances, palpitations are due to benign premature beats rather than to serious arrhythmias. Likewise with his atypical chest pain, Louis was encouraged to begin thinking of possible, alternative benign causes of this sensation (e.g., increased intercostal muscle tension, overexertion, anxiety) and to consider the relative likelihood of these benign events as compared with coronary heart disease, given the negative results of his extensive cardiac workup.

As we examined the process of somatic appraisal and attribution, Louis began to see the role confirmatory bias played in his belief that he had undiagnosed heart disease; that is, he was selectively focusing on bodily sensations and information that confirmed his worst suspicions (i.e., of lethal heart disease) and selectively ignoring disconfirmatory evidence (e.g., he did not notice all the times when he did not feel palpitations). He came to see that he had become caught up in a self-validating, self-perpetuating cycle of belief and perception whereby his belief that he was sick amplified his symptoms, which further convinced him that he was sick, and so on.

Finally, as Louis examined how thoughts, expectations, illness memories, and emotions can amplify benign bodily distress, he became more open to considering a new model to explain his symptoms—a model of sensory nervous system dysfunction rather than of organ pathology. He had noted early in therapy, "The doctors keep telling me what I don't have, but no one tells me what I do have." His statement illustrated the point that hypochondriacal patients cannot be reassured without being offered an alternative explanation for their symptoms. Simply telling patients that no serious medical disease is present is inadequate; they know that something is wrong, for they truly experience the symptoms they report. Hence, they need some explanatory model to fall back on. Here the model of cognitive and perceptual symptom amplification was helpful to Louis. I suggested an analogy to a radio whose volume has been turned up so high that the background static has become noxious. The notion was that the problem lay in the sensory nervous system rather than in the periphery. He began to see that some bodily sensations, although distressing, disturbing, and even disabling, were not necessarily due to disease. Indeed there are many symptomatic conditions for which modern medicine lacks a satisfactory pathological or pathophysiological explanation; low back pain and migraine headaches are two common examples of this. Louis found it helpful to realize that he was not alone in his predicament and that his problem was really not so different from that of many others.

As therapy progressed, it emerged that during his time as a restaurant owner Louis had invented several gadgets that worked well in his commercial kitchen to streamline cooking times and service. Now he began to wonder if any large restaurant chains might be interested in one of his devices, and he was eventually retained as a consultant by one of them. He had noted earlier in therapy that since his premature retirement, he had "too much time on [his] hands." "If I were busier, I don't think I'd spend so much time on my health." In our later sessions, more of our time was taken up with his excitement about his invention and less time was spent on his medical complaints and health concerns. When asked about his symptoms at one point toward the end of therapy, Louis responded, "When I stop to think about it, I still get that pressure in my chest sometimes. But I just don't think about it anymore." He also noted a decline in the number of medical visits he was making to specialists, commenting that he was just too busy and no longer had the time to seek out so many consultants.

During this later phase of therapy, Louis experienced one of several transient setbacks that are typical in the course of treating hypochondriasis. He developed an episode of chest pressure that seemed different in character to him and he went to an emergency department, wondering if this was "the big one." However, he was able to take some reassurance from the diagnosis of "heartburn" he was given in the emergency department, from a calming phone conversation with his primary care doctor the next day, and from the remission of the pain itself. Thus the course of improvement with CBT is generally one of intermittent, briefer and briefer relapses interspersed between longer and longer periods of improvement.

DISCUSSION

In my experience, Louis's case illustrates the typical outcome of CBT for hypochondriasis: not a definitive or complete cure of somatic symptoms, but rather a decrease in their noxious and bothersome quality; a reduction in the anxiety, fear, and frustration they arouse; and a marked improvement in role functioning. Life becomes more satisfactory, but the somatic symptoms do not vanish completely. Rather, they lose the grip they seemed to have on the patient's mind.

Although traditional, insight-oriented psychotherapy can be helpful for some hypochondriacal patients, many do not seem to derive much benefit from it. It is less focused and may be less economical than a CBT approach. The latter targets the hypochondriacal symptoms specifically and generally does not entail a long course of treatment; often, 8–12 weekly or biweekly sessions suffice. These may be followed by booster sessions as needed if relapses occur over the ensuing months and years. Louis was seen weekly, then biweekly, and finally monthly, for a total of 14 sessions over an 8-month period. This is the typical course for treatment of hypochondriasis.

Pharmacological treatment of hypochondriasis is an area that remains largely unexplored at this time. There is a high prevalence of comorbid depressive or anxiety disorder with hypochondriasis, and many hypochondriacal patients respond positively to pharmacotherapy for these comorbid conditions. In primary hypochondriasis (hypochondriasis unaccompanied by another major Axis I disorder), the efficacy of these agents remains unclear. However, anecdotal case reports and small studies suggest that serotonin reuptake inhibitors (e.g., fluoxetine) and/or dual reuptake inhibitors (e.g., venlafaxine) may have some role in the treatment of primary hypochondriasis.

Louis's therapy was fairly typical in my experience. There are, however, a number of hypochondriacal patients who find the CBT therapeutic approach unhelpful and cannot be engaged in it. For these patients, the treatment approach seems utterly nonsensical because they are firmly convinced they have an undiagnosed medical illness that only medical or surgical interventions can address. As one patient put it, "I don't need to talk about this. I need to find a doctor who will take me seriously enough to repeat that CT scan." But for those hypochondriacal patients who acknowledge that their anxieties and worries about their health, their reactions to their symptoms, and their beliefs about what is wrong are contributing to their distress, CBT can be helpful.

REFERENCES

Barsky AJ, Wyshak G, Klerman GL: Psychiatric comorbidity in DSM-III-R hypochondriasis. Arch Gen Psychiat 49:101–108, 1992

Keeley R, Smith M, Miller J: Somatoform symptoms and treatment nonadherence in depressed family medicine outpatients. Arch Fam Med 9:46–54, 2000

Noyes R, Reich J, Clancy J: Reduction in hypochondriasis with treatment of panic disorder. Br J Psychiat 149:631–635, 1986

Thomas L: The Lives of a Cell. New York, Bantam Books, 1975

SUGGESTED READING

Barsky AJ: Clinical crossroads: a 37-year old man with multiple somatic complaints. JAMA 278:673–679, 1997

Barsky AJ, Ahern DK: Cognitive behavior therapy for hypochondriasis: a randomized controlled trial. JAMA 291:1464–1470, 2004

Looper KJ, Kirmayer LJ: Behavioral medicine approaches to somatoform disorders. J Consult Clin Psychol 70:810–827, 2002

Mayou R, Bass C, Sharpe M: Treatment of Functional Somatic Symptoms. Oxford, Oxford University Press, 1995

Starcevic V, Lipsitt DR: Hypochondriasis: Clinical, Theoretical and Treatment Aspects. New York, Oxford University Press, 2000

Taylor S, Asmundson GJG: Treating Health Anxiety: A Cognitive-Behavioral Approach. New York, Guilford, 2004

CHAPTER 21

"I Look Like A Monster"

Pharmacotherapy and Cognitive-Behavioral Therapy for Body Dysmorphic Disorder

Katharine A. Phillips, M.D.

Katharine A. Phillips, M.D., is Professor of Psychiatry at Brown Medical School and Director of the Body Dysmorphic Disorder and Body Image Program at Butler Hospital in Providence, Rhode Island. Dr. Phillips has conducted research into and treated patients with body dysmorphic disorder (BDD) since 1990; her work has involved approximately 900 individuals with this disorder. Her pioneering work, which has focused largely on BDD's psychopathology and treatment, has brought this disorder to the attention of the public and professionals alike. In addition to her many articles on BDD in scientific journals, she has written and edited several books on BDD and body image, including *The Broken Mirror: Understanding and Treating Body Dysmorphic Disorder* (1996; revised edition 2005).

ROB WAS A 27-YEAR-OLD, single, Caucasion, unemployed man who lived with his parents. His chief complaint was "I look like a monster." He referred himself to me for treatment after reading about body dysmorphic disorder (BDD) and thinking he might have this disorder. At the same time, he doubted that this diagnosis applied to him because, as he explained, he had read that people with BDD actually look normal, whereas he was truly ugly.

Rob was extremely anxious at his first session. He explained that he was convinced that he looked like a monster, stating, "People tell me I look normal, but they're just trying to be nice. I know what I see when I look in the mirror." Rob believed that other people stared at his supposed physical deformities and recoiled in horror. Because of these beliefs, he was unable to work or even leave his house. In reality, Rob was a handsome young man who looked entirely normal, although his appearance was notable for his shaved and penciled in eyebrows, unusually dark tan, and a baseball cap that was pulled down to cover his forehead.

HISTORY

Rob had had a normal developmental history, had done well in school, and had many friends until he was age 13, when a friend called him "big nose." "No one else ever said I had a big nose, but that was it. I looked in the mirror, and all I could see was this gigantic nose. How did I never notice it before?" Rob also began to worry that he looked abnormal in other ways. He thought his eyebrows were "too big and bushy," his eyes were "small and beady," his skin was too pale, and his hair "stuck out all bizarre" and was the wrong color (it was actually blond but he thought it was gray). He thought about these perceived appearance flaws "all day long," stating, "I couldn't stop thinking about it—that I looked really ugly. I thought all the kids were laughing at me and I felt really self-conscious. I just couldn't get it out of my mind." Rob started checking his appearance in mirrors and other reflecting surfaces from several inches away for hours a day. He frequently compared his appearance with that of other people, such as models in men's magazines and actors on television, thinking everyone looked better than he did. He spent hours a day frantically combing and styling his hair, trying to get it to "look right"; because he was never satisfied, he covered it with a hat. He spent more than $50 a week on hair products that never worked. Rob also spent several hours a day plucking and shaving his eyebrows, trying to "even them up and get them in the right shape." He felt too self-conscious to go outside to tan, so he had his parents build a tanning booth in their home so he could darken his "pale" skin.

Rob was so distressed over his appearance and his belief that other people stared and laughed at him that he dropped out of high school and could not work, see his friends, or date. He left his house only on rare occasions to do an errand or buy hair products or street drugs. He had begun to abuse alcohol and a variety of drugs, stating that alcohol, benzodiazepines, and opioids offered him some relief from his tormenting obsessions. By age 20, after becoming convinced that his body was too "puny" and inadequately muscular, he began using illegally obtained anabolic steroids.

In his mid-20s, at his family's insistence, Rob sought psychiatric treatment. He tried many medications, including the serotonin reuptake inhibitors (SRIs) paroxetine (20 mg/day for several weeks), sertraline (100 mg/day for 2 months), and citalopram (up to 60 mg/day for 7 weeks). He also tried several antipsychotic medications but discontinued them after a brief trial because he could not tolerate their side effects. None of these medications were helpful. He also received cognitive-behavioral therapy (CBT), which partially diminished his symptoms and enabled him to leave the house more often, but he eventually stopped the therapy because, in his words, he was lazy, meaning that he did not want to put in the effort (e.g., doing the homework) that CBT required. His condition subsequently relapsed. Fluoxetine up to 80 mg/day for about 1 year substantially improved his BDD symptoms, depression, and functioning, but after Rob stopped taking the medication because of related gastrointestinal discomfort and decreased appetite, he relapsed again. Rob had previously made three suicide attempts, citing his BDD symptoms as the motivation for these attempts. One attempt, an overdose that led to hospitalization in an intensive care unit, occurred several months before I started treating him.

DIAGNOSIS

Rob had correctly diagnosed his illness; he had severe, classic BDD. His symptoms met criteria for BDD because he was preoccupied with nonexistent defects in his appearance (BDD can also be diagnosed if the appearance flaws are slight), and his appearance preoccupations caused him clinically significant distress and impairment in functioning. Although BDD-related repetitive and safety behaviors (e.g., excessive mirror checking, camouflaging) are not required for the diagnosis, virtually all patients perform one or more of them (Phillips 1996, 2001). Rob's poor functioning and suicidality were also characteristic of BDD. Functioning and quality of life are poor for most BDD patients (Phillips et al. 2005b); approximately 80% of these patients have lifetime suicidal ideation and 22%–28% attempt suicide (Phillips et al. 2005a). Substance use disorders are also common among this population, and many patients report using substances to relieve the dysphoric feelings caused by their BDD symptoms (Grant et al. 2005).

Rob was also diagnosed with major depressive disorder. In the past, he had been diagnosed with obsessive-compulsive disorder, but all of his obsessions and compulsive behaviors were related to his appearance, making BDD the more accurate diagnosis.

An interesting and complex diagnostic issue was whether Rob should be diagnosed with delusional disorder, somatic type, which is classified in the schizophrenia and other psychotic disorders section of DSM-IV-TR. DSM-IV-TR actually allows patients like Rob, whose appearance beliefs reach delusional proportions, to be diagnosed with both BDD and delusional disorder. This convention is somewhat awkward, because it entails two different diagnoses being applied to the same symptoms. On the other hand, this double coding reflects available evidence suggesting that BDD's delusional and nondelusional forms are probably the same disorder—in other words, BDD may be characterized by different degrees of insight, ranging from good insight (realizing that one's appearance beliefs are not accurate) to poor insight to no insight (i.e., being delusional).

BDD is underrecognized and underdiagnosed in clinical settings (Phillips 2001). Patients may not volunteer their symptoms because they are too ashamed and worry the clinician will consider them superficial or vain. Many are too self-conscious to draw further attention to the "defects" by discussing them. BDD is often misdiagnosed as another disorder, such as major depressive disorder, obsessive-compulsive disorder, social phobia, agoraphobia, psychotic disorder not otherwise specified, or even schizophrenia. If BDD is not targeted in treatment, the treatment may fail. Indeed, Rob had received several medication trials that were reasonably adequate for depression but probably not for BDD and that did not diminish either his BDD or his depressive symptoms.

TREATMENT

Choice of Treatment

Essential Ingredients

Patients with BDD can be very difficult to engage in treatment. Many are too embarrassed and anxious about how they look to even come to the clinician's office. Others, believing that they have actual physical deformities, prefer surgery, dermatologic treatment, or other nonpsychiatric medical treatment for their perceived appearance flaws (Phillips 1996, 2001). The first critical step in treatment is for clinicians to convey that they take a patient's appearance concerns seriously. It is also important for clinicians to avoid agreeing with patients' view of their appearance, arguing with them over how they actually look, or simply reassuring them that they look normal. It is more helpful to focus on the psychiatric treatment's potential to diminish their suffering, improve their functioning, and help them enjoy their lives. Psychoeducation about BDD and its treatment will provide essential groundwork for the treatment. For the treatment to succeed, it is important to focus specifically on BDD in addition to any comorbid disorders.

Medications

SRIs are currently considered the first-line medication for BDD (Phillips 2002). Results from two controlled studies, four open-label trials, and case reports and series consistently indicate that SRIs are often efficacious for BDD (Hollander et al. 1999; Phillips 2002; Phillips et al. 2002). Although the data are very limited, other medications, including non-SRI antidepressants, appear to be less effective than SRIs (Hollander et al. 1999; Phillips 2002). Of note, SRIs as single agents appear effective not only for nondelusional BDD but also for delusional BDD (patients who are completely convinced that they look abnormal and who would receive a diagnosis of delusional disorder in addition to BDD) (Hollander et al. 1999; Phillips 2002; Phillips et al. 2002). This approach might sound counterintuitive, as psychotic symptoms in other disorders are usually treated with antipsychotics. Very little data are available on the efficacy of antipsychotics for BDD, but these data (which are largely retrospective) suggest that typical neuroleptics alone are ineffective, even for delusional patients (Phillips 2002).

BDD appears to often require relatively high SRI dosages; in my clinical experience, patients usually receive dosages that are too low. Although no studies have compared different SRI dosages, in a chart-review study from my clinical practice, the average SRI dosages were fluoxetine 66.7±23.5 mg/day, fluvoxamine 308.3±49.2 mg/day, paroxetine 55.0±12.9 mg/day, sertraline 202.1±45.8 mg/day, and clomipramine 203.3±52.5 mg/day (Phillips 2002). Average dosages of citalopram were 66 ± 36 mg/day and of escitalopram were 29 ±12 mg/day. Some patients respond only to dosages higher than the maximum recommended dosage for SRIs. Even with fairly rapid titration of an SRI, BDD symptoms usually require an average of 4–9 weeks to respond; an SRI should be tried for 12 or even 14 weeks before a clinician can determine if it is working. If BDD is not recognized and only depression is diagnosed, patients may receive too low an SRI dosage or too brief a trial, as did Rob.

Psychotherapy

Although the research on psychotherapy for treating BDD is limited, results from clinical series and several studies that have compared CBT with a no-treatment waiting-list condition have indicated that CBT is often effective for BDD (Veale et al. 1996; Wilhelm et al. 1999). CBT is currently considered the first-line psychotherapy for BDD (Neziroglu and Khemlani-Patel 2002). CBT for BDD usually consists of both cognitive and behavioral components: *cognitive restructuring* teaches patients to identify and evaluate their negative appearance-related thoughts and beliefs, identify cognitive errors, and develop more accurate and helpful beliefs; *response (ritual) prevention* helps patients resist performing excessive repetitive or safety behaviors (e.g., mirror checking, camouflaging); and *exposure* helps patients gradually face avoided situations (e.g., social situations). Exposure is usually combinated with *behavioral experiments* in which patients design and carry out experiments to test their BDD beliefs to determine if they are accurate. An additional CBT technique that may be helpful is *mirror retraining*, which helps patients learn to look at their entire face or body (not just the disliked areas) in the mirror and objectively (rather than negatively) describe their body. *Habit reversal*, an established treatment for trichotillomania, may be helpful for skin picking, hair plucking, and body touching. It consists of awareness training, learning a competing response, relaxation, and rewarding oneself for not picking, plucking, or touching the body area. *Mindfulness skills*, which involve observing and being aware of one's thoughts and emotions by focusing on them "in the moment" in a nonjudgmental way, and *refocusing*, or gently focusing one's attention and thoughts on what is happening in the environment rather than on BDD thoughts, may also be helpful. More severely ill and poorly functioning patients may benefit from *activity scheduling* and *scheduling pleasant activities*.

The optimal number and frequency of CBT sessions is not known. Sessions may range from 50 minutes to several hours and take place anywhere from daily to weekly. Some patients respond to CBT within several months whereas others need much lengthier treatment (e.g., a year). From a clinical perspective, more severely ill patients require more frequent sessions and a longer treatment duration. Homework is an essential part of CBT, as this enables patients to learn and practice CBT skills between sessions. Treatment also includes relapse prevention, which focuses on helping patients maintain the gains they made in treatment; booster sessions may be helpful after the treatment has ended.

Initial Phase of Treatment

When I first met with Rob, I completed a comprehensive psychiatric evaluation and encouraged him to tell me about his appearance concerns, including how they affected his life and how he had tried to cope. I told him that he had correctly diagnosed himself and that he had many classic BDD symptoms. I provided psychoeducation about BDD, telling him that it is a relatively common and treatable body image disorder and explaining what is known about its symptoms, possible causes, and effective treatments. I also recommended reading about BDD. I did not reassure him that he looked normal, because many patients interpret reassurance as an attempt to trivialize or minimize their worries and suffering. I also didn't say something like, "Well, your nose is slightly larger than average, but it isn't *that* big!" because well-intended statements like this can plunge patients into despair or even trigger suicidal thinking, as patients usually view them as a confirmation of their belief. I also did not focus on or argue over whether his defects were real, as such discussions are usually fruitless. Instead, I simply noted that I and other people viewed Rob's appearance differently than he did for reasons that are not well understood. I then focused on the potential for treatment to alleviate his suffering and improve his functioning and enjoyment of life.

Because Rob was considering a rhinoplasty, I told him that no one can predict how an individual patient will respond to surgery, but that such treatments appear to be usually ineffective for BDD and can even worsen appearance concerns (Phillips 1996). I explained that psychotropic medication and therapy are much less risky, would likely help him feel better, and were worth a try. Rob reluctantly agreed to put his rhinoplasty plans on hold and to try psychiatric treatment, although he was somewhat discouraged by his past treatment "failures." I agreed that he had tried many medications that had not helped, but I noted that an SRI plus CBT had been fairly effective for him and that these treatments were worth trying again. I told him that I could not guarantee that he would improve but said that I was very optimistic because most people with BDD do get better with adequate treatment. I also met with Rob's family to provide psychoeducation about BDD, discuss the treatment plan, answer their questions, and offer them hope that Rob would improve.

Because Rob had recently attempted suicide, I initially focused on his safety, including developing a safety plan that involved his family, and having his parents keep his medications for him, given his recent overdose. I emphasized the need for Rob to stop all street drugs and alcohol and recommended additional treatment focused specifically on his substance use. However, Rob replied that he had successfully stopped using alcohol and drugs in the past without treatment and was convinced that he could stop again on his own. We discussed restarting fluoxetine, but Rob was against using this medication. I decided to try escitalopram; even though citalopram had not been helpful, his trial on the medication had been too brief to determine its efficacy. Because he had a history of poor medication tolerance, I titrated the dosage a little more slowly than usual. I ordinarily would start at about 10 mg/day of escitalopram for several weeks, then increase the dosage to 20 mg/day for several weeks and then to 30 mg/day, as tolerated. Although it is unclear whether adding an antipsychotic to SRI therapy diminishes BDD symptoms per se, in my clinical experience antipsychotics can be invaluable for BDD-associated agitation and anxiety. Rob had poorly tolerated many antipsychotics in the past; I decided to try the atypical antipsychotic ziprasidone, starting at 10 mg/day. Several weeks after starting these medications, Rob still felt anxious, agitated, and distressed and had moderately severe insomnia, so we discussed adding an anxiolytic/hypnotic. We considered many nonbenzodiazepine options, all of which Rob had tried without success except for the antiepileptic gabapentin. We reached a dosage of 1,200 mg/day and saw modest improvement in his anxiety. Rob then wanted to try alprazolam, which had been helpful in the past, although I expressed concern about this option, given his past benzodiazepine abuse. However, Rob said that he had not used any street drugs for some time and would not abuse it (his urine toxic screens had been negative). I thus prescribed alprazolam 0.25 mg bid, which significantly improved his anxiety and insomnia.

We also began weekly CBT, which initially focused on psychoeducation about CBT, and developed a model of Rob's BDD symptoms (e.g., how his repetitive behaviors and avoidance reinforced his preoccupations) and his goals for treatment. We attempted to do cognitive restructuring as well as response prevention focusing on his mirror checking and other behaviors. However, Rob was too severely depressed to do CBT homework and did not make much progress. I used some motivational interviewing techniques as described by Miller and Rollnick (1991) for other disorders, but this had little effect. (This included techniques such as expressing my belief that Rob was capable of making positive changes and helping him elucidate the pros and cons of engaging fully in CBT and doing homework.) In fact, Rob was so depressed that he was spending most of his days in bed. I then changed his treatment to focus more on providing support, activity scheduling, and scheduling pleasant activities (e.g., cooking, spending time on the computer). Because I was concerned that his treatment was not sufficient, I encouraged him to consider a higher level of care. However, Rob refused, saying that he would not be able to tolerate being in the hospital where people would look at him. In the past, he stayed in a day treatment program for only 1 day, leaving after he had looked in the mirror and thought that he looked like a monster. Although I was concerned that the treatment I was providing was not optimal, I understood his reluctance to enter a higher level of care and continued to treat him.

After several months of treatment, and reaching doses of escitalopram 40 mg/day, ziprasidone 20 mg/day (the highest dosage he could tolerate), gabapentin 1,200 mg/day, and alprazolam 0.5 mg/day, Rob felt less obsessed, anxious, and depressed and could better resist some of his repetitive behaviors. He was not abusing alcohol or drugs and was spending less time in bed. We estimated that his BDD symptoms were about 30% better overall. He had passive suicidal ideation but denied any intent or plan. However, after staring at his face in the mirror for several hours one day, he was so distressed that he bought some over-the-counter medication, overdosed, and was hospitalized. This was upsetting and discouraging for both me and Rob's family. At this point, Rob, his family, and I again considered various treatment options. I strongly recommended that Rob attend a residential treatment program in another state that would focus on his BDD. However, Rob was petrified of this option, thinking he would be unable to tolerate being around other people (even though I noted that this "built-in" exposure would be helpful); he was also concerned about being so far from his family. We also discussed the possibility of obtaining outpatient treatment in the state mental health system, which would be able to provide more intensive treatment (e.g., case management). However, Rob insisted that he was feeling better, that he had had "just one 1 bad day," and that he wanted to continue treatment with me. He stated that he was not currently suicidal, he realized how much his suicidal behavior had frightened and hurt his family, and that he would not make any further suicide attempts. I was concerned, as I had been in the past, about Rob's not accepting my recommendation for what I considered optimal treatment, even after I conveyed my worry that he would not improve without more intensive treatment and after exploring his reluctance. The dilemma for me was whether I should insist he follow my recommended plan and tell him I would not continue to treat him if he did not, or whether I should instead provide potentially "good enough" treatment. At this point, we decided that I would continue to treat him but that if he did not clearly improve within 3 months or if he tried to harm himself again he would go to the residential program. He also made a commitment to a safety plan.

Later Phase of Treatment

After a 14-week trial of escitalopram, it was time to consider the next medication step, because this trial was adequate in terms of both dosage and duration. Rob was now taking 40 mg/day of escitalopram (several weeks on 50 mg/day and then 60 mg/day was not more efficacious than 40 mg/day, so I lowered the dosage to 40 mg/day, which he was tolerating well). I decided to continue and augment the escitalopram rather than switch to another SRI because Rob was clearly better. Few data are available on SRI augmentation strategies for BDD; although buspirone augmentation appears to often be helpful, Rob had not been able to tolerate buspirone in the past and did not want to retry it. I decided to add venlafaxine to the escitalopram, as it has prominent serotonergic properties and, in my experience, can improve BDD symptoms. I started it at a low dosage and gradually titrated the dosage upward while I continued to monitor Rob carefully and watch for possible symptoms of serotonin syndrome (although I have never observed this with an SRI-venlafaxine combination). I also continued the alprazolam, gabapentin, and ziprasidone. I tried several times to stop the ziprasidone to replace it with another antipsychotic, but Rob's obsessions and depression clearly worsened each time, so I continued it. After about 6 weeks on the venlafaxine, Rob noticed a definite improvement in his BDD and depressive symptoms. He continued to improve as I gradually raised the dosage up to 450 mg/day, which seemed the most efficacious dosage for him. When I tried decreasing the dosage to determine whether a lower dosage might be equally effective, both his BDD and depressive symptoms worsened.

As Rob further improved, he was able to get out of bed more often and was now more motivated to participate in CBT. To learn cognitive restructuring, Rob completed thought records to better identify his negative thoughts (e.g., "Everyone at the store will think I look totally ugly.") and the feelings his thoughts generated. He then learned how to identify cognitive errors (e.g., mind reading, fortune telling, catastrophizing), evaluate the evidence for and against his beliefs, and generate more accurate and helpful beliefs (e.g., "I can't read people's minds and I don't really know what they will think; they'll probably be thinking about the groceries they need to buy."). Rob also started doing exposure combined with behavioral experiments to test his beliefs and gather evidence as to whether they were accurate or not. For example, he started walking around his neighborhood and collecting evidence as to whether people seemed to take special notice of him, stare at him, or recoil in horror when they saw him. He prepared his thoughts ahead of time (by completing a thought record and doing cognitive restructuring) and then tested a specific belief (e.g., "I believe 80% of people will laugh at me or stare at me with at least a brief look of horror on their face."). We then reviewed the evidence from the exposure/behavioral experiments and discussed whether the expected outcome had occurred and what he had learned. Much to his surprise, Rob found that the evidence did not support his beliefs. He had never realized that people did not take special notice of him, because when he did go out of his house, he was so certain that people were staring at him that he did not look up at anyone and just assumed this was happening. Once he felt more comfortable walking around his neighborhood, he tried more anxiety-provoking exposures, eventually even going to the shopping mall. Rob also learned response (ritual) prevention, first reducing the behaviors that would cause him the least anxiety to resist. For example, he gradually cut back on checking his face in a pocket mirror when he went out, and he pushed his hat back farther and farther. Eventually, he stopped wearing the hat altogether once he realized that nothing terrible happened when he went out without it. He cut back on and eventually stopped comparing himself with other people and unnecessarily checking mirrors, which greatly diminished his anxiety. With mirror retraining, he learned to look at himself in the mirror without zeroing in on and scrutinizing his flaws or berating himself about how awful he looked. Using response prevention, Rob also gradually tanned less, and, with habit reversal, he was able to shave and pluck his eyebrows less often. Doing homework regularly enabled Rob to learn and consolidate his skills.

Although Rob was still symptomatic, he continued to gradually improve. He was no longer housebound, and he went out to shop, do things with his family, and see his friends. One day he said that he was planning to apply to college. I was thrilled to hear this and expressed strong support of his goal, although we both had some concern about his taking too big a step too quickly; we discussed possible transitional steps he might take first, such as volunteering or attending school on a part-time basis.

DISCUSSION

Rob received both the first-line pharmacotherapy (an SRI) and the first-line psychotherapy (CBT) for BDD, both of which appeared to contribute to his improvement. It is not currently known whether combining CBT and an SRI is more effective than using either treatment alone. However, for more severely ill patients like Rob, it makes good clinical sense to combine them. For patients with severe BDD, especially very depressed, delusional, or suicidal patients like Rob, in my view it is best to always use an SRI to diminish their symptoms and suicide risk. In addition, improvement with an SRI can improve patients' motivation and enable them to do the work (e.g., homework) required to learn CBT skills. However, some patients may improve with CBT alone and others may improve with an SRI alone. Many patients will improve, at least partially, with the first SRI they try, whereas others may need multiple SRI trials and various SRI augmenters before they finally improve. The decision to try an SRI and/or CBT depends on factors such as how severely ill the patient is, whether there is additional comorbidity that requires treatment, the patient's preferences, and the availability of these treatments. Some patients may also benefit from additional treatment that focuses on issues such as problematic life stressors or life transitions. Much more research is needed on how to effectively treat BDD. Nonetheless, available evidence from efficacy trials and the "real world" of clinical practice suggests that most patients—even very ill patients—will ultimately improve with treatment as long as the patient and clinician work together and persist at finding the treatment that works for them.

REFERENCES

Grant JE, Menard W, Pagano ME, et al: Substance use disorders in individuals with body dysmorphic disorder. J Clin Psychiatry 66:309–311, 2005

Hollander E, Allen A, Kwon J, et al: Clomipramine vs desipramine crossover trial in body dysmorphic disorder: selective efficacy of a serotonin reuptake inhibitor in imagined ugliness. Arch Gen Psychiatry 56:1033–1039, 1999

Miller W, Rolnick S: Motivational Interviewing: Preparing People to Change Addictive Behavior. New York, Guilford, 1991

Neziroglu F, Khemlani-Patel S: A review of cognitive and behavioral treatment for body dysmorphic disorder. CNS Spectr 7:464–471, 2002

Phillips KA: The Broken Mirror: Understanding and Treating Body Dysmorphic Disorder. New York, Oxford University Press, 1996 (Revised and Expanded Edition, 2005)

Phillips KA: Body dysmorphic disorder, in Somatoform and Factitious Disorders. Edited by Phillips KA (Review of Psychiatry Series, Vol 20; Oldham JM and Riba MB, series eds). Washington, DC, American Psychiatric Publishing, 2001, pp 67–94

Phillips KA: Pharmacologic treatment of body dysmorphic disorder: review of the evidence and a recommended treatment approach. CNS Spectr 7:453–460, 2002

Phillips KA, Albertini RS, Rasmussen SA: A randomized placebo-controlled trial of fluoxetine in body dysmorphic disorder. Arch Gen Psychiatry 59:381–388, 2002

Phillips KA, Coles M, Menard W, et al: Suicidal ideation and suicide attempts in body dysmorphic disorder. J Clin Psychiatry 66:717–725, 2005a

Phillips KA, Menard W, Fay C, et al: Psychosocial functioning and quality of life in body dysmorphic disorder. Compr Psychiatry 46:254–260, 2005b

Veale D, Gournay K, Dryden W, et al: Body dysmorphic disorder: a cognitive behavioral model and pilot randomized controlled trial. Behav Res Ther 34:717–729, 1996

Wilhelm S, Otto MW, Lohr B, et al: Cognitive behavior group therapy for body dysmorphic disorder: a case series. Behav Res Ther 37:71–75, 1999

PART IX

Factitious Disorders

CHAPTER 22

The Search

Psychosocial Treatment of Factitious Physical Disorder

John Q. Young, M.D., M.P.P.
Stuart J. Eisendrath, M.D.

John Q. Young, M.D., M.P.P., is Clinical Instructor of Psychiatry in the Department of Psychiatry at the University of California, San Francisco. He serves as the Assistant Director of the Adult Psychiatry Clinic and the Associate Director of the Residency Training Program. He directs the pharmacotherapy clinics at the Langley Porter Psychiatric Hospital and Clinics and oversees the teaching of psychophathology, diagnosis, and therapeutics in the residency program. He has a long-standing interest in the diagnostic and treatment challenges presented by abnormal illness behavior. He also has an active interest in cognitive therapy for schizophrenia. His current research focuses on the impact of the Medicare Part D benefit on patients who have both Medicaid and Medicare.

Stuart J. Eisendrath, M.D., is Professor of Clinical Psychiatry at the University of California, San Francisco. He is also Director of Clinical Services at Langley Porter Psychiatric Hospital and Clinics. He has a long-standing interest in somatoform and factitious disorders and has developed therapeutic strategies for this challenging population. He also serves as Director of the Depression Center at Langley Porter, which is devoted to developing evidence-based treatment programs for major depression.

ANNIE, A 34-YEAR-OLD, single, Asian, female pharmacist, was transported by ambulance to the emergency department of the hospital where she worked. Her evaluation in the emergency department noted a mild delirium that cleared shortly after she was admitted to the medical inpatient unit of the hospital. Laboratory studies confirmed her third episode of life-threatening pancytopenia (i.e., deficiency in blood cells) within the past 6 months. The hematology staff recommended a bone marrow transplant. However, Annie was reluctant to pursue this, stating she did not deserve such a costly treatment. Because Annie was noted to be tearful and depressed and reported recent minimal food intake, the hematology staff requested a psychiatric consultation.

HISTORY

The hospital chart revealed that Annie had her first episode of pancytopenia 6 months prior to this admission. A bone marrow biopsy had shown severe hypocellularity, which was initially attributed to a viral syndrome. She experienced a spontaneous remission soon after the diagnosis, which was atypical for such cases. However, 2 months later, the pancytopenia recurred. A repeat bone marrow biopsy led to a diagnosis of aplastic anemia. Treatment included antithymocyte globulin, methylprednisolone, cyclosporine, erythropoietin, granulocyte colony-stimulating factor (G-CSF), and transfusions. She responded to these measures. However, 3 months later, she experienced a sudden relapse of pancytopenia (her third episode in 6 months), leading to loss of consciousness and her current admission.

When the illness course was reviewed with her hematologist, he noted several atypical features. He was first puzzled because a sudden relapse in aplastic anemia is unusual. He was also puzzled by Annie's account that she had a period of alopecia, which he had never seen in aplastic anemia cases. This is, however, commonly seen in patients on chemotherapeutic agents.

During the psychiatric consultation, it was noted that Annie's illness enabled her to avoid sexual intimacy with her boyfriend. Her psychiatric history included two hospitalizations for anorexia, dramatic fluctuations in weight (ranging between 87 and 150 pounds), and a documented history of laxative and diuretic abuse. She admitted that she had enjoyed deceiving the nurses by continuing to engage in bingeing and purging behavior during these hospitalizations. During one admission, it was reported in Annie's chart that she had expressed a desire "to be taken care of like a child." At the time the aplastic anemia was diagnosed, she was in outpatient psychotherapy with a social worker to whom she revealed that as a child, while being physically and emotionally abused by her mother, she had made a suicide pact with her sister to die by poison ingestion by her thirty-fifth birthday.

Annie described frequent hospitalizations for pneumonia as a child. She had enjoyed the hospital care as a reprieve from her mother's abuse. She received not only positive attention from the medical staff but also from her otherwise abusive parents. During college, she acknowledged that she had ingested excessive aspirin to induce hematemesis and anemia, which required hospitalization. She also acknowledged once having taken furosemide (a strong diuretic) prior to running a marathon to induce hypovolemia. She collapsed during the race. She reported feeling like "I was committing suicide in front of all those people while everyone watched and no one knew what I was doing."

Annie lived alone and had never been involved in a sexual relationship, although she did have a boyfriend. Annie's sister was contacted and confirmed that their mother had been abusive towards both of them during childhood. The sister also reported that, in the month prior to Annie's most recent illness, one of Annie's colleagues had been diagnosed with leukemia and two of her friends had died, one by suicide. Around this same time, Annie's boyfriend had begun to pressure her for sexual intimacy. They were now estranged, after he accused her of causing her illness through careless occupational exposure. Annie denied using alcohol and nonprescription drugs. Her family history revealed the probability of bipolar disorder in her mother.

The psychiatric consultant called Annie's psychotherapist. The therapist disclosed that Annie had revealed to her that she had ingested busulfan at the time of the initial diagnosis of an anemia problem. The nonmedical therapist did not realize that busulfan was a bone marrow ablative medication used in chemotherapy, and Annie had minimized the significance of the ingestion in her discussion with her. Annie also misled the therapist into believing that the hematologist had been informed of the busulfan ingestion.

DIAGNOSIS

As the consultation unfolded, factitious disorder with predominantly physical signs and symptoms emerged as the most likely diagnosis for Annie. This case highlights the crucial role that collateral information often plays in the diagnosis of factitious disorder. Collateral information was especially helpful in determining that Annie's symptom production was conscious and willful. By speaking with Annie's therapist, the consultant had discovered historical data suggesting the intentional (and hidden) production of a physical disorder—in this case, severe bone marrow suppression by ingestion of a chemotherapeutic agent. In addition to the information regarding busulfan, Annie's history contained a number of features that commonly indicate the conscious production of symptoms (Eisendrath and McNiel 2002). The course of the physical illness had been atypical. Her illness repeatedly did not follow the natural history of the presumed disease, with spontaneous remission and then recurrence after successful treatment. Annie also demonstrated physical signs, such as alopecia, that were inconsistent with the presumed disease process. As we saw later in the case, physical evidence of a factitious etiology (e.g., syringe, surreptitious medication) was discovered. In some cases of factitious disorder, direct observation of illness-inducing behavior is made. In the absence of this kind of data, the patient's intentionality is inferred after a long process of diagnostic and treatment interventions have failed to find any physiological explanation for the symptoms.

Other factors associated with factitious disorder were also evident in Annie's case. Descriptive studies have identified two variants of factitious disorder: Munchausen syndrome and a non-Munchausen variant. Munchausen syndrome refers to the much less common (less than 10% of those with factitious disorder) but more famous variant. These patients are mostly male, socially isolated, and unemployed; have antisocial traits; and serially present at one hospital after another with fantastic tales. The non-Munchausen variant is much more common and usually less striking in presentation. These patients are typically employed, educated, and socially connected. Like Annie, they are typically women in their third or fourth decade of life with a history of a health-related occupation (Krahn et al. 2003). Patients often have a symptom model—a prototype that informs the psychological generation of the condition (e.g., Annie's co-worker who was recently diagnosed with leukemia). In addition, patients with factitious disorder frequently have a history of recent loss (e.g., the death of Annie's two friends), multiple somatic complaints that are unexplained or out of proportion to the presenting biomedical disease, prior factitious disease (e.g., Annie's aspirin-induced hematemesis or furosemide-induced hypovolemia), and childhood illness with primary gain (e.g., Annie's frequent pneumonia requiring tertiary care and resulting in positive attention from otherwise abusive parents). It is not uncommon for an intimate associate of the patient to express suspicion about the disease etiology, as did Annie's boyfriend.

As we will explore in more depth, Annie's motive centered around the primary gain of experiencing the psychological benefits of the sick role. External incentives (secondary gain) such as economic gain or avoiding legal responsibility did not appear to be present in Annie's case; if they were, the diagnosis would be malingering rather than factitious disorder. The process of distinguishing primary from secondary gains is not always straightforward. For example, Annie's avoidance of sexual activity might have constituted a primary or secondary gain, depending on the context. In Annie's case, she used factitious behavior to manage her psychological conflicts around sexual intimacy, which constitutes primary gain. The malingering patient generally will not endure significant secondary loss, such as invasive medical procedures or permanent disability (Eisendrath 1996). In contrast, factitious disorder patients will endure significant secondary loss, including somatic dysfunction and loss of a self-esteem–enhancing career. For these patients, the primary gain (e.g., permanent sick role with dependency gratifications) outweighs the secondary losses (e.g., bilateral avascular hip necrosis from corticosteroid treatment) (Eisendrath and McNiel 2004).

TREATMENT

Eventually Annie was discharged to a new psychotherapist familiar with medical problems who collaborated with a psychiatrist in managing her care. The therapist's familiarity with medical problems facilitated 1) collaboration with the multiple medical specialists involved, 2) recognition and appropriate treatment of psychologically generated physical complaints, and 3) effective advocacy for restraint and caution among medical specialists who may have deemed it necessary to subject Annie to unnecessary medical interventions. Several important themes emerged from Annie's case: symptom production to meet dependency needs and avoid sexual intimacy, and reenactment (of childhood trauma in the form of illness production) to master the trauma.

The treatment for factitious disorder has developed significantly over the past decades. Shortly after Asher (1951) identified Munchausen syndrome, case reports became more and more common. The idea of maintaining a blacklist of Munchausen patients emerged that would allow hospitals and clinics to exclude these patients from care. For ethical reasons, this idea never became a major tool in managing these disorders.

For most factitious disorder patients, psychological interventions are necessary. The literature suggests that these are rarely effective for the severe end of the factitious disorder spectrum (Munchausen syndrome) but offer more success for the less severe and more common non-Munchausen cases. Annie, who did not have the extensive wandering from specialist to specialist, the sociopathy, and the continuous patienthood of Munchausen syndrome, appeared to represent a non-Munchausen factitious disorder case. Moreover, she had a stable social system and job, which are also uncommon in Munchausen syndrome.

The evidence for the effectiveness of treatments in dealing with factitious disorders is limited. No randomized trials have been undertaken to date. Most of the data available are drawn from retrospective chart reviews and case histories. Some experts advocate nonpunitive confrontation (Hollender and Hersch 1970). In one variation of this approach, the primary physician reveals the diagnosis of factitious disorder to the patient. After reviewing the findings that led to this conclusion, the physician suggests that the patient must be experiencing great distress to use this coping strategy. The psychiatrist then interprets the patient's factitious behavior as a cry for help. Finally, psychiatric treatment is offered to provide the patient with a more adaptive way of coping with his or her stressors. Some patients have benefited from intensive psychoanalytically oriented psychotherapy (Plassman 1994; Schoenfeld et al. 1987). These therapies often use the factitious physical symptoms as metaphorical communications from the patient, with less emphasis on detecting the origin of the symptom (Mayo and Haggerty 1984).

Although this and other similar approaches have some merit, clinical experience has suggested that these approaches are not effective for most patients. Even when presented with incontrovertible evidence, most patients will not admit to the factitious nature of their disorder. For example, in one of the larger case series reported, Reich and Gottfried (1983) noted that less than one-sixth of the patients admitted the factitious etiology after being confronted with evidence of the disease, and only a small fraction of those patients appeared to have benefited from the confrontation in long-term follow-up. A recent retrospective case review of 93 patients with factitious disorder replicated these findings (Krahn et al. 2003); that group reported that 76% of patients in their cohort were confronted and only 17% of those confronted acknowledged their role. Many patients will experience the confrontation as humiliating and terminate treatment soon thereafter.

A role for confrontation does exist, however, in the treatment of factitious disorders. Nonconfrontational approaches are not practical in emergent situations. Some patients may create a life-threatening disorder that demands authoritative intervention. In Annie's case, there was insufficient time for the nonconfrontational approaches, which are described in detail below. Instead, the psychiatric consultant organized a multidisciplinary team meeting including representation from hematology, nursing, social work, and the hospital attorney. Because of concerns that Annie might have continuing access to bone marrow ablative agents, a decision was made to confront her and ask permission to search her room. When she was confronted with the information that had been obtained, Annie admitted to having ingested 4 mg of busulfan before her first emergency room visit and then feigning compliance with outpatient granulocyte colony-stimulating factor therapy by injecting herself with saline. She consented to a room search that revealed some syringes with benzodiazepines. She later revealed that she had obtained busulfan from the medical floor on which she was employed and ingested 10–12 $mg{\cdot}kg^{-1}{\cdot}day^{-1}$ over a period of many months. The ablative dose is 16 $mg{\cdot}kg^{-1}{\cdot}day^{-1}$ for 4 days. She also disclosed that she had been surreptitiously using oral and intravenous furosemide to regulate her weight and fluid retention.

In this case, the confrontation was both necessary and effective in medically stabilizing the patient's condition and averting a life-threatening situation. Annie reacted well to the confrontation with some apparent sense of relief that her secret was out. Her admission was somewhat anticlimactic because she was so critically ill. Her illness also precluded the possibility of her leaving the hospital, unlike some patients who might have been physically able to leave. In nonemergency situations, strategies that emphasize saving face over confrontation are often more effective. These strategies encourage the patient to relinquish the factitious symptom but allow the patient to do so without admitting to the fabrication (Klonoff et al. 1983–1984). The treatment team does not argue with the patient about the origins of the symptom (e.g., paraplegia, seizures) but accepts the symptom as needing treatment (Solyom and Solyom 1990). Positive reinforcements for the factitious behavior are minimized and healthy behavior is rewarded. Regular medical visits that are not contingent on symptoms are one example of this approach (Smith et al. 1986). A treatment is offered to allow the patient to gain control over the symptom, such as biofeedback or massage.

Other nonconfrontational approaches have been described in the literature, including inexact interpretations and "double binds" (Eisendrath 1989). Inexact interpretations are correct, but incomplete, in that they capture much of the psychodynamics of the patient's abnormal behavior without identifying the factitious nature. For example, one female patient was guilt ridden as a consequence of childhood sexual abuse. Whenever her romantic relationships turned sexual, she developed abdominal pain; however, multiple medical workups identified no organic etiology. During an inpatient evaluation, her boyfriend proposed marriage. That night she developed unexplained septicemia, as she had on two prior hospitalizations. The psychiatric consultant suggested to her that "she might feel a need to punish herself when good things, like the engagement, happened in her life." The patient readily agreed with the interpretation. Several days later, she revealed that, because of her guilty feelings, she had injected a foreign substance intravenously after her boyfriend proposed. She then entered outpatient psychotherapy that increased her capacity to tolerate intimate relationships with less guilt (Eisendrath and Young 2005).

The therapeutic double bind represents a similar nonconfrontational technique. The team offers the patient another intervention, such as a new medication or minor procedure (e.g., split thickness graft for a nonhealing wound, hypnosis, biofeedback). The offer includes a bind. The patient is informed that the factitious disorder is now in the differential diagnosis and if the patient does not respond to this treatment, the team will have to conclude that the disorder is factitious. If, on the other hand, the illness responds to the intervention, this diagnosis will not be made. Many patients, when given this choice, will stop the factitious behavior after the intervention rather than have their disorder be labeled factitious.

It is important to note that the interventions discussed do not address the underlying intrapsychic and interpersonal pathology. Rather, these interventions have the much more limited goals of symptomatic improvement and engaging the patient in treatment. Once the patient is engaged, either through confrontation or nonconfrontation, the foundation has been laid for the longer-term goal of psychotherapeutic change.

Patients with factitious disorder often have concurrent Axis I disorders such as a major depressive, anxiety, substance abuse, or eating disorder. The presence of major depression improves the likelihood of the patient's being responsive to treatment (Earle and Folks 1986). In our case, once medically stabilized, Annie was transferred to the inpatient psychiatry department for treatment of the depression that had become manifest during her medical treatment. She was given a selective serotonin reuptake inhibitor and her depression remitted.

Longer-term treatment uses psychodynamic, cognitive, and behavioral approaches in helping the patient to understand the underlying conflicts and needs that lead to the factitious-illness behaviors and then learn more adaptive ways of meeting those needs. Factitious disorder patients often have comorbid cluster B personality disorders (i.e., antisocial, borderline, histrionic, and narcissistic personality disorders) and use mastery, masochism (self-destructive behavior), and dependency as defenses.

DISCUSSION

Careful attention to countertransference is critical in treating patients with factitious disorder. The patient gains the attention of the caregivers by assuming the sick role, a role sanctioned by society for people who have a disease and want to recover. When the health care team discovers that the patient has violated this contract, the patient, not the disease, becomes the antagonist. In Annie's case, once the diagnosis had been confirmed, the treatment team experienced intense emotions, including betrayal about the deception and resentment over the time and resources expended to treat Annie. If these feelings are not acknowledged, normalized, and contained, it is more likely that the staff will act out the countertransference through premature discharge or inappropriate medical decisions. In this case, the psychiatric consultant organized several team meetings in which staff were invited to explore and ventilate feelings of anger, betrayal, and resentment. The other physicians and nurses were educated about factitious disorder as a disease, which helped the staff to view the patient as having a serious psychiatric disease.

Gains made by patients undergoing treatment for factitious disorder are often modest. Over the 5 years after the diagnosis of factitious disorder and undergoing the interventions described above, Annie did not again intentionally induce aplastic anemia. This life-threatening factitious illness behavior stopped. However, other types of factitious disorder behavior continued. She had at least three hospitalizations for polymicrobial sepsis. The microbiology results strongly suggested these were the result of fecal contamination of her central line.

This case also illustrates how the long-term sequelae of factitious behavior are often severe. After the diagnosis of factitious disorder, Annie was hospitalized 20 times for treatment of the complications related to factitious aplastic anemia, including bilateral hip replacement due to avascular necrosis from corticosteroid treatment. The total cost of Annie's medical treatment for aplastic anemia and its sequelae exceeded $1 million.

REFERENCES

Asher R: Munchausen's syndrome. Lancet 1:339–341, 1951

Earle JR, Folks DG: Factitious disorder and coexisting depression: a report of successful psychiatric consultation and case management. Gen Hosp Psychiatry 8:448–450, 1986

Eisendrath SJ: Factitious physical disorders: treatment without confrontation. Psychosomatics 30:383–387, 1989

Eisendrath SJ: When Munchausen becomes malingering: factitious disorders that penetrate the legal system. Bull Am Acad Psychiatry Law 23:471–481, 1996

Eisendrath SJ, McNiel DE: Factitious disorders in civil litigation: twenty cases illustrating the spectrum of abnormal illness-affirming behavior. J Am Acad Psychiatry Law 30:391–399, 2002

Eisendrath SJ, McNiel DE: Factitious physical disorders, litigation, and mortality. Psychosomatics 45:350–353, 2004

Eisendrath SJ, Young JQ: Factitious physical disorders: a review, in Somatoform Disorders. Edited by Maj M, Akiskal H, Mezzich J, et al. New York, John Wiley & Sons, 2005

Hollender MD, Hersh SR: Impossible consultation made possible. Arch Gen Psychiatry 23:343–345, 1970

Klonoff EA, Youngner SJ, Moore DJ, et al: Chronic factitious illness: a behavioral approach. Int J Psychiatry Med 13:73–83, 1983–1984

Krahn LE, Hongzhe L, O'Connor MKL: Patients who strive to be ill: factitious disorder with physical symptoms. Am J Psychiatry 160:1163–1168, 2003

Mayo JP, Haggerty JJ: Long-term therapy of Munchausen's syndrome. Am J Psychother 38:571–578, 1984

Plassmann R: Inpatient and outpatient long-term psychotherapy of patients suffering from factitious disorder. Psychother Psychosom 62:96–107, 1994

Reich P, Gottfried LA: Factitious disorders in a teaching hospital. Ann Intern Med 99:240–247, 1983

Schoenfeld H, Margolin J, Baum S: Munchausen syndrome as a suicide equivalent: abolition of syndrome by psychotherapy. Am J Psychother 49:604–612, 1987

Smith GR, Monson RA, Ray DC. Psychiatric consultation in somatization disorder: a randomized controlled study. N Engl J Med 314:1407–1413, 1986

Solyom C, Solyom L: A treatment program for functional paraplegia/Munchausen syndrome. J Behav Ther Exp Psychiatry 21:225–230, 1990

PART X

Dissociative Disorders

CHAPTER 23

Melinda Who?

Treating Dissociative Identity Disorder

Richard P. Kluft, M.D.
Richard J. Loewenstein, M.D.
Daphne Simeon, M.D.

Richard P. Kluft, M.D., is Clinical Professor of Psychiatry at Temple University School of Medicine. He practices psychiatry and psychoanalysis in Bala Cynwyd, Pennsylvania. He has treated over 160 dissociative identity disorder patients to the point of integration. He founded and directed the Dissociative Disorders Program at The Institute of Pennsylvania Hospital (1989–1996). Dr. Kluft has authored over 200 publications on the natural history, diagnosis, and treatment of dissociative identity disorder; the nature and stability of the process of integration; the accuracy and management of traumatic memories; and many other dissociation-related topics. He has developed numerous techniques now widely used in the psychotherapy of dissociative identity disorder. He edited *Childhood Antecedents of Multiple Personality* and (with Catherine G. Fine, Ph.D.) *Clinical Perspectives on Multiple Personality Disorder*. He was formerly the Editor-in-Chief of *Dissociation* and is currently the Clinical Forum Editor for the *International Journal of Clinical and Experimental Hypnosis* and is Advisory Editor for the *American Journal of Clinical Hypnosis*.

Richard J. Loewenstein, M.D., is a senior psychiatrist and the Medical Director of the Trauma Disorders Program at Sheppard Pratt Health Systems, Baltimore, Maryland, which was ranked by U.S. News and World Report as one of America's 10 top psychiatric facilities. He is also Associate Clinical Professor of Psychiatry and Behavioral Sciences at the University of Maryland School of Medicine. He is a graduate of the University of California, Berkeley and Yale University School of Medicine, where he did his residency. After a research fellowship at the National Institute of Mental Health in Bethesda, Maryland, he spent 5 years at the University of California, Los Angeles and the West Los Angeles VA Medical Center.

Dr. Loewenstein is the author of over 50 papers and book chapters on sleep disorders, consultation-liaison psychiatry, dissociation, dissociative disorders, and trauma disorders. He has written a chapter on treatment of dissociative amnesia and fugue for the American Psychiatric Association's second and third editions of *Treatment of Psychiatric Disorders*. He is coauthor of the section on dissociative disorders in *Kaplan and Sadock's Comprehensive Textbook of Psychiatry*, 8th Edition. He is the founder and Director of the Trauma Disorders Program at Sheppard Pratt Hospital, including a 20-bed inpatient unit, a day hospital program, an outpatient program, a postdoctoral fellowship program, and research, consultation and teaching components.

Daphne Simeon, M.D., is Associate Professor of Psychiatry at the Mount Sinai School of Medicine, New York. She has conducted extensive research in the field of dissociative disorders. After graduating from medical school and completing her psychiatric residency at Columbia University in New York City, she received a National Institute of Mental Health–sponsored research fellowship at Columbia University/New York State Psychiatric Institute. She is also a graduate and faculty member of the Columbia Psychoanalytic Institute. In 1994 she joined the Mount Sinai School of Medicine faculty, where she served as Director for Medical Student Education in Psychiatry until 2000.

For over 10 years Dr. Simeon has conducted clinical research in the field of dissociation. She currently cochairs an international task force appointed by the International Society for the Study of Dissociation that will generate new recommendations for the DSM-V classification of dissociative disorders. She is an internationally recognized expert in depersonalization disorder and is author of *Feeling Unreal: Depersonalization and the Loss of Self* (2006).

HISTORY

Carole, a 36-year-old, married, Caucasion, speech-language pathologist, began outpatient treatment with me (R.P.K.) after she had a series of baffling and medically serious suicide attempts by massive ingestions, each resulting in psychiatric hospitalization. Carole had no recall of the attempts or their precipitants; the first occurred shortly after her daughter's third birthday. Carole described experiencing several weeks of tearfulness, early morning awakening, and reduced appetite prior to each attempt but did not recall feeling suicidal. She reported that her marriage was stable, she enjoyed her lovely daughter, and she was pleased with her career. As her inpatient psychiatrist, I could neither engage her in treatment nor persuade her to accept a comprehensive medical and neurological workups. She never followed up with recommended outpatient care.

I was genuinely surprised when Carole made an appointment for psychotherapy. At the appointment, her customary pleasant and smiling demeanor rapidly crumbled. Crying and trembling, she said she believed she was going crazy and that her world was coming apart. She found the thought of sex intolerable, which led to stress in her marriage. She was uncomfortable bathing and dressing her daughter. Carole had unwelcome "flashes" of her daughter's being sexually violated and was disgusted to find herself experiencing the urge to touch her daughter's genitals. Men's attention toward herself made her feel she was "dirty," "a whore and a slut." Friends confronted her about forgetting what she had said to them, arrangements she had made with them, and things they had done together. She was mortified that a handsome neighbor had blown her a kiss.

DIAGNOSIS

My psychiatric evaluation of Carole elicited a wide range of depressive symptoms. It was easy to make the diagnosis of major depressive disorder, recurrent, moderate intensity. Carole agreed to psychopharmacology and was begun on fluoxetine 20 mg/day.

The revelation that Carole was experiencing recurrent episodes of dense amnesia suggested to me that she might have a chronic but previously covert dissociative disorder. The inexplicable changes in Carole's behavior toward her daughter raised the possibility that Carole may have been involved in some disremembered activities of a sexual nature. Carole's being flooded by disruptive sexual images and ideas and afflicted with both avoidant and intrusive symptoms with sexual themes raised concerns that she had experienced some form of sexual mistreatment and might be developing the delayed onset of posttraumatic stress symptoms. Overall, Carole's presentation suggested to me that she should be evaluated for a posttraumatic state with profound dissociative symptomatology, long clandestine, but currently decompensating and becoming overtly symptomatic.

I asked her some screening questions. Did she have experiences of watching herself as she went through life events? Had she ever felt she did not look like herself in the mirror? Had she ever found articles among her possessions she did not recall acquiring? Reluctantly, she acknowledged such experiences.

To help clarify her situation, I administered the Dissociative Experiences Scale (Bernstein and Putnam 1986), which measures the extent to which patients experience 28 dissociative phenomena. Scores of 30 or more are typically found in patients with dissociative identity disorder (DID) and related forms of dissociative disorder not otherwise specified (DDNOS). Carole scored 37.

Patients with DID and those forms of DDNOS that are similar to DID but that fail to meet its full diagnostic criteria are highly hypnotizable. I checked Carole's Spiegel Eye-Roll score; high scores on this measure co-occur with high hypnotizability (Spiegel and Spiegel 1978). The eye-roll is scored from 0 to 4 based on how much of the iris is visible when a patient, having looked up as if looking through the top of his or her head, is asked to let his or her eyelids flutter down and close. If the iris is completely visible when the lids begin to descend, the score is 0. If only sclera, the white part of the eye, is visible, the score is 4. Carole's received the maximum score of 4, suggesting the presence of high hypnotizability.

I administered the Structured Clinical Interview for the Diagnosis of DSM-IV Dissociative Disorders, Revised (SCID-D-R; Steinberg 1994). Carole's scores for amnesia, depersonalization, derealization, identity confusion, and identity alteration were at the maximal level. For example, she was aware of inner voices, which she experienced as originating within her own head, and reported that at times other people had addressed her by different names as if they had known her by those different names. Carole reported that while at a convention, she returned to her hotel room to find a dozen long-stemmed red roses in a vase with an accompanying note thanking "Melinda" for a wonderful time. She was puzzle, mortified, and irate. "Melinda!" Carole raged, "Melinda who?"

Several times people she did not know had addressed her as Melinda.

She associated one of the voices she tried to block out with "Melinda." During the SCID-D-R, Carole's face underwent striking transitions, including assuming very angry, very fearful, and frankly seductive expressions. She also reported feeling "unreal" and "outside of her body" and had limited recall of the content of the interview.

These findings were strongly suggestive of DID or a related form of DDNOS. We discussed the likely dissociative disorder diagnosis and its treatment implications (an overall consent that included the use of hypnosis and imagery should it appear to be useful). As part of my obtaining Carole's informed consent for treatment, we discussed the controversies that surround dissociative disorders. Carole understood my opinions that DID occurred naturalistically but could worsen and be complicated by inappropriate interventions, but that in view of her repetitive serious disremembered suicide attempts, the risk that she might die of an untreated dissociative disorder argued strongly for proceeding.

TREATMENT

Carole did not want to acknowledge having any mental disorder, but she was worried. We agreed to meet weekly, keep a supportive focus, and manage medications for her moderate recurrent major depression. After 3 weeks of her taking fluoxetine 30 mg/day, her depressive symptoms were largely in remission. It soon became clear that other alternate identities ("alters"), without acknowledging their activities and without being elicited or confronted by me, were making appearances in sessions. Usually Carole would begin to have a headache and then an apparent transition ("switch") would follow. When Carole regained awareness of her circumstances after a period of amnesia, she would feel headachy, confused, anxious, and uncertain about what had occurred.

During one session, after Carole had complained about finding a bright yellow (and uncharacteristically revealing) outfit in her closet, she seemed to fade away, stating, with a flirtatious demeanor and different voice, "It's my color. And it looks better on me." As Carole resumed her usual demeanor, she shook her head sadly and told me, "I keep trying to tell myself she can't be real. I'm so ashamed that she is part of me. I guess you just met Melinda." Within minutes, Carole was insisting that there was no such person as "Melinda" and no such condition as DID. She cancelled her next session.

When she returned a month later, Carole steeled herself to tell me some facts she had always remembered but tried to push out of her mind. As a youngster she had masturbated compulsively, even in public, despite being disciplined by teachers and ridiculed by her classmates. She had been reproached for initiating sexual explorations with male classmates. She had been sent to a doctor about this.

A few weeks later Carole switched to another alter and told me, "That thing about the doctor's office—it was about what Carole did to her grandfather. Well, actually Melinda did it." This identity stated that Carole had been seduced by her father, who encouraged her to initiate sexual encounters with him to show how much she loved him. Melinda developed as the alter who would contain these experiences and perform these activities. While visiting her maternal grandparents, Melinda had made repeated efforts to unzip her grandfather's fly. Her grandparents shared their concerns with Carole's family doctor, who brought the whole family together in his office. Carole was asked if anything was bothering her, but she remained mute. In our session, Carole said she thought she remembered being in a doctor's office with her parents and grandparents but being unable to speak.

Some of Carol's alters maintained that the visit to the doctor's office was an actual memory that linked what she always recalled about her childhood sexual behavior to the frightening possibility that she had been the victim of incestuous sexual abuse. Other alters ridiculed the idea that any abuse had occurred. Carole wanted to know the truth before plunging into treatment. As Carole equivocated on this issue, she began to have painful flashbacks of incestuous trauma and soon complained of recurrent traumatic nightmares about father-daughter incest. In addition, she tried to avoid all matters and experiences related to sexuality. Her concentration deteriorated, her sleep became disrupted, and she developed a vigorous startle reaction. She developed additional trauma spectrum symptoms as well. Within 6 weeks, Carole fulfilled diagnostic criteria for posttraumatic stress disorder, delayed type.

We discussed the pluses and minuses of prescribing additional medications for her escalating posttraumatic symptoms and sleep disruption. We also discussed nonpharmacological alternatives. Carole was very afraid of taking additional medications. She had witnessed her mother's long-term misuse of prescription tranquilizers and sedatives and had decided against taking such medications in her own treatment. She was taught relaxation techniques and used them with moderate success.

I tried to help Carole appreciate that the purpose of therapy is healing, not investigation, and that the exploration of memory in treatment has to proceed with the realization that apparent memory can be a mixture of the recalled and the reconstructed and is vulnerable to distortions and compromised accuracy in the registration, retention, and retrieval of autobiographical events. Therapy routinely deals with materials of unknown accuracy.

I understood that defensive self-interest might render Carole's parents questionable informants. As an only child of two only children, there were no siblings or cousins who might be useful resources. Carole's grandparents were deceased and her parents were divorced. Her father had broken ties with the family when he remarried. Carole had severed her relationship with her alcoholic mother after her mother drained Carole's bank account of her tuition money, forcing Carole to drop out of school.

I learned enough about the doctor's office from Carole's alters to determine its location. With Carole's permission, I telephoned the doctor. Now near retirement, he recalled meeting with Carole's family 40 years earlier. At the time he had believed Carole was being mistreated, but without an actual accusation or admission, he felt unable to act. The family rapidly left his practice.

Carole was now willing to proceed with therapy and we formed an unusually solid therapeutic alliance. We discussed the three-stage model of trauma treatment and its application to dissociative disorders. We agreed to begin strengthening and stabilizing her and trying to contain dysfunctional behaviors (stage 1). Once this was accomplished, we would explore her recollections of her life and process whatever we found (stage 2), aiming to reduce disruptive and intrusive symptomatic manifestations of the past to the status of painful memories.

When this material was no longer interfering with her functioning and disrupting her life, we would consider pursuing integration (stage 3). I reviewed the potential benefits and liabilities of the use of hypnosis and imagery as adjunctive modalities and again obtained informed consent from Carole for their use. We discussed the fact that although treatment itself might provoke some crises and the consequential risk of self-harm to Carole, in the absence of such treatment it was likely that Carole's serious suicide attempts would continue, with grave risk of her being successful in her self-destruction. Carole agreed to go forward, even while hearing her father's voice inside her head cursing and threatening to hurt her if anything negative about him was said.

Carol's agreement to pursue psychotherapy was reluctant and grim. She understood that she needed a treatment that would expose her to what she had spent her life avoiding. She wanted to deny that she had ever been abused and convince herself that she had had a normal and loving family, but she knew this wish was challenged by facts she could not deny. She appreciated that treatment might be difficult and painful.

We agreed to meet for two 45-minute sessions each week and to schedule occasional double sessions when we were working with painful and potentially destabilizing issues. It is very difficult for most DID patients to feel safe and move forward with a single, conventional-length session per week. Problems in their contemporary lives must be addressed and intervals of a week or more between sessions while working on traumatic material often leaves them feeling overwhelmed, without sufficient support or continuity. This is especially true in the beginning stages of treatment for patients whose alters are involved in dysfunctional behaviors that threaten the patients' safety and stability.

We began to bring additional alters into the therapeutic alliance and develop self-soothing and self-protective techniques. Additional historical and traumatic material continued to emerge spontaneously. Whenever possible, we deferred its exploration, lest we inadvertently precipitate an intense abreaction, revivification, or period of disruptive flashbacks.

Carole learned cognitive and autohypnotic techniques to ground herself when she felt she was slipping into an altered state, dialog with alters whose concerns were beginning to be expressed by intrusive symptoms or painful memories, ask for assistance from other alters in resolving contemporary memory gaps, create "safe place" imagery so that alters whose responses to current issues were unsettling could imagine themselves safely removed from contemporary stressors, and put unsettled self-states to sleep in a safe place if their emotional reactions or impulses to take action were problematic.

Carole practiced these techniques until she could use them rapidly and efficiently. She showed a tenacity uncommon in DID patients, many of whom panic and feel helpless when urged to master self-soothing approaches and are upset when they find that these methods are neither instantaneously nor inevitably successful. These techniques gradually increased Carole's sense that she could achieve mastery over her difficulties.

Often in the treatment of DID, the therapist elicits material from alters that are cooperative with treatment only to have those alters that oppose the treatment, often identified with persons in the patient's life thought to be abusive or iconic representations of evil intent (e.g., the devil, Nazis) punish the cooperative alters by attacking the body, setting the patient up to be exploited or injured, or sabotaging therapeutic and self-soothing efforts.

Therefore, I tried to build rapport with these apparently more negative alters and avoided eliciting materials or evoking affects (such as shame) that would trigger their aggression. These alters were based on

Carole's father and other vaguely identified men who claimed to own Carole and to have the right to make her do anything they wanted her to do. They denied the realities of the victim's helplessness and identified with the aggressor. Feeling distress often prompted them to reaffirm their power and strength by (psychically) hurting other alters and/or the patient's body.

For months we discussed these negative alters' defensive needs. Gradually they realized that they were experiencing flashes of other alters' pain and reassuring themselves by imagining themselves violating several young alters based on Carole as a child or exploiting Melinda. My empathizing with the threats they perceived facilitated their giving permission for the treatment to proceed and contracting not to punish parts working in treatment.

Early in work with these alters, I mapped Carole's system of alters. Some believe that mapping is suggestive and may create iatrogenic complexity, but therapists who are highly effective in treating DID regard mapping as a safety measure. By using mapping, therapists hope to learn what they are up against in terms of the structure and composition of the alter system to allow them to conduct a safer and more circumspect psychotherapy. If beginning trauma work with known alters triggers additional reactions in others as yet unknown, the patient's stability may be jeopardized.

Carole was asked to write her name in the center of a blank piece of paper. I then requested that the other alters either write their names or instruct Carole to write their names (or an "X" or dash, respectively, if alters were nameless or unwilling to give their names) next to the names or parts they experienced as most similar and close to themselves. Ultimately there were 19 names or marks. There were alters based on Carole's father, some "bad men," a good mother, a bad mother, and comforting idealized versions of both maternal grandparents. In addition, there was the sexually aggressive Melinda and a more passive sexual alter, Alice, who believed she must be very sexual because she had been told that she made men want to be sexual with her. Most of the remainder were traumatized child alters that experienced what had befallen them as devastating and abusive. However, one self-state, 3-year-old "Little Carole," believed her parents loved her and that she had never been abused.

I interviewed all of the alters willing to talk to me and asked them to share their stories. Each one offered its own subjective individual history. Many stories were incompatible; for example, Melinda represented herself as her father's willing lover, but several child alters said they had been brutalized to make them submit to the father's demands.

Once I was better informed about the personality system and spectrum of alleged abuses, I asked whether an alter(s) was willing to discuss and process its experiences. Processing a traumatic experience may involve intense discussion, facilitated abreaction, and/or the use of specialized techniques such as hypnosis or eye-movement desensitization and reprocessing. The traumatized child alters were eager to be rid of their pain. It is my practice to start, whenever possible, with an alter that is not carrying as much traumatic material as others, as processing painful material may have unexpected complications. Starting with what appears to be the least amount of potentially disruptive material is a safeguard. Also, beginning trauma work does not mean an exclusive focus on trauma that might overwhelm the patient and neglect contemporary issues. With Carole, perhaps one out of three sessions prioritized trauma work.

In a typical trauma processing session, we briefly reviewed Carole's current situation and requested that any alters aware of concerns that were being overlooked or requiring more urgent attention so inform me. Absent contraindications, I accessed the alter(s) with whose issues we were working. Others would be invited to listen in or turn their attention elsewhere, depending on the clinical circumstances. If an alter that was to work had been hypnotically put to sleep between sessions, hypnosis might be used to access it. We then would begin an emotionally intense processing, often experienced as recurring in the present. The last third of the session was reserved to review and discuss the material and evoked feelings and restabilize the patient. I typically would use hypnotic suggestions to put the alters doing the trauma work and/or those who were disrupted by the trauma work to "sleep" between sessions, thus restoring executive control to the alter that was present at the beginning of the session.

Carole's personalities told and processed their stories. Most shared and worked with apparent experiences of physical, sexual, and psychological mistreatment by Carole's father. We learned that each suicide attempt was correlated with Carole's daughter's reaching the age or encountering a circumstance associated with the initiation or escalation of Carole's own abuse. Toward the end of this process, one alter described sexual misuse by her mother at her father's insistence and had images of Carole's father and other men watching sexual acts between herself and her mother. Although it was not clear whether these referred to actual historical events, these episodes of abuse were processed as well. When personalities that were close to one another had processed their experiences, they tended to begin to integrate into one another and into Carole herself. Sometimes they blended spontaneously, but others required hypnotic suggestions (using imagery of joining) to integrate.

With Melinda and Alice, I first worked toward their developing a better understanding of their origins and defensive purposes and making efforts to reduce their shame and guilt. As a child, Carole came to understand that her father would not be dissuaded from exploiting her, that he would use force if she tried to refuse him, and that he wanted Carole to act in accordance with the rationale he voiced, that it was good for fathers to love their little girls and that little girls should enjoy loving their fathers. Therefore, both alters represented themselves as enjoying sex, and Melinda developed a pattern of being aggressively sexual to reduce the likelihood of being hurt and to exert some degree of control over what occurred. Of course, once this pattern was established, the notion that Alice enjoyed sex convinced her that the sex occurred because she was sexual and wanted it. Thereby her father's exploiting her was reframed as his response to her sexuality, and the idea that her father was good was preserved defensively.

Melinda and Alice initially resisted these reformulations by acting out sexually, including Melinda's behaving provocatively toward me. Over a period of months, this behavior was curtailed. These alters explored the genesis of their behavior patterns, learning about the association between the pain Carole and other alters had been experiencing and the way their own adaptations attempted to mitigate that pain, however dysfunctionally. For example, by taking the stance that the sexual events were pleasurable and of her own free choice, through Melinda and Alice, Carole denied the helplessness of her own circumstances and the full depth of her father's betrayal of her.

The alters based on abusers tried to retain their stance of being completely separate from Carole and others who saw themselves as being mistreated. However, with empathic confrontation, they were able to face and process the experiences that led them to disavow their connection with Carole. Once their apparent memories were processed, they increasingly identified with Carole and other alters.

Some DID patients' alters integrate one by one or in small groups, whereas others' alters remain separate until all or almost all are ready to join together. In Carole's case, there was no spontaneous integration until the material concerning her mother was processed. Thereafter most alters joined spontaneously. Integration of the remaining alters was facilitated by hypnotic suggestion using congenial imagery (streams flowing together).

After 4 years of twice weekly treatment, Carole was integrated and stable. Her marriage was improving. She was pleased with herself and the outcome of treatment. Sessions became weekly, and we anticipated tapering her sessions further. Her fluoxetine had been reduced to a maintenance level of 10 mg/day.

One evening Carole called me. She was very distressed and clearly had been drinking. At the request of her mother's 12-step counselor, Carole had agreed to meet with her mother. As her mother "worked her program," she felt she had to make amends to Carole. Her mother apologized for failing Carole, especially for being unable to protect Carole from her husband's sexual mistreatment and for succumbing to her husband's pressure to perform sexual acts with Carole while he watched. She reminded Carole that her father's work often took him to the Far East, where he was able to engage in sexual acts with children and combinations of partners, and that he tried to recreate these opportunities at home.

Until that moment, Carole had assumed that her painful memories about her mother were merely fantasies. Although these memories had already been processed and no longer disrupted or disturbed her, she had never acknowledged them as real. She accepted her mother's apologies and tried to comfort her. She then told her mother that she recently had begun to have vague recollections of sexual acts between the two of them being performed while other men watched. Carole asked her mother if she knew why she (Carole) might be having them. Her mother hung her head, wept, and said she couldn't make herself talk about it—her therapist told her that she would go crazy if she did.

After talking to her daughter, Carole's mother immediately began to drink again and decompensated. In a letter, she told Carole that for her own mental health, she would not have any further contact with Carole. Carole and I resumed twice weekly therapy sessions. Carole was very distressed. Additional alters were discovered, associated with the experiences noted above. Her fluoxetine was once again titrated upward to 30 mg/day. The next year was spent working through the information obtained from her mother. As we did so, her alters integrated. Then therapy and medication were tapered. She is currently being seen every 3 months in follow-up and continues to take fluoxetine 10 mg/day.

DISCUSSION

Carole experienced considerable turmoil in the course of her treatment, but she appreciated that she was reclaiming herself from the chaos of her illness. Disruptive impulses gradually were relegated to the realm of thought and fantasy, no longer enacted by the various alters. As Carole's alters shared, neared, and joined, Carole found herself able to think more clearly, with fewer blocks and disruptions. She tolerated experiencing her emotions more directly and completely. She never lost the opportunity to remind me that this was a mixed blessing—increased awareness had its benefits but meant difficult matters and painful feelings could not be easily put aside or avoided.

It is always painful to treat someone like Carole. As gratifying as it was to free Carole from the burdens of her past, my empathizing with her pain; her mortification, confusion, acting out under stress, and struggle to sort out how to understand important relationships; and the difficulties associated with what to make of her traumatic memories were challenging, sometimes to the point of being ordeals. As Carole wondered what to make of her memories, I too struggled with the vicissitudes of memory, always trying to avoid imposing premature closure on her uncertainties and doubts and to be cautious and circumspect lest I seem to be imposing a particular conclusion upon her.

Carole's treatment was typical for DID patients with the strength to engage in definitive rather than supportive psychotherapy. However, in five respects there were differences. First, Carole's comorbid conditions were easily manageable. Her affective disorder remained in remission with psychopharmacology and her posttraumatic stress disorder symptoms resolved along with her DID. Second, although most DID patients demonstrate a degree of parasuicidal behavior, such as self-mutilation, Carole, except for her severe suicide attempts, channeled her distress almost exclusively into sexual behaviors. Third, once committed to the work of the therapy, Carole was less avoidant of facing trauma than most DID patients, many of whom persist in trying to distance themselves from painful material. Fourth, starting treatment with external evidence suggesting that abuse has occurred is not common; it is also uncommon to obtain a perpetrator's confession of abuse and reasonably solid documentation of recovered memories during the course of treatment. Fifth, Carole and I were able to develop an excellent therapeutic alliance and a minimum of negative transference, probably because the external information available early in treatment kept Carole's focus on her relationship with her parents and inhibited developing typical negative transferences to me.

I attribute Carole's rapid and excellent outcome to her strong motivation, her high level of ego strength, the mildness of her comorbidities, and the strong therapeutic alliance that she formed with me. She dedicated herself to recovery and stayed the course despite its inherent discomfort.

REFERENCES

Bernstein E, Putnam FW: Development, reliability, and validity of a dissociation scale. J Nerv Ment Dis 174:727–735, 1986

Spiegel H, Spiegel D: Trance and Treatment: Clinical Uses of Hypnosis. New York, Basic Books, 1978

Steinberg M: Structured Clinical Interview for DSM-IV Dissociative Disorders, Revised. Washington, DC, American Psychiatric Press, 1994

SUGGESTED READINGS

Brown D, Scheflin A, Hammond D: Memory, Trauma Treatment, and the Law. New York, Norton, 1997

Kluft RP: Treatment of multiple personality disorder. Psychiatr Clin North Am 7:9–29, 1984

Kluft RP: Applications of hypnotic interventions. Hypnos 21:205–223, 1994

Kluft RP: Reflections on the traumatic memories of dissociative identity disorder patients, in Truth in Memory. Edited by Lynn S, McConkey K. New York, Guilford, 1998, pp 304–322

Kluft RP: Current issues in dissociative identity disorder. Journal of Practical Psychiatry and Behavioral Health 5:3–19, 1999

Loewenstein RJ: An office mental status examination for complex chronic dissociative symptoms and multiple personality disorder. Psychiatr Clin North Am 14:567–604, 1991

Putnam FW: Diagnosis and Treatment of Multiple Personality Disorder. New York, Guilford, 1989

PART XI

Sexual and Gender Identity Disorders

CHAPTER 24

Chemical Castration

Treatment for Pedophilia

Richard B. Krueger, M.D.
Meg S. Kaplan, Ph.D.

Richard B. Krueger, M.D., is a psychiatrist and the Medical Director of the Sexual Behavior Clinic at New York State Psychiatric Institute. He is Associate Clinical Professor of Psychiatry in the Department of Psychiatry, Columbia University College of Physicians and Surgeons. He received his medical degree from Harvard Medical School in 1977. He consults on sex offenders for the New York State Office of Mental Health. Dr. Krueger's research interests include the study of individuals arrested for crimes against children over the Internet and psychopharmacological treatment of compulsive and aggressive sexual behavior.

Meg S. Kaplan, Ph.D., is a psychologist and the Director of the Sexual Behavior Clinic at the New York State Psychiatric Institute. She is Associate Professor of Clinical Psychology in Psychiatry at Columbia University College of Physicians and Surgeons. She received her doctorate in Human Sexuality from New York University in 1984 and has conducted clinical research in psychosexual disorders since then. Dr. Kaplan was a parole officer for the State of New York for 10 years. Dr. Kaplan was previously on the Board of the Association for the Treatment of Sexual Abusers and is the current Director of the Special Classification Review Board at Avenyl Correctional Facility in New Jersey. She is a reviewer for numerous publications and has authored 50 publications in the sexual disorders field.

ERIC, NOW AGE 37, HAS BEEN a patient of ours for over 20 years. At the time of the initial evaluation, he was age 17 and had been referred to us from a local hospital for treatment of pedophilia. His case is being presented as an illustration of a young man with extraordinary motivation and courage in his long struggle with pedophilia and as someone who has been helped a great deal in this struggle over the last 10 years by antiandrogen medication therapy.

HISTORY

Eric had a troubled childhood. The product of an unwanted pregnancy, he was placed in foster care immediately after birth where he was sexually and physically abused. He was eventually adopted by another family at age 5, where he was also abused. Due to problems that occurred during his delivery, he experienced developmental delays in walking and speaking. His intelligence testing revealed an IQ of 80. Eric was placed in special classes and finished school through the tenth grade.

Eric's inappropriate sexual behavior began at a very young age. From age 5 to 10 years, Eric repeatedly exposed his genitals to his peer-aged adoptive cousins, both male and female. Eric started puberty at age 12; at age 13 he began sexually abusing his younger adoptive brother, age 2 years. This continued repeatedly for 3 years and consisted of fondling his brother's buttocks and performing oral sex on him, at times masturbating to ejaculation during these episodes. This was discovered when Eric reported it to a school counselor, apparently out of guilt. Child Protective Services investigated and reported to the authorities and a decision was made not to prosecute if Eric was admitted to a psychiatric hospital, which occurred when Eric was age 16.

After being hospitalized for 8 months, Eric was discharged to home, where he promptly sexually abused his adoptive parent's biological daughter, age 2. This abuse consisted of fondling her genitals while masturbating to ejaculation. He was arrested, pled guilty, and was sentenced to a juvenile lock-up facility for 3 years, where he sexually abused a 14-year-old male inmate (too impaired to give consent) by performing oral sex on him. At that time, in 1985, specialized therapy was not available in Eric's community and so, at age 17, he was referred to us for an evaluation and consultation.

Prior to beginning our evaluation, we discussed with Eric the limits of confidentiality, indicating that we were mandated to notify child protective services if he disclosed any current abuse of a child. We also indicated to him that he should not mention specifics of prior sexual abuses that were currently unknown to the authorities in a way that could lead to his identification and prosecution.

DIAGNOSIS

During our evaluation, Eric, then age 17, reported that for the past several years he had experienced intense recurrent sexual fantasies, urges, and behaviors involving sexual activity with both male and female children of various ages. Eric also disclosed several past victims unknown to the authorities in addition to those already known.

Our evaluation consisted of interviews, psychometric testing, and objective measurement. Eric underwent penile plethysmography, a procedure in which a male's erectile response is measured as he is presented with a variety of visual or auditory stimuli. The results indicated Eric had significant responses to stimuli involving young children, both male and female, but had a much stronger arousal to young boys. He had much less of a response to teenage and adult males and females.

During the evaluation, Eric also reported for the first time that his foster father had sexually and physically abused him between the ages of 3 and 5 years, once or twice per week, by tying him to a bed and forcing him to place his mouth on his penis. Eric's foster father also engaged in anal penetration, which on one occasion required Eric to have rectal stitches. Eric disclosed that his adoptive mother would routinely beat him with a yardstick, force him to bathe in bleach and on one occasion gave him a black eye. He was also physically abused by his adoptive father by being thrown against a wall, which resulted in a fractured arm, and by being hit on the head. Various studies suggest a high number of child molesters were themselves the victims of child molestation (Finkelhor 1986), and this has been thought to often have etiologic significance. Often male patients who have been sexually abused are exceedingly reluctant to disclose their own abuse, as was the case with Eric. He also reported nightmares and frequent intrusive memories of his own sexual abuse.

Eric also had moderate symptoms of depression that did not fulfill full criteria for a major depressive episode. Because Eric was an adolescent, we decided not to diagnose him as having pedophilia but instead indicated that he had inappropriate sexual interest in young boys and girls. (Because there is no known "cure" for a paraphilia, a patient will carry such a diagnosis throughout his or her life and therefore we are conservative in giving this diagnosis to teenagers. Adolescence is a time of sexual experimentation, and sexual behaviors and interests can change.)

As an adult, however, Eric's sexual interests did not change and we made the following diagnoses: pedophilia, depressive disorder not otherwise specified, posttraumatic stress disorder, and borderline intellectual functioning.

TREATMENT

Cognitive-Behavioral Treatment

Despite his history of molesting children, Eric had an ingratiating and sympathetic quality and a capacity to find caregivers who would look after him. One such caregiver, a psychologist, took an interest in Eric and expressed an interest in learning about cognitive-behavioral therapy (CBT) treatments of sex offenders; subsequently, he and Eric read about CBT modalities used with this population. These modalities were first developed under a National Institute of Mental Health grant to assess and treat child molesters; a manual describing the use of CBT techniques with this population was developed through research (Abel et al. 1984). Some of these techniques are described briefly below.

Eric continued to be hospitalized for the next several years in his local hospital, but he and his psychologist consulted and periodically met with us to receive an assessment and further instruction in CBT treatment. For a year, Eric used these techniques in his local hospital. For example, he learned and used masturbatory satiation, a technique that taught him to use his deviant fantasy postorgasm in a repetitive manner to the point of satiating himself. This treatment is self-administered, tape recorded, and checked by a therapist. Patients find that by masturbating with the deviant fantasy in mind in a repetitive way after ejaculation has occurred, the deviant fantasy is reduced or even becomes boring or repulsive (Abel et al. 1992).

Eric also learned covert sensitization, a technique that involves having the patient imagine various feelings or behaviors that precede a deviant fantasy or behavior and then immediately bring to mind aversive images and negative consequences. This sensitizes the patient to the onset of deviant urges to disrupt the pattern and pair antecedent emotions or behaviors with negative consequences. For example, in one session, Eric described being at home, feeling lonely, and subsequently molesting his landlord's son who had knocked on his door. Eric was then asked to pair these feelings and behaviors with an aversive consequence, such as his landlord walking in, finding him with the landlord's son, and calling the police. This had the aim of helping him recognize and interrupt the urge to abuse a child.

Eric also received instruction in sexual education, cognitive restructuring (a process of confronting and correcting rationalizations that sexual abusers use to justify and maintain their behavior, such as the notion that having sex with a child is a good way for an adult to teach a child about sex), social skills and assertiveness training, and relapse prevention (a self-control program taught to offenders to help them anticipate and cope with high-risk situations that lead to relapse and then to develop strategies to avoid these situations). For example, he was taught to avoid situations that would bring him into the proximity of children, such as schools or playgrounds, and never to be alone with a child, with instructions to leave a room if a child entered it. These are standard CBT techniques that are used to treat paraphilias (Abel et al. 1992).

Most individuals with paraphilias are difficult to treat because they deny their sexual interests, have little or no motivation to change, and seek evaluation and treatment only because of a court mandate. In the case of Eric, we were elated that we finally had a patient who admitted his crimes and his problem, wanted to change, and was remorseful for his previous actions. This dynamic helped him in that we became and remain involved in his treatment despite infrequent contact and his distant location from us.

Two years later, at age 19, Eric was again discharged to live in an apartment complex, but promptly sexually abused his landlord's 14-year-old son by performing oral sex on him. He informed his case manager and was again hospitalized. Eric then remained in a psychiatric hospital for the next 6 years. He practiced behavioral treatments and was seen periodically in consultation by us. He continued to report sexual fantasies about and high arousal toward children as well as toward adults. Both hospital authorities and Eric were fearful of his lack of control and the likelihood that he would continue to victimize children should he be released into the community.

Many individuals with paraphilias try to control their behavior; some succeed but many do not. Although there is no cure for pedophilia or for any sexual preference, because such sexual interests or preferences are extremely difficult to modify, the CBT and relapse-prevention techniques described earlier have as their goal helping individuals reduce and control unwanted sexual impulses and avoid relapse. For some patients, these techniques work well, but for others, even with the best of intentions, they fail. In this regard, these patients are not dissimilar to those who abuse alcohol or other substances and have the best of intentions on discharge from the hospital to refrain from substance use but are unable to control their choices once in the community.

Eric's attempts to control himself were quite remarkable in that despite numerous failures and adverse consequences, he refused to give up. Most patients with pedophilia find their atypical sexual interest and behaviors to be quite pleasurable and ego-syntonic and are extremely reluctant to relinquish them. Indeed, many never do. For others, as with substance addictions, it takes a series of negative consequences to bring them to a point of deciding that they should relinquish such interest and behavior and make their elimination a target of therapy. Earlier in his career, Eric had had many victims and had developed "grooming" routines to acquire victims (i.e., behaviors that sex offenders develop, such as befriending children to gain their confidence and set them up to be victimized later). However, he eventually found that such behavior was ultimately associated with extremely negative consequences (in his case, his chronic confinement to psychiatric facilities), and thus he became motivated to control his behavior.

During the next 6 years, while hospitalized, Eric, through his own efforts and those of his mental health attorney, became aware of "chemical castration" or antiandrogen treatment. He had approached his local hospital caregivers repeatedly for treatment with antiandrogens, but they had indicated that they had no knowledge of or expertise involving these agents and were unwilling to administer them. Finally, Eric initiated a lawsuit to force the hospital to treat him with antiandrogens. To avoid the consequences of the lawsuit, the hospital authorities agreed that Eric be transferred to a hospital where we could evaluate him for antiandrogen treatment.

Initiation of Antiandrogen Treatment

Eric was evaluated for antiandrogen treatment at age 27 in an inpatient setting. This evaluation consisted of a thorough psychiatric history, physical examination, intelligence and neuropsychological testing, a computed tomography scan, karyotyping (which had not been previously done to evaluate his mild mental retardation), a complete blood count, blood chemistries, a urinalysis, and an electrocardiogram, all of which confirmed that he had no unrecognized medical illnesses or contraindications to antiandrogen therapy. The main contraindication to antiandrogen therapy with gonadotropin-releasing hormone (GnRH) analogues is a history of hypersensitivity to GnRH, GnRH agonist analogues, or any of the excipients in the particular preparation used. (The use of GnRH analogues here is described for male patients only. We are not aware of any use of GnRH analogues for this indication in female patients, and the possibility of pregnancy while a female patient is receiving this drug is a contraindication to its use.) In our practice, we also perform a bone density evaluation of patients to assess for the presence of osteopenia (a condition of decreased bone mineralization and density that is a precursor to osteoporosis) or osteoporosis. These entities are relative contraindications, as GnRH agonists can create or worsen them; evaluation and treatment of these disorders might be required before GnRH agonists are administered.

Although several antiandrogen agents are available, a decision was made to use depot leuprolide acetate, which is one of several available GnRH analogues. These agents have been widely used in general medicine for 20 years, principally to reduce sex hormones in patients with cancers that are sensitive to them (e.g., prostate cancer), for various gynecological indications (e.g., endometriosis), or to treat the premature onset of puberty by reducing puberty-related sex hormones. GnRH analogues have the advantage that they can be administered as a depot injection. Various time-release preparations are available that have a duration of action of 1, 3, 4, and, more recently, 12 months.

GnRH analogues work by reducing the release of luteinizing hormone (LH) and follicle-stimulating hormone from the anterior hypothalamus. LH drives production of testosterone by the Leydig cells in the testes; GnRH analogues reduce LH release, which in turn reduces testosterone to essentially castration levels. Concomitant with the reduction in testosterone, there is a reduction in sexual drive and sexually motivated behavior. Side effects are more modest than with earlier available agents, such as estrogen or progesterone, and include mainly hot flashes and hypogonadism (a generic term referring to loss of libido, diminution of an ability to have erections and ejaculations, and a decrease in testicular size and ejaculate volume). It is also important to note that for about the first 2 weeks after the initiation of such therapy, there is a testosterone surge that can be associated with hypersexuality; to prevent this, Eric was treated with flutamide, an antiandrogen, for his first month of therapy. Others have not taken this precaution and reported no problem with initial hypersexuality (Rosler and Witztum 1998). Caution should be exercised in the use of flutamide as it has many side effects, including hepatotoxicity (fatal hepatic necrosis has been reported with this medication). As for all medications discussed in this case, the manufacturer's product labeling and description should be consulted for details and new information.

Within a month, Eric was delighted with the results of this medication. He reported that before the medication, if he saw a child, he rated his control over his sexual urges or behavior at 15% (with 0% representing no control and 100%, total control). He stated that after being on the medication for a month, he felt as though a weight had been lifted from his shoulders and reported 100% control over his behavior. He also reported that before the medication he had an ejaculatory frequency of 14–21 times per week and had sexual thoughts all day long. After receiving the GnRH medication, he reported having 0–1 ejaculations per week and only infrequent sexual thoughts.

Eric was also diagnosed during this hospitalization as having a borderline personality disorder. In fact, he had a history consistent with this diagnosis, with numerous suicidal gestures and attempts, a tendency to be overly dramatic and to exaggerate, and emotional lability, among other things.

Outcome and Follow-Up

We have seen Eric every 2 years since his antiandrogen treatment was initiated. After being on leuprolide acetate for 5 years, Eric was found at age 32 to have developed mild osteopenia (men require testosterone to maintain bone mass just as women require estrogen for the same purpose). This was not recognized in the literature as a significant risk at the time that he was initially treated, but has subsequently been reported in many populations. A recent article has discussed the increased fracture rate in men treated with GnRH agonists (Shahinian et al. 2005).

Eric was started on alendronate sodium, which inhibits bone resorption, and his bone demineralization stopped and then improved. Eric has been followed by his local medical doctor who prescribes the alendronate, measures his testosterone levels, and performs bone density evaluations every year. Eric's testosterone levels have continued to remain low and his osteopenia has improved. Eric initially gained approximately 70 lb over a several-year period (one of the side effects of antiandrogen therapy is weight gain) but has recently lost 40 lb.

For the past 10 years that Eric has been on leuprolide acetate, he says he has continued to have "100% control" over his sexual impulses. He reports that he has not sexually abused anyone since he has been on leuprolide acetate, and there are no reports or suggestions that he has had any other victims. He reports that he has had several girlfriends with whom he has been sexual, inasmuch as he has had an erection and engaged in sexual intercourse, but he has been unable to have an ejaculation for several years. He was discharged from the hospital and has lived in several halfway houses. He has been rehospitalized several times, not for issues of sexual acting out but instead for being suicidal or physically threatening a girlfriend.

Eric continues outpatient therapy at a local mental health clinic and intermittently in structured work or activity situations. Other medications, including various antidepressants, mood stabilizers, and antipsychotics have been tried to treat his mood lability and other aspects of his borderline personality disorder, but have had no significant effect.

Aside from his hospitalizations and progression to discharge, Eric has not had any restrictions on his activity for several years. He continues to receive his leuprolide acetate and is now receiving an injection every 4 months. He reports that he is grateful for this medication and says that he intends to remain on it for the rest of his life. He says that it has saved him from a life of inpatient hospitalization and from victimizing other children. He reports that he has no sexual interest in children, a claim that we have found to be believable. He says that he may notice a child now, but that he is not drawn to him or her. Eric has not found the need to engage in behavioral treatments for many years; sex offender–specific group treatment, which is indicated for patients like Eric, is still not available in the area in which Eric lives, so leuprolide acetate is the main modality of treatment.

DISCUSSION

Eric initially presented as an adolescent who had sexually abused several young children. Although many clinicians will react with revulsion to such a person, Eric has a personality that is likeable and engaging. He was also a sexual and physical abuse survivor and has coped with severe social, intellectual, and psychological limitations. He had not actively chosen to become sexually attracted to children but instead found himself drawn to them and unable to control his urges to abuse them or impaired peers. This behavior and attraction became very ego dystonic and he sought help for his pedophilia. All of these factors engendered positive feelings on our part toward him.

Another aspect of our motivation in working with Eric has been that the treatment of pedophilia, when successful, results in less victimization. Although many in our society are of the opinion that pedophiles should be kept away from society indefinitely, there is a huge cost to warehousing such individuals, and effective treatment is available for some individuals, such as Eric (Fagan et al. 2002).

Eric has had a long and difficult struggle and has so far succeeded in controlling his impulses. We are respectful and admiring of his strength in the face of many limitations, as is the psychologist who has continued to work with him for 20 years. We have been very gratified by Eric's response to leuprolide acetate. We receive periodic letters from him that update us as to his life and in which he reports his various successes and failures, and we look forward to these letters and to our periodic meetings.

REFERENCES

Abel GG, Becker JV, Cunningham-Rathner J, et al: Treatment Manual: The Treatment of Child Molesters. Atlanta, GA, Abel Screening Inc., 1984

Abel GG, Osborn C, Anthony D, et al: Current treatment of paraphiliacs, in Annual Review of Sex Research: An Integrative and Interdisciplinary Review, Vol III. Edited by Bancroft J, Davis CM, Ruppel J, et al. Allentown, PA, The Society for the Scientific Study of Sex, 1992, pp 255–290

Fagan PJ, Wise TN, Schmidt J, et al: Pedophilia. JAMA 288:2458–2465, 2002

Finkelhor D (ed): A Sourcebook on Child Sexual Abuse. Newbury Park, CA, Sage, 1986, pp 102–104

Rosler A, Witztum E: Treatment of men with paraphilia with a long-acting analogue of gonadotropin-releasing hormone. New Engl J Med 338:416–422, 1998

Shahinian VB, Kuo Y-F, Freeman JL, et al: Risk of fracture after androgen deprivation for prostate cancer. New Engl J Med 352:154–164, 2005

SUGGESTED READING

Abel GG: Paraphilias, in Comprehensive Textbook of Psychiatry, 5th Edition. Edited by Kaplan HI, Sadock BJ. Baltimore, Williams & Wilkins, 1989, pp 1069–1085

Abel GG, Becker JV, Cunningham-Rathner J, et al: Multiple paraphilic diagnoses among sex offenders. Bull Am Acad Psychiatry Law 16:153–168, 1988

Association for the Treatment of Sexual Abusers: Professional Code of Ethics. Beaverton, OR, Association for the Treatment of Sexual Abusers, 2001

Bradford JMW: Organic treatment for the male sexual offender. Behav Sci Law 3:355–375, 1985

Gijs L, Gooren L: Hormonal and psychopharmacological interventions in the treatment of paraphilias: an update. J Sex Res 33:273–290, 1996

Krueger RB, Kaplan MS: The paraphilic and hypersexual disorders: an overview. J Psychiatr Pract 7:391–403, 2001

Krueger RB, Kaplan MS: Behavioral and psychopharmacological treatment of the paraphilic and hypersexual disorders. J Psychiatr Pract 8:21–32, 2002

Krueger RB, Kaplan MS: Treatment resources for the paraphilic and hypersexual disorders. J Psychiatr Pract 8:59–60, 2002

CHAPTER 25

"I'm Half-Boy, Half-Girl"

Play Psychotherapy and Parent Counseling for Gender Identity Disorder

Kenneth J. Zucker, Ph.D.

Kenneth J. Zucker, Ph.D., is Professor of Psychiatry and Psychology at the University of Toronto. He is Psychologist-in-Chief at the Centre for Addiction and Mental Health and Head of the Gender Identity Service in the Child, Youth, and Family Program. His major academic interest pertains to psychosexual differentiation and disorders. Dr. Zucker was a member of the DSM-III-R and DSM-IV Subcommittees on Gender Identity Disorder. He is the current President of the International Academy of Sex Research and Editor of *Archives of Sexual Behavior*.

AFTER SEEING A TELEVISION program on which I appeared discussing gender identity problems in children, Brian's father called me in tears, stating that he was concerned about his son.

Brian was a 5-year-old boy (IQ 104) living with his parents and three sisters (two older, one younger). Both his parents were professionals. The father worked full time and the mother remained at home. I conducted a family interview (with the younger sister absent), a joint parental interview, and interviews with each parent and Brian. I also conducted psychological testing of Brian, and his parents completed various questionnaires.

For the family interview, Brian brought along a bag containing his array of female dolls. There were so many of them that he had trouble hauling the bag into the interview room. I recall feeling amused at the sight of Brian struggling to carry the bag; at the same time, I was acutely aware that it was of obvious importance to him that he have his dolls with him. At the outset, I was immediately taken by the high level of familial anxiety. Indeed, the parents and sisters cried at different points (connected to their deep sense of guilt that they had caused Brian's gender identity problem).

Brian struck me as an acutely anxious youngster who tried to contain his anxiety by ordering his parents not to talk. When I began the interview by asking the parents why they had come to see me, Brian exclaimed, "Don't say it!" Later, when I met with Brian individually, I had to resort to monetary incentive to get him to talk about difficult topics and to provide answers other than "I don't know." The reward of one penny for each question answered worked beautifully and Brian was quite proud in earning 25 cents.

HISTORY

At age 18–24 months, Brian began to cross-dress in skirts and was enamored with, and attempted to emulate, idealized female characters such as Snow White and Ariel from The Little Mermaid. His parents felt that Brian had been exposed to a largely female peer group, including his sisters and their girlfriends. Regarding same-age peers, however, the parents said that Brian played with both boys and girls. If he were teased by other children for his cross-gender interests, Brian's general strategy was to fight back verbally by making comments such as, "Oh, they're just stupid." In talking about his peers, Brian commented, "I don't know what boys really do." When asked if he would like to know, he said, "I don't know." As a toddler, one of Brian's older sisters had cross-dressed him (in a ballet tutu) on occasion, which Brian's mother described as "being cute at the time." Brian's mother tearfully commented that his problem was partly her fault because she had not wanted him to be into Ninja Turtles and guns. His father reported that he often overheard Brian stating to himself, "I am a girl," and both parents reported that Brian would frequently declare that he was "both a boy and a girl." I asked Brian's mother to ask him if he wanted to be a girl, to which he replied, "I don't know about that one."

As Brian's cross-gender identification persisted, it became an increasing source of worry for the parents; at the same time, they reported that they had been preoccupied with various other stressors and thus had not addressed it in any formal or systematic way. Brian's mother noted that Brian's cross-gender behavior, at times, made her mad: "There was too much of [it]....I already have girls. I want a boy." At the same time, she expressed ambivalence about his behavior, commenting, "Why if he's a male...is it wrong?"

Regarding the family history, Brian's parents elaborated on familial stressors, including the family's large size, their living in a small home, their serious financial problems, illness in the extended family, the mother's difficult fourth pregnancy (which she believed made her less accessible to Brian), and the father's chronic depression. The father's life history indicated that he had labile self-esteem and was very self-critical. During a period of severe financial difficulty when Brian was a toddler, he admitted, "I sunk into my own private hell. I was just glad that these girls [sic] would look after him." Brian's mother indicated that the various stressors had left her feeling quite impatient and critical, particularly toward her son.

During my meeting with the parents as a couple, they agreed that for the first several years of Brian's life, his primary attachments were to his mother and older sisters (along with his female dolls). He was reluctant to spend time with his father, who indicated that he preferred this because of his own preoccupations, saying, "[I] let him down."

The parents expressed their concern that Brian "is" (not "would be") gay or transsexual. His mother indicated that she would be comfortable if Brian grew up to be gay and that she would help him to be well adjusted. At the same time, she professed anxiety about this because of AIDS and social discrimination. Brian's mother commented that she had the feeling that the situation with Brian was ominous: "I want to grab you by the shirt and [have you] tell me he's normal....[I think] he's pretty messed up."

The parents noted that Brian had poor fine motor skills. He was the only left-handed member of the family and was said to have always been clumsy. Brian reached general developmental milestones within normal limits. Although Brian's mother described him as being quite a stubborn (behaviorally rigid) and defiant child, the parent ratings on the Child Behavior Checklist indicated a youngster with a predominance of internalizing as opposed to externalizing difficulties. My clinical impression was that Brian had a lot of general anxieties, reminiscent of a youngster with behavioral inhibition, as described by Kagan (1989).

DIAGNOSIS

When I met with Brian individually, he was able to answer some questions, but was generally inhibited and avoidant, particularly around his gender-related feelings. He indicated a desire to spend more time with his father, but commented, "He's sort of very busy." He claimed that his mother did not do anything with him, that "she just does things with herself." He said that she used to play with him, but that "was a long time ago." The parents had remarked that Brian seemed quite bothered by the birth of his younger sibling as he no longer felt he was the center of attention.

In my individual interview with Brian, I administered a structured Gender Identity Interview (Zucker et al. 1993). His initial responses were all, "I don't know." With monetary incentive, he was somewhat more responsive, and his answers suggested a fair bit of gender identity confusion. For example, when asked if he were a boy or a girl, Brian said, "That is a really hard question. I am both." When asked if he would grow up to be a mom or a dad, he said, "Both." He indicated that, in his mind, he had thoughts of wanting to be a girl and was confused about himself, not really being sure if he was a boy or a girl. In his dreams, he was both a boy and a girl. When asked if he ever thought that he really was a girl, Brian, after a long pause, said, "I don't know....I have no idea."

For reasons of space, I will not provide information about the parents' own backgrounds, but will note the following. The parents were quite intelligent. They had a good marital relationship, although it was compromised by the various stressors noted above, including the father's psychiatric difficulties. Brian's mother was a resilient individual, although the various stressors had depleted her personal resources.

In my view, Brian's symptoms were consistent with the DSM-IV-TR diagnosis of gender identity disorder. Regarding the A criterion, "strong and persistent cross-gender identification," he manifested at least four of the five indicators: a repeatedly stated desire to be the other sex, a preference for cross-dressing, a preference for cross-sex roles in fantasy play, and a preference for cross-sex toys. I was less certain about his peer affiliation preferences. Regarding the B criterion, "persistent discomfort with his or her sex or sense of inappropriateness in the gender role of that sex," Brian was clearly averse to rough-and-tumble play and showed no real interest in stereotypical masculine toys and activities (which, at his age, could be interpreted as a "rejection" of them).

My case formulation was as follows:

1. Brian presented as a temperamentally sensitive and anxious youngster.
2. He was extremely clumsy, which made it difficult for him to engage in various physical activities often engaged in by boys.
3. His cross-gender identification emerged in the context of increased maternal unavailability and chronic paternal unavailability. He was "mothered" by his older sisters and, for various reasons, overidentified with them. The female dolls to which he was tenaciously attached (e.g., carrying them around wherever he went) seemed to function as transitional objects, perhaps replacing his mother who was overwhelmed with parenting the other children and going through a difficult pregnancy with his younger sister.
4. During the toddler and preschool years, Brian's cross-gender behavior was tolerated, if not reinforced (e.g., by his older sister cross-dressing him).
5. Brian seemed to view female individuals as being quite powerful. Also, because of his father's psychological unavailability, he did not have much of a relationship with him during the early years of his cross-gender identification. At the time of the assessment, he seemed quite ambivalent about his status as a boy, even finding it difficult to acknowledge that he was a boy.

TREATMENT

I recommended weekly play psychotherapy for Brian, in which we would explore his internal gender representations and address his generalized anxiety, and periodic counseling sessions for his parents. I also made recommendations for helping Brian in his naturalistic environment, including more exposure to same-sex peers, setting clearer limits on his cross-gender behavior, and more one-on-one time with his father.

In my view, my recommendations were consistent with a variety of approaches that have been identified in the treatment literature (Coates and Wolfe 1995; Zucker 2001; Zucker and Bradley 1995). It differed, however, rather substantially from one competing paradigm, which takes the position that "gender variance" is not a mental disorder, that children such as Brian should be accepted as they are and that therapists, such as myself, "who advocate changing gender-variant behaviors should be avoided" (Menvielle et al. 2005).

Because Brian's parents were comfortable with my recommendations for treating Brian in his naturalistic environment, I did not feel that the parents required more intensive, direct treatment. In addition, because Brian's father was already in psychoanalysis, I did not feel it appropriate for me to spend a lot of time exploring his issues; however, because his chronic depression was still quite apparent after years of treatment with a nonmedical analyst, I gave him my frank opinion that I thought that he deserved to be seen by a physician for an opinion about pharmacological approaches. In part because of his dependent personality style, the father complied with this recommendation. He saw his family physician, who prescribed nefazodone (Serzone). He responded quickly to it and terminated his analysis several months later.

Treatment of Brian

Over a 39-month period, I saw Brian for 101 individual sessions (with breaks during the months of July and August and during school recess, etc.). Because the family lived a fair distance from the office, I would frequently meet with the parent who brought Brian for a brief session in addition to formal therapy sessions with both parents. In total, I saw the parents 82 times.

In play psychotherapy, the therapist can be interested in at least two elements of the process: 1) the manner in which the child relates to the therapist and the ensuing way in which the therapeutic relationship affects the course of treatment (as one 3-year-old boy remarked to me years later, "You were my first friend"), and 2) how the child uses play (or other forms of communication) to provide a window into his internal world.

After reviewing my handwritten notes from each session, I identified three therapeutic issues or themes that seemed to characterize the treatment: 1) helping Brian master his general anxieties and inhibitions, 2) addressing Brian's astonishing use of an array of dolls and action figures (Barbie, Bionicles, Digimon, Megazords, Pokémon, Power Rangers, Star Wars characters, X-Men, etc.) to master his gender identity confusion, and 3) helping Brian regulate intense sexual and aggressive feelings. Regarding Brian's use of dolls and action figures, he taught me more about who was who and who did what than any child I have ever worked with. He literally knew by heart the names of several hundred of these characters.

Brian's general anxiety and inhibition were most salient in the first 10 sessions or so. In session 1, for example, Brian could only say that he did not know why he was coming to see me, as he scratched himself and tugged at his ear lobes. After he sat down, he commented softly, "I wonder what's next." In play psychotherapy, the general therapeutic approach is to tell the child, "You can do whatever you want: play, draw, talk, tell me about your dreams." As standard an approach as this is, it proved difficult for Brian. He often asked me what I wanted to do and was very resistant in doing what he wanted to do. I remember that this made me feel very anxious because the standard approach was not working and Brian was rather tenacious in insisting that I had to decide what we were going to do. After fumbling with this for a while, in session 10, I came up with the idea of writing down on pieces of paper a number corresponding to the various play options in the office (e.g., toy boxes, Magic markers) and then having Brian pick, at random, one of the numbers. This seemed to help him settle into play and, I think, Brian could sense that I was nonjudgmental about what he chose to do.

By session 14, Brian started to bring his own dolls and action figures to the sessions. He did this regularly throughout the treatment. In reviewing my notes, I was struck by how this was the primary medium through which Brian was able to allow me access to his internal world. Not surprisingly, Brian was initially much more focused on the female characters (e.g., Barbie, Queen Amidala [Padmé] from the movie "Star Wars," the female Power Rangers) than the male characters. Of course, what interested me more was what exactly it was about these female characters that was of importance to him. In my judgment, the salient issue was that of power, of feeling overwhelmed by the power of females. This, I think, was related to his experience of relative ineptness in relation to his more competent older sisters, his rambunctious younger sister, his mother's critical attitude, and some dominant, controlling girls at school who petrified him. He was also drawn to many of the dolls that had powerful, transformative properties (e.g., the Power Rangers). Thus I think that the central underlying issue was to help Brian believe that he could transform himself from feeling weak and inept to being a more powerful and competent "boy person."

In session 21, Brian identified strongly with Queen Amidala (Padmé). In session 30, he identified with a female morphing character, exclaiming, "I have the power." In session 32, Brian was thoughtful in trying to decide whether or not the female or male action figures were "meaner" and therefore "had the power." (Indeed, in session 49, when I reflected to Brian his belief in females having "all the power," he replied, "I don't want to think about it.") In session 35, I observed that Brian was starting to focus more on the male characters from Star Wars and, when he played with them, he seemed happier, humming to himself throughout the session. Moreover, he was actually talking more in the sessions. In contrast, his play with the female characters had an obligatory quality, in which he seemed to be working through the issue of why they had "the power." Nonetheless, and not surprisingly, his relative attention to the female versus the male characters continued to vacillate for many months.

On the relatively rare occasion when Brian talked spontaneously about his "real life" rather than reflecting it in his play, he identified a girl in his class (who had been bullying him) as "public enemy number one." At the same time, he spent the entire session playing with the Green Power Ranger (a male figure), albeit one that had its arms broken off. To me, this reflected nicely the inadequacy Brian felt as a male. Brian was always thrilled when I showed him the new dolls and action figures I had purchased for the office. When, in session 56, I showed him a new set of Power Rangers (both males and females), he was ecstatic, exclaiming that he could play with me all day.

After 21 months of treatment, I told the parents that, based on their and my observations, Brian appeared to have consolidated a more comfortable identity as a boy and that we might think about ending therapy or at least reducing its frequency. The parents were surprised by my comment and, as it turned out, I continued to see Brian for another 18 months. Indeed, when Brian's father talked to him about the idea of ending the sessions, Brian became tearful and angry and referred to me as "Dr. Dementor."

It was clear that the suggestion of termination (or even tapering) our sessions made the parents and Brian feel anxious; for a period after I made this suggestion, Brian was uncharacteristically aggressive toward me. For example, in session 62, he shot me with a laser gun and, in session 67, he engaged in a lot of "anal" talk and talk about "balls" and he kicked, hit, and threw things at me. I observed that this period of aggressiveness also coincided with renewed parental stressors. I think I helped Brian master his anxiety about us ending our sessions by telling him all of the things that I would miss about him. I recall being rather surprised at how aggressive he was toward me, but I was not sure that he appreciated that he was actually hurting me. When I responded by being firm ("It's okay to be angry at me, but I will not let you hurt me"), but not angry, Brian settled down rather quickly and his aggressive behavior became more playful.

After a summer break, Brian presented in session 80 as being very glad to see me. He was relaxed, burped noisily after drinking his 7-Up, and farted loudly with clear pleasure. He was clearly much less inhibited than the Brian I had first met! A week later, I saw Brian right after the events of September 11, 2001. We talked about the terrorists and Brian equated Osama Bin Laden, the purported leader of the terrorist group Al-Qaeda, with Saruman, a character from "The Lord of the Rings." At session 93, I told Brian that I would now see him every other week, to which he commented that he "could come back [more frequently] if [there were] any troubles." In session 94, Brian commented, somewhat philosophically, "The power can be held in the smallest of things." He left the session saying, "See you in 2 weeks."

As we neared the termination of our sessions, Brian's interest in action figures had clearly shifted to a predominant interest in male figures. In our last session, shortly after his ninth birthday, he proudly showed me his birthday gifts, which included various Star Wars characters, Power Ranger comic books, and a realistic Obi-Wan Kenobi doll. As his father remarked, "He seems more like a boy than ever."

Parent Counseling

The parents were able, with relative ease, to work on Brian's issues in the naturalistic environment. In part, I think this was because they were not ambivalent about instituting changes and were eager to help Brian feel better about being a boy. In session 1, the mother reported that starting to set limits on Brian felt "very good." She also remarked, "I don't understand why I bought (female) things for him," although, in part, she related her actions to a comment from her pediatrician when Brian was age 3 years to not worry about his proclivity for female toys. Many months later, in session 52, his mother commented, "I bought him a Barbie Dreamhouse for his third birthday. I must've been out of my mind." She reported that Brian initially responded to the limit setting by saying he was "too nervous to change" and beginning to cry. However, she reported that he settled down fairly quickly and was very happy with the new toys that they purchased for him (e.g., Transformers), exclaiming, "This is like Christmas!" She felt that he was thriving because he was receiving more attention from his parents and was becoming less oppositional and defiant. In an interesting revelation, Brian told his mother that he could remember liking to play with toy cars when he was age 2 years and she reflected, "It's almost like we had him back a little bit."

From the parents' reports during these sessions, Brian appeared to make steady gains, although there were certainly many occasions in which he showed his female interests and identifications. As his mother said in session 2, he progressed "two steps forward, one step backward." She said that when he played with boys, "You wouldn't think anything is wrong." When in the company of girls, however, he would become quite immersed in playing with Barbie dolls. This helped his mother recognize the importance of encouraging play time with other boys. Indeed, as early as session 3, Brian's mother reported that at school Brian had clearly increased his interaction time with other boys. In this session, his mother was more cognizant of his motoric clumsiness (comparing him to a noodle) and how this caused him to be wary about involving himself in more boisterous activities. She was also now more aware of how he used female dolls as a transitional object ("hanging onto Belle for dear life"). In session 5, Brian's mother reported that Brian was nervous about joining the Beavers (a group much like Cub Scouts, but for younger children), but was happy that his father was there as one of the leaders. In session 6, the mother said that one of Brian's teachers reported he was more confident with his peers and called out to them from across the classroom.

The parents generally believed that Brian became more feminine when the family was under stress. At these times, Brian could be very open with his father and could describe his dual gender identification well: "Part of me is a boy, part is a girl.... My penis is a boy, but my bum is a girl." In session 13, the parents reported that Brian drew an imaginary line down the middle of his body, saying, "That's how I grew up, half-boy, half-girl." In session 20, the father talked about Brian's fascination with a commercial by the clothing manufacturer GAP in which a boy and girl blend together: "That's just like me," he said. The parents talked about his struggle with dominant, controlling girls at school, but, at the same time, they also felt that Brian was becoming more assertive. In session 15, the parents reported that Brian remarked, "I used to play with cars, but then you abandoned me and I was acting like a girl." Speaking to his father, he continued, "Now you're back." In session 19, the father reported that one of Brian's older sisters was teaching him how to catch a ball and, with remarkable insight, commented, "He is struggling with who he is." In session 27, the father reported that he asked Brian if he knew why he was coming to see me, to which Brian replied, "It's because I am confused." In session 28, the parents reported Brian's extreme distress after hearing a girl at school say, "Girls go to college because they have knowledge. Boys go to Jupiter because they are stupider." Yet Brian was affiliating with other boys who were excluding girls from their play (a common characteristic of gender segregation in the peer group).

In session 29, the father reported Brian's increased affiliation with boys, noting that this represented a big change and that Brian seemed a lot happier. Brian's mother subsequently wrote me a note in which she reported that Brian had brought his red Power Ranger (a male figure) for show and tell: "At the end of the day, he came running out of school with a very happy and pleased smile on his face, saying, 'My show and tell was a big success.'" All of the boys had gathered around him to inspect this toy. "I was so popular, Mom! You were right, Mom. When I share my inside with people, they get to know me and like me. Why did it take me so long to do it?" In session 39, Brian's father reported that Brian had become intensely anxious when reading to him about a female Star Wars bounty hunter who could "change identities at will."

Shortly after I raised the prospects of termination (session 42) with the parents, the father's mental health deteriorated. He had stopped taking his Serazone and became more depressed. At this juncture, I referred him to a psychiatrist colleague, who began seeing him in therapy and reinstituted the Serazone. My colleague eventually diagnosed him with bipolar disorder and placed him on risperidone (Risperdal).

In session 56, the parents reported that Brian had, with anxiety, joined a baseball team. He turned out to be a pretty good hitter and seemed to enjoy the camaraderie with the other boys. In session 60, the father reported that Brian shared with him that his "boy side" had increased. However, Brian still talked about having boy and girl angels on his shoulders and that there was a struggle over who was stronger; he professed to his father a desire for the "boy side" to win. Brian cried and asked why he was like this, to which his father replied, "Maybe your father was not very strong."

In session 69, I met with Brian's mother and older sister, who was, in my view, astonishingly perceptive about family dynamics and her brother. She noted that he was quite jealous of her and her friends and, at these times, would try and mimic them to "be part of us."

In session 64, the parents reported that, with great anxiety, Brian was learning how to skate, but that he needed concrete rewards to persevere. His mother could see that he was gradually gaining more confidence in areas in which he was quite behind other children. In session 70, the father reported that Brian had said to him that the "b-o-y" had won the battle; that is, that Brian was now feeling much more like a boy.

In my last two sessions with the parents before termination, they reported that, as far as they were concerned, Brian was over his gender identity problems. He was relating very well to other boys and would say that the "half and half doesn't exist anymore." In a follow-up session with the parents 5 months after I had stopped seeing Brian (he was now age 9½ years), his father said, "He's definitely cured of his gender identity disorder." The father also reported that Brian's oldest sister was also of the view that her brother had changed. They reported he had formed a strong bond with other boys, noting how the boys would hug each other and give each other "high fives." With pride, they noted Brian's interest in Harry Potter, the male characters from "The Lord of the Rings," BeyBlades, and his Yugioh cards. These were his new (gender) transitional objects: "He always carries something around," they said. He had become more independent and mature and no longer wanted his mother to hover over him while he did his homework.

In working with Brian's parents, I experienced one big surprise. In session 30, they reported a lot of sexualized behavior on Brian's part (he was age 7 at the time). He would rub his parents' buttocks, touch his mother's breasts, and rub his father's penis "up and down." Indeed, the father reported Brian approaching him and fondling him, with Brian stating that he was "stimulated." The parents also reported that they often walked in the nude around all of the children. For intelligent parents, I was taken aback, as they seemed to be astonishingly naïve at how their own behavior could overstimulate Brian (a youngster who was struggling with regulating affect). I told them that their behavior was not helpful for Brian, that they should not allow him to touch their nude bodies, and they should stop walking naked around the house. Because they were "compliant" parents who listened to authority, they changed their behavior immediately and Brian stopped "coming on" to them. In retrospect, I am sure that I did not explore this issue completely with them (e.g., that the father's allowing Brian to touch him was a naïve compensatory maneuver for his own harsh upbringing pertaining to sex matters).

DISCUSSION

I think that the treatment helped Brian resolve his cross-gender identification and gender dysphoria. His anxiety and inhibition also improved, and he seemed to develop a solid alliance with other boys. These clinical impressions are consistent with the parent reports on questionnaires. For example, on the Gender Identity Questionnaire for Children, a parent-report measure (Johnson et al. 2004), Brian's score moved from solidly in the range of gender-referred boys at assessment to the control range for boys 15 months after treatment began and at termination. On the Child Behavior Checklist, his internalizing T score moved from the clinical range at assessment to the nonclinical range at the two follow-up administrations of the questionnaire.

It is reasonable to ask to what extent this treatment case is representative of all gender-referred children who are seen in therapy. This remains a difficult question to answer because there is a dearth of systematic outcome studies on this population (Zucker 2001). From a clinical perspective, I believe that Brian was representative of youngsters who do show systematic changes in their gender identity, but I would not want to argue that this is true for all children who receive treatment. On this point, a great deal of therapeutic research remains to be done.

REFERENCES

Coates S, Wolfe S: Gender identity disorder in boys: the interface of constitution and early experience. Psychoanalytic Inquiry 15:6–38, 1995

Johnson LL, Bradley SJ, Birkenfeld-Adams AS, et al: A parent-report gender identity questionnaire for children. Arch Sex Behav 33:105–116, 2004

Kagan J: Unstable Ideas: Temperament, Cognition and Self. Cambridge, MA, Harvard University Press, 1989

Menvielle EJ, Tuerk C, Perrin EC: To the beat of a different drummer: the gender-variant child. Contemporary Pediatrics 22:38–46, 2005

Zucker KJ: Gender identity disorder in children and adolescents, in Treatments of Psychiatric Disorders, 3rd Edition, Vol 2. Edited by Gabbard GO. Washington, DC, American Psychiatric Publishing, 2001, pp 2069–2094

Zucker KJ, Bradley SJ: Gender Identity Disorder and Psychosexual Problems in Children and Adolescents. New York, Guilford, 1995

Zucker KJ, Bradley SJ, Lowry Sullivan CB, et al: A gender identity interview for children. J Pers Assess 61:443–456, 1993

PART XII

Eating Disorders

CHAPTER 26

Be Careful What You Wish For

A Case of Bulimia/Anorexia After Gastric Bypass Surgery

Melissa Arbuckle, M.D., Ph.D.
Philip R. Muskin, M.D.

Melissa Arbuckle, M.D., Ph.D., is an Instructor in Clinical Psychiatry and Assistant Director of Residency Training for the Department of Psychiatry at Columbia University Medical Center and the New York State Psychiatric Institute. She is also Director of the long-term psychodynamic psychotherapy training and research clinic at the New York State Psychiatric Institute. Dr. Arbuckle completed a residency in adult psychiatry in the New York State Psychiatric Institute/Columbia University Medical Center program. She received her medical degree from the University of Oklahoma along with a doctorate of philosophy in the field of pathology.

Philip R. Muskin, M.D., is the Chief of Consultation-Liaison Psychiatry at the Columbia University Medical Center of the New York-Presbyterian Hospital; Professor of Clinical Psychiatry at Columbia University College of Physicians and Surgeons; and a faculty member of the Columbia University Psychoanalytic Center for Training and Research. Dr. Muskin's research and publications have examined mood disorders and AIDS, the psychodynamics of the failure of empathy toward AIDS patients, panic disorder, medical presentations of psychiatric disorders, treatment of anxiety and depression in medically ill patients, maladaptive denial of physical illness, personality disorders in the primary care setting, the role of religiosity in patients' decisions regarding do-not-resuscitate status, the psychodynamics of physician-assisted suicide, and the impact of intercessory prayer on medical outcomes.

Dr. Muskin was the editor of *Complementary and Alternative Medicine and Psychiatry* (2000). He is Past President of the Association for Academic Psychiatry and the Society for Liaison Psychiatry. He has been a member of the Scientific Program Committee of the American Psychiatric Association (APA) since 1990, serving as the Committee Chair for the 2001 and 2002 annual meetings. He is currently the head of the APA Council on Psychosomatic Medicine.

THE PSYCHIATRIC CONSULT request form read, "History of morbid obesity. Status-post–gastric bypass complicated by persistent nausea and vomiting. Binges and purges. Weighs 95 lb. Also depressed." Maria, a 31-year-old married woman, was admitted to the medical service for severe malnutrition. Emaciated with temporal wasting and thinning hair, Maria looked much older than her stated age. Although her taut face had the haunting appearance of starvation, her arms and legs were draped in excessive folds of skin.

HISTORY

Maria weighed 170 lb by age 16, having reached her adult height of 5′3″. She reported chronic overeating and numerous failures with diet and exercise programs to control her weight. At age 29 and at a weight of 340 lb, she elected to undergo gastric bypass surgery.

The initial months after her gastric bypass were largely uneventful. Although Maria underwent fairly rapid weight loss and was pleased with the changes that she saw in her body, she became increasingly frustrated with the restrictions of her postgastrectomy diet. Although her husband (weighing close to 300 lb himself) could eat "normal" meals, she was limited to small portions and specific types of food. She gradually began binge eating and ignored all dietary restrictions despite the physical consequences of nausea, vomiting, and diarrhea.

Maria's history suggested that she did not tell her doctors about her noncompliant eating behaviors. Approximately 6 months after the surgery, she underwent an extensive workup for intractable nausea and vomiting. The studies, including an exploratory laparotomy, did not reveal any abnormal findings. A gastrostomy tube was placed in the remnant antrum of her stomach to provide her with supplemental nutrition because she could not tolerate an oral diet. She reported compliance with the dietary restrictions and tolerance of self-administered tube feedings for another 6 months. She became non-adherent because she became "tired of it" and stopped. Her binge eating habits returned, along with the chronic nausea, vomiting, and diarrhea.

At the time Maria was seen by the consultation-liaison psychiatry service, almost 2 years after her bypass surgery, she weighed only 95 lb. She was noted to be pancytopenic (presenting with abnormally low levels of white blood cells, hematocrit, and platelets) with numerous electrolyte abnormalities, an elevated coagulation profile, and hypoalbuminemia. Along with numerous metabolic abnormalities, Maria was amenorrheic. She reported several symptoms of depression, including low mood and frustration, tearfulness, difficulty sleeping, and low energy but denied anhedonia or suicidal ideation. Her mental status exam was most notable for a concrete thought process with very poor insight into her eating disorder–related behaviors and subsequent health consequences.

DIAGNOSIS

Maria's eating disorder most closely fell into the category of eating disorder not otherwise specified (DSM-IV-TR, 307.50). Her illness had many features that resembled anorexia nervosa, but she failed to meet the full criteria for the disorder. With a body mass index of 16.8 kg/m^2, she was clearly less than 85% of her ideal body weight. Although anorexic patients generally report an intense fear of becoming fat, Maria denied concerns about gaining weight and acknowledged that she was "too thin." These atypical features are not entirely uncommon and have been previously reported in 17% of anorexic patients in eating disorder programs (Strober et al. 1999). Despite her denial, Maria was clearly distressed about the process of gaining weight and exclaimed, "I'm getting fat!" although she remained emaciated. She consistently demonstrated extremely poor insight into the serious and life-threatening nature of her eating disorder. Her body distortion was further evident in the fact that she was seemingly unaware of her dramatic decline in weight. In fact, she reported that she was shocked when she discovered just how low her weight was. These body image changes have been previously reported in patients after bariatric surgery and are reminiscent of the "phantom limb" syndrome (Segal et al. 2004).

After Maria's bariatric surgery, it was important for her to eat several small meals throughout the day. Due to the dramatic decrease in her stomach size, she was also instructed to limit her fluid consumption at meals (drinking liquids 30–60 minutes before or after meals). As part of her postgastrectomy diet, she was taught to avoid high-fat, fried foods; fatty meats; and concentrated sugars. On the other hand, given her body's new limited ability to absorb nutrients, it was important that she continued to consume adequate amounts of protein and vitamins. Although Maria did not specifically restrict her food intake, she would not eat small frequent meals as she was instructed. Despite being hungry during the day, she would instead "wait for dinner." In addition, if she were served food that she did not like, she would state that she was not going to eat it and would rather starve. On the other hand, she consistently ate food that was not compatible with her altered gastrointestinal anatomy (both in the type of food she chose and the amount, with her often overeating). Although she did not self-induce vomiting or misuse laxatives, diarrhea and vomiting were the natural consequences of her eating behaviors.

Although Maria had several features of depression, she did not have enough symptoms to justify a diagnosis of major depressive disorder or dysthymic disorder.

TREATMENT

There were many important considerations for managing Maria's eating disorder. As with any medical or psychiatric patient, establishing and maintaining a therapeutic alliance was a primary objective. Our treatment goals in the acute medical phase were focused primarily on restoring her healthy weight, treating her physical complications, setting behavioral limits, and encouraging Maria to participate in treatment.

Maria's severe malnutrition resulted in multiple medical consequences. At the time of admission, she was pancytopenic with numerous metabolic abnormalities (including low electrolytes, an elevated coagulation profile, and low albumin levels). Initial treatment focused on her medical stabilization. A thorough medical evaluation and hematology/oncology consultation ruled out potential medical causes for her complex symptom presentation other than starvation. A gastroenterology evaluation revealed that she did not have a malabsorption syndrome. Her gastrostomy tube was found to be functional, and she was begun on tube feeding as a supplement to her oral diet.

It was difficult to build and maintain a working alliance with Maria. She demonstrated limited insight into her illness, was concrete in her thought process, and did not see a need for psychiatric treatment. Any discussion of ongoing psychiatric care was met with much resistance. Attempts to remind her of the serious nature of her illness and potential consequences resulted in Maria saying that her medical team need to be more "positive and encouraging". The concern of the medical team took the form of chastising Maria for non-adherence rather than complimenting her when she followed the plan or gained weight. In addition to Maria's lack of insight into her need for treatment, she was unable to provide seemingly simple details regarding her history as recent as 6 months prior to her presentation. It was quite difficult for her to provide a coherent time line regarding the sequence of events after her gastric bypass, and she could not name a single person who had been previously involved in her medical care. These cognitive limitations were particularly striking given her history of a college education and previous employment as a special education teacher. Cognitive deficits have been reported in patients with anorexia nervosa. Although some investigators attribute cognitive abnormalities to malnutrition, refeeding does not always restore normal cognitive functioning (Kingston et al. 1996). It is unclear if cognitive deficits precede and contribute to the development of eating disorder–related behaviors (Lena et al. 2004) or if persistent cognitive deficits are a long-lasting consequence of malnutrition.

Without the structure and staff of an inpatient psychiatric unit, the psychiatric consultant has limited ability to enforce behavioral changes on a medical ward. Early in her hospital course, Maria had difficulty in complying with prescribed limitations. The hospital staff reported that she stole food from other patient's trays and ate food brought in by her family that was not within the prescribed diet. Maria hoarded food in her room, a behavior frequently seen in patients after semistarvation (Keys et al. 1950). She became very upset when she was told that she could not have extra food in her room, claiming she was saving food for her family. Later Maria admitted that she ate the food herself.

The treatment team responded to Maria's repeated nonadherence to behavioral limitations and treatment (e.g., at times Maria refused electrolyte repletion) with anger and frustration. Coordination of care; collaboration among the nursing, medical, and psychiatric staff; and education were particularly crucial in this setting, in which the primary medical treatment team had little training or experience in treating eating disorder patients. Because of Maria's exceedingly low weight, her treatment team was initially very encouraged by her eating. Thus the real problem, her overeating, was missed. She almost exclusively ate improper food and in amounts that resulted in nausea, vomiting, and diarrhea. In the setting of starvation, it seemed counterintuitive to everyone to encourage her to eat less.

Maria's clinical treatment focused on restructuring her eating behaviors toward small frequent meals. In addition, Maria was encouraged to keep a diary of everything she ate during the day. Although the nausea and vomiting continued, it gradually reduced from three to four times daily to once daily.

In addition to educating Maria regarding healthy nutrition and eating patterns, it was important to address the associated psychiatric conditions to her eating disorder behaviors. Maria did not meet diagnostic criteria for depression, but there was a consensus among her treatment providers that depressive symptoms contributed to her eating disorder–related behaviors.

The use of medications in the treatment of eating disorder patients is an area under much investigation. Some research on anorexia nervosa has suggested that it is best to assess the need for antidepressant medication after weight gain, when the psychological effects of malnutrition are resolving (American Psychiatric Association 2000). In bulimic patients, antidepressants such as selective serotonin reuptake inhibitors have been shown to reduce binge eating and vomiting even when the patients are not depressed (Goldstein et al. 1995). Eating disorder specialists are increasing their use of low-dose, second-generation antipsychotic medications in combination with selective serotonin reuptake inhibitors in treating highly obsessional and compulsive patients with anorexia nervosa, although there are few data to support the effectiveness of this strategy (American Psychiatric Association 2000). Case reports of patients treated with olanzapine suggest that antipsychotic medications may be helpful in encouraging weight gain, decreasing agitation and anxiety, and improving sleep, general functioning, and overall compliance with treatment (Boachie et al. 2003; Cassano et al. 2003). Early in the hospitalization, Maria was treated with paroxetine-CR 12.5 mg/day (an antidepressant) and quetiapine (a second-generation antipsychotic medication) 50 mg qhs. She reported some improvement in depressive symptoms and denied significant side effects.

During the acute phase of treatment, the efficacy of specific psychotherapeutic interventions for facilitating weight gain remains uncertain. Attempts to conduct formal psychotherapy with malnourished patients with cognitive impairment may be ineffective. Given Maria's clear cognitive limitations, psychotherapy sessions were focused toward support and encouragement. Because problems in family relationships may contribute to the maintenance of eating disorders, enlisting family support and providing family counseling is also important.

The psychosocial interventions with Maria were informed by a psychodynamic understanding of her relationships (American Psychiatric Association 2000). It was surprising that Maria acknowledged little awareness of her dramatic decline in weight, and it was almost incomprehensible that her husband had failed to notice the disfiguring changes caused by her weight loss. Further evaluation revealed that there were important aspects of their relationship that contributed to her ongoing eating disorder–related behaviors. Maria described their early courtship as evolving around food and going out to dinner on dates. She described their mutual love of food as something that they shared, a special connection that she missed after the gastric bypass. She felt that they could not even enjoy watching movies together anymore because she could not eat popcorn. It appeared that her eating restrictions were isolating her more and more from her husband. Despite her dietary limitations, she continued to cook full meals for her husband and their 9-year-old daughter. She became increasingly jealous of her husband's ability to eat normal food and gradually stopped compliance with her postgastrectomy diet. Maria's husband seemed to have minimal awareness of how his behaviors influenced her. In fact, while in the hospital, she reported that he brought in a hamburger and french fries and proceeded to eat them in front of her.

Conducting a family meeting was a critical component of Maria's treatment. It was important to educate her husband on the severe nature of her symptoms and enlist his support in helping her recover. During this meeting, he said that he would work on his own diet, and he and Maria agreed to try to incorporate new activities into their social life so that they could begin to do non–eating-related social activities together again.

Maria was hospitalized for a total of 2 months to medically stabilize her condition. Although weight gain is the typical indicator of recovery, Maria demonstrated significant edema. She gained approximately 50 lbs in the first few weeks, largely from fluid overload in the setting of low albumin levels. In addition, the excessive amount of skin she had made it difficult to assess exactly what was her ideal body weight. To track her progress, her white blood cell count and prealbumin levels were used as markers for recovery. Her pancytopenia was particularly persistent and did not improve dramatically until she was treated with filgrastim and erythropoietin (medications often used in cancer patients to increase white and red blood cell production after chemotherapy). Over time she was gradually tapered off of gastric tube feeds and encouraged to incorporate liquid protein supplements into her diet. At the time of her medical discharge, all her electrolyte abnormalities had resolved and her albumin was in the normal range. She was maintaining her weight with oral intake alone and had no vomiting.

Throughout Maria's medical care, there was substantial consideration of what psychiatric treatment options would be pursued after her discharge. It was clear from the beginning of treatment that Maria needed long-term psychiatric care and would benefit most from a structured inpatient setting. Finding an appropriate program proved to be quite complicated. There is some evidence that patients treated in eating disorder inpatient specialty units have better outcomes than those treated in general psychiatric inpatient settings (Palmer and Treasure 1999). In fact, it is rare for general psychiatric units to be able to provide the intensity of care needed by such patients. General psychiatric units declined to admit her because they felt they were not adequately qualified to address her specific psychiatric needs. On the other hand, the psychiatric units specializing in eating disorder patients did not have adequate medical services readily available and felt that Maria presented considerable risk for future medical complications, particularly given her ongoing need for a gastrostomy tube. Interactions with the team took on an adversarial quality at times. The team wanted her out of the hospital but was afraid to send her home. The catch-22 of the team being unwilling to remove her gastrostomy tube and inpatient psychiatric units being unwilling to take her with the tube led to heated discussions of the problem with psychiatrists. Both the surgical and medical teams felt that Maria lacked the physiological reserve to make removing the gastrostomy tube at the time of discharge a viable option. If she did not respond to further psychiatric treatment, she was at high risk for medical relapse and would need reinitiation of tube feedings. In addition, given her altered anatomy, removal and subsequent replacement of the gastrostomy tube would require significant surgical interventions.

An appropriate inpatient eating disorder program was ultimately identified, but Maria consistently refused an inpatient psychiatric hospitalization, particularly after 2 months of inpatient medical care. Maria was eventually referred to an intensive day treatment program specializing in eating disorder patients. Inpatient hospitalization would have been ideal, offering Maria the best chance for weight maintenance and relapse prevention. Because Maria claimed she had never been in psychiatric treatment, it was unclear to us that inpatient treatment was absolutely necessary. She could not be admitted against her will, and she had not failed outpatient treatment. We knew that there was evidence that compared with an inpatient setting, outpatient treatment could provide equivalent outcomes and improve overall compliance (Crisp et al. 1991). It was not possible to ascertain what, if any, psychiatric evaluation was done preceding her gastric bypass surgery or what psychiatric evaluation or intervention was attempted in prior medical care in other hospitals.

DISCUSSION

Maria's case was somewhat unusual in the spectrum of anorexia nervosa cases encountered by most clinicians. Most anorexic patients are brought to the attention of clinicians at an earlier stage in their illness than was Maria; she demonstrated the extreme consequences of malnutrition. She was also unique given her history of obesity and the evolution of symptoms after gastric bypass surgery. Postsurgical anorexia may represent a unique class of eating disorder (Segal et al. 2004). Whether the surgery unveils the anorectic component of the eating disorder or causes the eating disorder remains to be elucidated. A careful psychiatric evaluation prior to bariatric surgery may spare some patients from developing an eating disorder or other related psychiatric disorder. Understanding the psychological factors involved in the person's obesity might reveal risks related to altering eating behavior. As the popularity of bariatric surgery increases, it is likely that patients such as Maria will also be seen in increasing frequency.

REFERENCES

American Psychiatric Association: Practice Guideline for the Treatment of Patients with Eating Disorders, 2nd Edition. Am J Psychiatry 157 (suppl 1):1–39, 2000

Boachie A, Goldfield GS, Spettigue W: Olanzapine use as an adjunctive treatment for hospitalized children with anorexia nervosa: case reports. Int J Eat Disord 33:98–103, 2003

Cassano GB, Miniati M, Pini S, et al: Six-month open trial of haloperidol as an adjunctive treatment for anorexia nervosa: a preliminary report. Int J Eat Disord 33:172–177, 2003

Crisp AH, Norton K, Gowers S, et al: A controlled study of the effect of therapies aimed at adolescent and family psychopathology in anorexia nervosa. Br J Psychiatry 159:325–333, 1991

Goldstein DJ, Wilson MG, Thompson VL, et al: Long-term fluoxetine treatment of bulimia nervosa. Fluoxetine Bulimia Nervosa Research Group. Br J Psychiatry 166:660–666, 1995

Keys A, Brozek J, Henschel A, et al: The Biology of Human Starvation. Minneapolis, University of Minnesota Press, 1950

Kingston K, Szmukler G, Andrewes D, et al: Neropsychological and structural brain changes in anorexia nervosa before and after refeeding. Psychol Med 26:15–28, 1996

Lena SM, Fiocco AJ, Leyenaar JK: The role of cognitive deficits in the development of eating disorders. Neuropsychol Rev 14:99–113, 2004

Palmer RL, Treasure J: Providing specialized services for anorexia nervosa. Br J Psychiatry 175:306–309, 1999

Segal A, Kinoshita Kussunoki D, Larino MA: Post-surgical refusal to eat: anorexia nervosa, bulimia nervosa or a new eating disorder? a case series. Obes Surg 14:353–360, 2004

Strober M, Freeman R, Morrell W: Atypical anorexia nervosa: separation from typical cases in course and outcome in a long-term prospective study. Int J Eat Disord 25:135–142, 1999

CHAPTER 27

The Contract

Cognitive-Behavioral Therapy for Anorexia Nervosa, Binge Eating/Purging Type

Michael J. Devlin, M.D.

Michael J. Devlin, M.D., is Associate Professor of Clinical Psychiatry at Columbia University College of Physicians and Surgeons and Clinical Co-Director of the Eating Disorders Research Unit at the New York State Psychiatric Institute. His major academic interest is in the treatment of patients with eating disorders, and he has recently completed work on a study funded by the National Institute of Mental Health on psychotherapy and medication treatment for overweight patients with binge eating disorder. He served recently as the psychotherapy supervisor at the Columbia site of a federally funded multisite clinical trial examining medication augmentation of cognitive-behavioral therapy for anorexia nervosa. In addition to conducting research, he is active in medical student education and in training and supervising psychiatric residents, particularly in cognitive-behavioral therapy. He is a member of the Work Group on Eating Disorders for the upcoming revision of the American Psychiatric Association Practice Guidline. He was the 2004–2005 President of and is still an active member of the Academy for Eating Disorders.

KIM FIRST PRESENTED to me as a 29-year-old single woman who had just been discharged from a specialized eating disorders treatment program at a major academic medical center. At a height of 5′1″, she weighed 116 lb, which translated to a body mass index of 21.9 kg/m^2, well within the normal range. She was looking forward to returning to her job as an assistant marketing specialist at a film production company and described the job as "all I have." Her employers had been supportive of her in the past, allowing her time for treatment and reserving her job when she was absent due to hospitalization, but they had informed her that henceforth it would be essential for her to remain well to keep her job. She lived with a roommate, Robin, with whom she shared a close and long-standing friendship, and although she had occasionally dated, she had not been in an ongoing romantic relationship for approximately 10 years.

From the first meeting, Kim struck me as a particularly engaging and spirited woman and one who very much needed to be appreciated. In addition to her marketing job, she was a published writer whose humorous essays drew on her own, often painful, experiences for inspiration. From the referral history, I knew that Kim had a long and complex eating disorder history and that she was at a high risk for relapsing. With great interest and considerable concern for Kim's long-term prognosis, I obtained the following history.

HISTORY

Kim's childhood had not been an easy one. After her parents' separation when she was a young girl, she and her older sister remained with their mother, a well-meaning young woman whose own childhood had been scarred by her mother's suicide. Kim's mother remarried Sonny, a man several years her junior, who entered the family when he was in his early 20s. Sonny alternated between flirtatious and abusive behavior toward his stepdaughters, at times holding them roughly or striking them. Although he did not have sexual intercourse with Kim, he often violated her privacy when she was unclothed (e.g., coming into the bathroom while she was bathing) and making derogatory remarks about her body. Kim was able to obtain Sonny's approval by performing physical services (e.g., massage) for him when asked. Kim had no history of major depressive disorder but did report depressive symptoms and suicidal ideation in connection with her worsening eating disorder symptoms. Her mother's unstable alcohol dependence, with alternating periods of abstinence and relapse, was an additional source of worry.

During her childhood and teenage years, Kim had been normal weight to overweight, reaching a maximum weight of 170 lb at age 15 years and maintaining a weight of 160 lb through high school and the beginning of college. Kim still had several painful memories of those years that were associated with intense feelings of shame. On one occasion, she was kissed by a boy, only to find out that her "friends" had paid him to do so. In an attempt to fit in with her friends, she began smoking, drinking, and experimenting with sex, all of which she later characterized as "fat Kim" behaviors. Just prior to the onset of her anorexia nervosa, Kim had her first love affair with Charlie, a young man she still remembers with a great deal of affection. Although she loved and trusted Charlie, Kim found herself unable to engage in sexual intercourse with him, which she found too upsetting. Kim ultimately ended the relationship with Charlie because of his continued drug use.

At age 20, during her junior year of college, Kim "discovered" anorexia nervosa. Her weight loss began innocently, with her deciding to attend a weight control program and subsequently reducing her weight to 125 lb, with much encouragement from friends and family. She had difficulty complying with the part of the program that encouraged her to "cheat" on weekends. Although she was advised to stay at 125 lb, she continued to lose weight. At a weight of 120 lb, she became amenorrheic and remained so for the next decade. Kim also began at that time to induce vomiting when she felt too full after eating, and, after about 3 months of vomiting, began binge eating objectively large amounts of food. She was able to stop purging after 6 months only by eating more and more restrictively and limiting her choice of foods to those whose precise caloric content she knew. The day after her college graduation, Kim was admitted to an eating disorders treatment program at a weight of 87 lb. She had difficulty adjusting to treatment on this unit and left prematurely at a weight of 103 lb. After leaving the program, she reinitiated binge eating, vomiting, and laxative misuse (up to eight suppositories each day), but her weight increased to 115 lb. To allow herself to stop purging, she began to exercise, arising at 5:00 A.M. and running five miles every morning. Her weight decreased to 95 lb. She became more obsessed with losing weight and reduced her weight to 81 lb, at which point she was once again admitted to an eating disorders inpatient program.

Kim spent the rest of her 20s essentially repeating this cycle, with a total of four inpatient admissions and several outpatient treatments with nutritionists and psychotherapists. Kim noted, "Once I get below 100 lb, I can't get my weight back up"; this indeed proved to be the case, with several periods of tenuous weight stability giving way to dips below 100 lb and then rapid downward spirals. Although Kim functioned at work during these years, she became known as "anorexic Kim," and her job advancement was adversely affected both by her deteriorating performance when she was symptomatic and her periodic absences for treatment. It was a tribute to Kim's talents, willingness to work hard, and likeability that she was able to keep her job despite her illness.

At age 29, Kim was admitted to a major teaching hospital–based eating disorders program at a weight of 87 lb. At this program, she was told that she must maintain a weight of 114–118 lb and, over the course of 2 months of behaviorally based treatment, she successfully increased her weight to within this range. She was discharged on a 2,500-kcal/day diet, but exercised intensively for at least 1 hour most days to prevent further weight gain.

Kim entered treatment with me as a participant in a newly initiated program of outpatient cognitive-behavioral therapy (CBT) for relapse prevention. Based on preliminary evidence of benefit in anorexia nervosa relapse prevention (Kaye et al. 2001), she was offered treatment with fluoxetine, a selective serotonin reuptake inhibitor, as an adjunct to psychotherapy, but she declined the medication.

DIAGNOSIS

Kim's diagnosis was clearly anorexia nervosa, binge-eating/purging subtype. Her case was classic in many respects. Although her age at onset was older than some, late adolescence is not uncommon for the onset of this disorder. The insidious progression from "normal" dieting to a frank eating disorder is frequently noted in patients with an eating disorder (Jacobi 2005), and the progression from restrictive eating to bingeing/purging behavior is also quite common (Sullivan 2002). A history of physical and sexual abuse is also not uncommon in patients with an eating disorder and, when present, as in Kim's case, has a profound impact on the patient's experience of illness and on the process of treatment (Brewerton 2005).

TREATMENT

The choice of CBT for Kim's relapse prevention was based on its theoretical appeal and on a recent study demonstrating its superiority to nutritional counseling in preventing relapse during the first year after hospitalization for anorexia nervosa (Pike et al. 2003). My initial treatment with Kim made use of a CBT manual for anorexia nervosa (Wilson and Pike 2001) and recently developed techniques for enhancing motivation in patients with this disorder (Vitousek et al. 1998). From the outset, we focused on the particulars of eating, exercising, and accompanying thoughts and feelings as well as on the larger issues of self-esteem and values, particularly Kim's dichotomous view of herself as either "fat Kim" or "anorexic Kim." Although an initial review of her food records revealed what appeared to be a healthy mix of foods, it soon became clear that Kim was adhering rigidly to the particular foods that felt safe and that the list of safe foods was gradually shrinking. In particular, each time Kim gained weight, even a small amount, she would attribute this weight gain to a particular food and then eliminate this food from her diet. Likewise, if Kim did more than the agreed-upon amount of exercise and did not lose weight, she assumed that she needed this exercise to maintain weight and thereby gradually increased her time spent exercising. Bingeing/purging episodes occurred infrequently and were deemed by the therapist and Kim to be much less worrisome than Kim's restrictive eating and excessive exercising. Not surprisingly, after about 2 months of weight maintenance, Kim began gradually and inexorably to lose weight.

During this phase of treatment, Kim was, as she often freely described herself, "a handful." In particular, although her overall weight trend was initially stable and then began to shift downward, when her weight occasionally fluctuated upward she was flooded by frustration and shame, feeling unfairly punished, despite her hard work. Nonetheless, I looked forward to sessions with Kim. She was engaged in the work of treatment and was increasingly able to appreciate, if not to actively address, the worrisome signs of relapse. She also initially made important efforts to develop a "healthy Kim" as an alternative to the "anorexic Kim" and "fat Kim," and to increase her involvement with friends and family and in other recreational activities. I remained optimistic about her, frequently finding myself after a session thinking, "She's really turned a corner this week." However, as time progressed and gradual weight loss continued, both Kim and I realized that she was losing ground. Like many therapists working with a patient with an eating disorder, I often felt frustrated by my patient's choices regarding eating and exercise and needed frequent reminders from my supervision group to support Kim in her struggle rather than endeavor to struggle against her. By the ninth month of treatment, Kim's weight had dropped to below 100 lb. Although she continued to struggle to regain lost ground, her weight loss continued. By the end of the year-long treatment program, Kim's weight had dropped to 96 lb. I strongly recommended rehospitalization and, although she was initially unwilling to pursue this option, Kim ultimately agreed to be admitted under pressure from her family and supervisors at work.

On the inpatient unit, Kim's target weight range was set at 118–122 lb. Although this represented approximately 100% of her ideal body weight according to the weight tables (in contrast to the unit's usual practice of setting the minimum acceptable weight as 90% of a patient's ideal body weight), she had in the past had normal menstrual cycling only when her weight was at least 120 lb.

After her successful weight regain and discharge, Kim reentered outpatient treatment with me. This time, however, we carefully negotiated a contract that proved to be a central component of our subsequent treatment. We agreed to meet twice a week in individual outpatient CBT sessions. However, in view of her chronic relapsing course, we also agreed that Kim would enter a 3-evening per week intensive outpatient program (IOP) if her weight dropped below 115 lb. If treatment at the IOP was not successful in restoring her weight to the agreed-upon range, she would enter day treatment or inpatient treatment for weight restoration. We further agreed that if Kim did not abide by the contract, our treatment would end. Kim initially believed that it was unlikely that her weight would dip. However, soon after discharge, her weight gradually declined and, after a quarrel with her roommate Robin, she resumed daily exercise at the gym. Her weight dropped more rapidly and, after 6 weeks, she met the criterion for IOP treatment. With great ambivalence, Kim agreed to enter the IOP, after which her weight stabilized at 105–110 lb.

When her coverage at the IOP ended, Kim met with me to discuss further treatment. At the end of her IOP treatment period, she had begun treatment with the atypical antipsychotic, olanzapine (5 mg/day), which has been found in preliminary studies to be helpful for some treatment-refractory patients (Powers et al. 2002); indeed, Kim found that it provided some help to her in avoiding "driven" activities, such as excessive exercise. She stated that she wished to continue outpatient treatment, but that her goals had changed. Her attempts to gain back to her goal range caused her to feel such intense self-loathing that it no longer seemed worthwhile. She felt that, despite the willingness of friends, family, and therapist to help, no one could help her bear the suffering of her body becoming larger. She was not concerned about her amenorrhea as she did not wish to have children and had not yet developed osteoporosis. Although she had not met the original weight goal, she felt that the IOP had been beneficial in helping her to stabilize her weight, cut back her exercise, and socialize more frequently with friends. Although I respected her dilemma, I felt it was crucial to adhere to Kim's initial intent and abide by the original contract, which stated that, under these circumstances, Kim would enter day or inpatient treatment.

A key cognition was Kim's belief that weight gain would be unbearable and that it would never be any easier once she reached her goal range. She also believed that she was not "sick enough" for day or inpatient treatment, despite my recommendation and that of her IOP therapists. I worked with Kim to analyze these thoughts and to complete a decision analysis. Although Kim recognized that there were treatment options, such as medication, that had not yet been fully explored and that she had not recently had the experience of remaining in her goal range for more than 1–2 months and therefore could not really predict what this would be like, she was ultimately unwilling to enter a day or inpatient treatment.

With the much-needed support of my supervision group, I ended treatment with Kim and provided carefully selected referrals. I explained to Kim that, although I believed that treatment directed toward harm reduction might be appropriate in some cases, that other therapists might well adopt such an approach with her, and that I might work in this way with other patients, our treatment was predicated on the goal of full recovery. She and I had put this in place as a nonnegotiable foundation of treatment, and the integrity of our treatment would be lost if we abandoned this goal. We ended treatment on good terms, and the door was left open for Kim to reenter treatment if she once again became willing to work toward recovery. The experience of ending treatment under these circumstances was one of the most difficult of my career.

Some months later, Kim contacted me. She had continued to lose weight and was now willing to reenter inpatient treatment. She once again increased her weight to within her goal range of 118–122 lb. As in the past, the inpatient staff noted the remarkable change in Kim's mood and thinking that accompanied weight gain. With weight gain, Kim went from being a woman single-mindedly obsessed with weight and calories to a bright, humorous, and much more future-oriented individual. Moreover, at the inpatient program, she found members of the inpatient staff with whom she felt particularly comfortable discussing painful experiences, both present (such as feelings when being weighed) and past. In addition, Kim began taking fluoxetine 80 mg/day. On discharge, she once again returned to outpatient treatment with me, and we agreed that our previous contract would remain in effect.

In the latter phase of her inpatient stay, Kim became interested in dating and began to make use of an online dating service. Shortly after her discharge from inpatient treatment, two key events took place. Kim's menstrual cycle returned, an event that she celebrated as a sign of health and normal womanly function. She also met and began dating Bill and, some months into the relationship, became sexually active for the first time in her adult life. At work, Kim began to shed the image of "anorexic Kim" and attained higher levels of achievement than she had ever previously attained. Another important development was that, for the first time, Kim committed herself to avoiding the gym and limited her exercise to walking and nonsolo activities like playing tennis with Bill or taking a dance class. Although in the course of her struggle to remain well Bill has been a valuable ally for Kim, she has avoided making him responsible for keeping her well and, in fact, continued to do well when they broke up for a period of time.

To the delight of patient and therapist alike, Kim has been able to maintain her weight for nearly 2 years at this writing. She is now living with Bill, spending more time with family and friends than ever before in her adult life, and taking particular pleasure in spending time with her nephew and niece now that she is no longer "sick Aunt Kim." Her weight maintenance has not occurred without considerable effort, though. Kim continues to struggle with flexibility in eating, and weight gains are still mildly upsetting to her, although much less so than they once were. Her bingeing/purging episodes continue to occur infrequently, but Kim consistently recovers quickly from these isolated lapses. During one period in which Kim's weight dipped briefly below the acceptable range, I met with Kim and Bill to discuss how they might work together to help her quickly get back into a healthy weight range; this meeting proved productive.

Although she continues to self-monitor her weight assiduously and set and follow through on goals, much of the work of treatment has shifted to Kim's relationships, particularly with Bill, and the ways in which this at times evokes painful core beliefs and old coping mechanisms. Over time, Kim has become much more able to discuss with me the shame-evoking memories of childhood and adolescence and to begin to view these from a more understanding and mature perspective. In addition, she is able to appreciate how these experiences continue to influence her relationship with Bill, and she has made a great deal of progress in identifying and asserting her needs in the relationship. The experience of discussing these issues with me has also provided an opportunity for a CBT-style discussion of transference—that is, we have discussed Kim's automatic expectations of how I would react to her revelations and examined the "reality check" of my actual response.

DISCUSSION

Now in her early 30s, Kim still struggles to maintain her health, but she is living life in a way that, for most of her adult life up to this point, had seemed beyond her reach. When asked about what has helped, Kim points to several aspects of treatment. Like many patients with anorexia nervosa, Kim believes that each episode of outpatient treatment and each hospitalization contributed something to her recovery, and that at a certain point she became able to put it all together in a way that allowed her to more successfully combat her illness. Although at times she is still preoccupied with the "fat Kim/anorexic Kim" dichotomy, the years of remaining out of anorexia's grasp have given her the time to develop a "healthy Kim" voice that combines her need to be strong and powerful and her need for indulgence and comfort. The contribution of fluoxetine treatment to her recovery is difficult to gauge, but both Kim and I believe it was helpful in ameliorating her rigidity in eating. Finally, the continued presence of the contract that once led to a cessation of treatment and may do so again has, perhaps paradoxically, brought a needed level of safety to the treatment. Kim and I have understood that the threat of losing this therapeutic relationship if she should refuse to take all steps necessary to maintain a healthy weight also represents a promise not to abandon the emerging "healthy Kim," even should anorexia nervosa once again cloud her vision of recovery.

REFERENCES

Brewerton TD: Psychological trauma and eating disorders, in Eating Disorders Review, Part 1. Edited by Wonderlich S, Mitchell J, deZwaan M, et al. Oxford, Radcliffe, 2005, pp 137–154

Jacobi C: Psychosocial risk factors for eating disorders, in Eating Disorders Review, Part 1. Edited by Wonderlich S, Mitchell J, deZwaan M, et al. Oxford, Radcliffe, 2005, pp 59–85

Kaye WH, Nagata T, Weltzin TE, et al: Double-blind placebo-controlled administration of fluoxetine in restricting- and restricting-purging-type anorexia nervosa. Biol Psychiatry 49:644–652, 2001

Pike KM, Walsh BT, Vitousek K, et al: Cognitive behavior therapy in the posthospitalization treatment of anorexia nervosa. Am J Psychiatry 160:2046–2049, 2003

Powers PS, Santana CA, Bannon YS: Olanzapine in the treatment of anorexia nervosa: an open label trial. Int J Eat Disord 32:146–154, 2002

Sullivan PF: Course and outcome of anorexia nervosa and bulimia nervosa, in Eating Disorders and Obesity: A Comprehensive Handbook, 2nd Edition. Edited by Fairburn CG, Brownell KD. New York, Guilford, 2002, pp 226–230

Vitousek K, Watson S, Wilson GT: Enhancing motivation for change in treatment-resistant eating disorders. Clin Psychol Rev 18:391–420, 1998

Wilson GT, Pike KM: Eating disorders, in Clinical Handbook of Psychological Disorders, 3rd Edition. Edited by Barlow DH. New York, Guilford, 2001, pp 332–375

PART XIII

Impulse-Control Disorders

CHAPTER 28

Hothead Harry, Gnome Assassin

Combined Treatment of Intermittent Explosive Disorder

Emil F. Coccaro, M.D.
Michael S. McCloskey, Ph.D.

Emil F. Coccaro, M.D., is the Ellen C. Manning Professor and Chairman of the Department of Psychiatry at the University of Chicago. Dr. Coccaro is a psychiatrist and clinical neuropsychopharmacologist whose National Institute of Mental Health–funded research in this area over the past 20 years has included work in the genetics, epidemiology, biology, neuroscience, and treatment of impulsive aggression.

Michael S. McCloskey, Ph.D., is Assistant Professor of Psychiatry at the University of Chicago Hospitals. He is a clinical psychologist who publishes research in the area of aggression and self-aggression. He has been the principal investigator on two National Institute of Health grants and three other foundation grants in these areas. Dr. McCloskey is currently developing a cognitive-behavioral treatment for intermittent explosive disorder.

HARRY, A 35-YEAR-OLD marketing director, called the anger and aggression treatment clinic after a heated argument with his fiancée. As Harry later explained, after being "nagged to death" by his fiancée to mow the lawn, he took a baseball bat and destroyed the couple's lawn gnome (his initial target was the lawn mower, but he thought the better of it). After this outburst, Harry's fiancée gave him the ultimatum to "get help or get lost."

Based on the phone information, I (E.F.C.) expected a bit of a "brute" and was a little surprised when a polite, slightly embarrassed man sheepishly introduced himself to me. Harry was clearly not a brute but a man acutely aware of how damaging his impulsive aggression was to him and others around him. It was easy to feel empathy for Harry as he described his personal history.

HISTORY

Harry stated that throughout his adulthood he has engaged in frequent aggressive outbursts including "heated arguments" and acts of property destruction ("too many to count"). He described several episodes in which he kicked in his television screen, smashed in a stranger's car window, and threw his cell phone at the wall—all in response to relatively minor provocations. Over the past few years, Harry estimated he had had approximately three arguments and one act of property destruction per week. In addition to jeopardizing his current relationship with his fiancée, his aggression had "ruined" past relationships, alienated his coworkers, and almost cost him his job. Harry explained that he became angry "at the drop of a hat...over anything...over nothing" and that the urge to be aggressive often felt overwhelming. Harry's eyes began to well up as he described the shame and remorse he felt following his aggressive acts, although he also reported feeling a huge sense of relief at the same time.

Difficulties with anger were not new for Harry or his family. Harry grew up in a middle class family living in the suburbs. His father, an accountant, although not physically abusive, "definitely had a hair trigger" and would often berate Harry in front of his friends for minor transgressions such as arriving home a few minutes late. Harry's sister and three brothers also had problems with verbal and physical aggression, so that family functions often turned into "war zones." Harry did quite well academically growing up, although he noted having difficulties getting along with classmates, which he attributed to his having low self-esteem. He described how his more severe aggressive acts emerged during childhood, when he would occasionally break small toys or school supplies when he was angry or frustrated.

Harry's impulsive aggression became more prominent in adolescence when he found himself becoming involved in frequent arguments (one to four a week) with friends, classmates, and family members. The frequency with which he would break items in anger (two to eight times a month) also increased. Eventually, his repertoire of property destruction included breaking dishes and punching holes in walls. Because he thought drinking "a few beers" would "mellow [him] out," he began drinking daily during adolescence. At its most severe level when Harry was ages 16–19 years, his drinking met criteria for alcohol abuse.

After graduating from high school, Harry left home to go to college where he obtained his bachelor's degree in marketing. He was also able to develop friendships and a few romantic relationships in college. However, his aggression difficulties continued unabated. His friend gave him the nickname "Hothead Harry" after an incident in which Harry responded to receiving a poor test score by kicking his chair and "accidentally" breaking it.

Harry began working for a marketing firm right out of college, but left the firm after 6 months because he "couldn't stand" how the company was run. He also admitted to not getting along with his coworkers, whom he considered "unprofessional idiots." Harry dated a woman for 3 years in his 20s until they broke up over his irritability and outbursts. Harry was clinically depressed for approximately a month afterward. During this time he considered seeking help but decided, "There is no pill to stop you from being an asshole."

Throughout his late 20s and early 30s, Harry worked at the same company. His dedication to his work helped offset his interpersonal problems; however, his verbal outbursts alienated his coworkers. This situation came to a head 3 years earlier when Harry grabbed and pushed a coworker (his only reported act of physical assault) after an altercation in which Harry yelled at the coworker for not completing a task. The coworker told Harry to "chill out and start drinking decaf." After the incident, Harry was mandated to see an employee assistance program counselor for five sessions. Harry did not find these sessions useful, explaining, "We didn't really do anything." Harry was introduced to his fiancée 2 years before I saw him. Their relationship was tumultuous, with Harry being warned on several occasions to control his anger after incidents in which he would yell or break objects. Harry described a pattern of his feeling guilty and angry with himself after his outbursts, after which he would attempt to apologize only to become defensive and verbally aggressive again when his fiancée expressed her anger at his overreaction. Harry was quick to add that he never threatened his fiancée nor put his hands on her in anger, stating "I am not that bad a guy, really. It is just my goddamned temper."

DIAGNOSIS

Harry's history of aggression was consistent with a diagnosis of intermittent explosive disorder (IED). Harry had a pattern of generalized reactive aggression that resulted in numerous acts of serious property destruction. The aggressive acts were not instrumental (i.e., they were not preplanned or used as a means to gain a tangible reward such as power or money). Rather, the aggressive behavior was an impulsive corollary to feelings of intense anger. Although Harry had a history of alcohol abuse and a previous major depressive episode, the aggressive behavior was not confined to either disorder, with most of his aggressive acts occurring in the absence of any comorbid Axis I disorder.

Harry's case illustrates clinical features common in IED. A number of his first-degree relatives also appeared to have problems with impulsive aggression. Studies show that up to 32% of first-degree relatives of IED patients also have IED (McElroy et al. 1998). Harry's symptoms appear to have first met full criteria for IED during adolescence, which is consistent with research showing the median age of onset for IED as mid-adolescence (Coccaro et al. 2005; McElroy et al. 1998).

Harry endorsed past alcohol abuse and major depression. Most individuals with IED have comorbid Axis I disorders. Among the more common are depressive disorders, anxiety disorders, and substance use disorders, with prevalence rates for each of these disorders over 50% in some IED population samples (Coccaro et al. 2005). The presence of these disorders would preclude a diagnosis of IED only if the aggressive behavior were better accounted for by the comorbid disorder. For example, if an individual becomes aggressive almost exclusively when intoxicated or during a depressive episode, then a diagnosis of IED should not be made. Although Harry had some obsessive-compulsive and paranoid personality traits, he did not have a personality disorder. Personality disorders are commonly comorbid with IED (Coccaro et al. 2005). Again, the existence of a personality disorder is only exclusionary when it appears to better account for the aggressive behavior. This distinction may be difficult to make in the case of individuals with antisocial personality and borderline personality disorders, both of which have anger and aggression as part of their criteria sets.

The outbursts described by Harry are also typical for individuals with IED. Aggressive outbursts in IED tend to have a rapid onset (McElroy et al. 1998), often without a recognizable prodromal period (Felthous et al. 1991; Mattes 1990). These episodes are usually short-lived (less than 30 minutes) (McElroy et al. 1998) and can involve verbal assault, destructive and nondestructive property assault, and physical assault (Mattes 1990; McElroy et al. 1998). The outbursts most commonly occur in response to a minor provocation by a close intimate or associate (Felthous et al. 1991; McElroy et al. 1998), although in some cases they can occur without any identifiable provocation (McElroy et al. 1998).

Two other facets of Harry's aggression common to IED, but not currently a part of DSM-IV-TR criteria for IED, are the frequent acts of verbal aggression and the distress and impairment caused by the aggressive acts. Harry reported engaging in over 3,000 heated arguments as an adult. Most individuals with IED also report clinically significant verbal aggression (i.e., greater than eight arguments a month) (Coccaro 2003). The ubiquitous nature of verbal aggression in IED has led Coccaro et al. (1998) to develop alternate research criteria that allow for the diagnosis of IED for individuals who have frequent acts of verbal aggression. Harry clearly identified his anger and aggression as being personally distressing as well as interpersonally and occupationally impairing. The DSM-IV-TR criteria for IED do not include evidence of distress or impairment. However, research has shown that IED is associated with substantial distress, impairment in social functioning, and occupational difficulty as well as legal or financial problems (Coccaro 2003; Mattes 1990; McElroy et al. 1998).

TREATMENT

During the assessment, Harry voiced a strong desire to reduce his aggressive outbursts. However, he refused an initial recommendation of a combination of medication and cognitive-behavioral therapy (CBT). Harry agreed to the medication but felt he could not comply with the demands of CBT. He was started on fluoxetine (20 mg/day for 4 weeks and then 40 mg/day thereafter) and was came to our clinic biweekly for follow-up.

As with many behavioral disorders, the treatment of IED may include psychopharmacological and/or psychosocial intervention. In mild-to-moderate cases of IED, patients should be encouraged to begin CBT augmented by medication, if necessary. In this case, Harry declined psychotherapy at first and accepted a medication-only treatment, mostly due to his perception of what was easier and more convenient. Medications such as fluoxetine have been shown to be effective in reducing aggression (especially verbal and object aggression) provided that the medication is continued for at least 6–12 weeks (Coccaro and Kavoussi 1997). Despite some improvement with this regimen, many patients continue to display aggressive behavior on "effective" doses and ultimately require psychosocial intervention so that strategies for dealing with environmental provocations may be learned and applied. In this regard, it is important to recognize that although medications appear to increase the threshold at which a patient with IED "explodes" through augmentation of central serotonergic activity, which in turn increases behavioral inhibition, medications do not address issues related to how patients could appropriately handle environmental provocations so that their threshold for exploding is never reached. For this, patients with IED benefit most from CBT.

Within 6 weeks, Harry's aggressive outbursts had decreased by 50%, and by 12 weeks he was having approximately one aggressive outburst per week. Although this represented a large improvement in his aggressive behavior, Harry realized that he was not doing as well as he would have liked. An increase in the fluoxetine to 60 mg/day did not reduce his aggressive behavior any further and only resulted in an increase in sexual side effects that, while tolerable on 40 mg/day po of fluoxetine, were not tolerable on 60 mg/day po of fluoxetine. Through our discussions, Harry realized that further improvement would require CBT if he wanted to reach a maximal level of symptom reduction. With that, Harry agreed to begin 13 weeks of CBT based on the treatment manual developed by Deffenbacher and McKay (2000). He was referred to my colleague (M.S.M.) for CBT.

Harry's initial refusal to engage in CBT suggested that his commitment to treatment may not have been sufficient to enable optimal results. Therefore the expectations and requirements of treatment were explained to Harry in even greater detail than usual. This meant first letting Harry know that although there is no empirically validated psychosocial treatment of IED (Galovski and Blanchard 2002), there is preliminary evidence to suggest that the 13-week course of CBT is effective in decreasing anger outbursts among IED patients (McCloskey et al. 2004). Harry smiled and replied, "So you think it works, but there are no guarantees." I (M.S.M.) thought, "So far so good, but here comes the hard part." The nature of the treatment was then discussed (i.e., 3 weeks of relaxation, 2 weeks of cognitive restructuring, and 7 weeks of combined relaxation, cognitive restructuring, and imaginal exposure). It was explained to Harry that for the treatment to be effective, it would require a strong commitment on his part, including his attending every session and completing all at-home assignments, which could take up to an hour a day. Harry suddenly stared at me and yelled, "This is stupid! You know I can't do this." My previous experience with anger patients helped me mute my immediate reaction of annoyance and frustration. We discussed what sacrifices he would need to make if he were to engage in CBT. We then discussed how his life would change if he could stop having regular aggressive outbursts. He decided that the difference would be well worth the 50- to 75-hour time investment, and his demeanor changed immediately. He was on board to undergo CBT treatment.

It might be assumed that IED patients will tend to be aggressive toward their therapist. However, although they can be argumentative, in our experience they are rarely threatening or in any way physically aggressive within the context of the therapeutic relationship. On the few occasions when this has occurred, it tended to be early in treatment and due to the therapist's failure to make the patient feel adequately understood. It is also important for the clinician to foster motivation early in treatment. IED subjects can be ambivalent about treatment early in therapy, especially if they are "forced" into treatment by a loved one's ultimatum. In this situation, a motivational enhancement strategy such as nonjudgmentally having the subject list the pros and cons of remaining aggressive or continuing therapy might be useful.

Harry had initial difficulty identifying the process by which his anger escalated into aggression. This was not disconcerting because IED individuals often initially feel their anger goes, as Harry stated, "from 0 to 100." To increase his awareness of the anger that preceded his aggression (and to document his progress), Harry monitored his anger and aggression throughout treatment using an anger log. This was also helpful in demonstrating the aggression cues of which Harry was not previously aware. For example, Harry noticed that after his fiancée's mother had called, he would often have an argument with his fiancée.

The first three sessions with Harry went smoothly. He quickly grasped the relaxation training skills (i.e., diaphragmatic breathing, muscle relaxation, and relaxation imagery) and was encouraged by his ability to use them to calm down after becoming angry. The use of relaxation training at the beginning of treatment often provides IED patients with a feeling of accomplishment and allows the therapeutic relationship to develop before work on cognitive restructuring begins.

The third session also included work on the use of "time out." The development of an escape strategy early in therapy is extremely important because the potential for violence is always present in individuals with IED. This can be accomplished after teaching a basic relaxation response, so that the patient has a beneficial behavior (rather than ruminating) to engage in during the time out. Harry initially balked at the use of a time out, stating that he would try it but felt he was being subjected to what he considered a child's punishment. I was impressed with Harry's ability to express a negative emotion without being overly hostile and his openness to try something with which he did not completely agree. That being said, I felt it important to address his impression of the time out strategy as being more appropriate for children. Harry was a sports fan, so the analogy of a coach's time out, which allows the players to "get out of the rut and get their heads together" was used. This had the desired effect, and Harry proceeded to rehearse using a time out during an argument with his fiancée.

By the fourth session, Harry was reporting a decrease in his anger and aggression. This was a relief as he was about to begin the treatment component that is often most difficult for IED patients—cognitive restructuring. Harry was able to identify automatic thoughts but had significant difficulty with the underlying cognitive distortion (i.e., blaming, misattribution, demanding/commanding, labeling, overgeneralizing, catastrophizing). However, his attitude in the sessions remained positive with little sign of the frustration he had evidenced at the outset of treatment. This was an unexpected treat and provided more evidence of Harry's commitment to treatment. With continued practice in sessions and at home, Harry gradually became quite adept at identifying his cognitive distortions.

Difficulty with cognitive restructuring, although frustrating for therapist and client alike, is not an insurmountable hurdle. It is helpful to proceed at a slow pace, using multiple examples and obtaining evidence that the client understands each step before moving on. However, the therapist must be cognizant of the low frustration tolerance of IED patients. Socratic questioning and rewarding partial success are useful in this regard.

By the sixth session, Harry reported with some pride that his coworkers had commented on his improved attitude. I was likewise pleased with his improvement. We began implementing cognitive and relaxation skills during imaginal anger exposure. Harry was asked to imagine a past provocation until he felt himself becoming angry again, then to use his cognitive and relaxation coping skills to regain his sense of calm. Harry was initially distressed about having to relive past anger situations and aggressive acts that he wanted to put behind him. I empathized with his desire to not reexperience his past anger and reframed the event as investing the anger toward developing skills that would lead to a calmer future. Harry was still skeptical but agreed to continue. After his first imaginal exposure, he reported that the experience, though unpleasant, was not as unpleasant as he had initially feared, and he volunteered that he might have catastrophized earlier.

Harry arrived at our eighth session quite distressed, stating that the treatment was not working. I immediately asked about the events of the past week. He reported that he had had a "huge blowup" with his fiancée who called him at work to discuss their wedding plans. During the argument he yelled and cursed at his fiancée and finally threw his cell phone, damaging it. Harry had made great strides in reducing his tendency to be overly harsh and blaming of others; however, dealing with his own fallibility was still difficult. Harry had presented me with the perfect opportunity to address this blindspot. As he talked I jotted down a few key statements. After a discussion about how and why his self-expectations might be a "hot button," we then went over the key statements I had noted (e.g., "If I were getting better, this wouldn't have happened") and identified the cognitive distortions involved. We then discussed relapse prevention, differentiating a slip from a relapse and examining how to learn from slips. This process is usually saved for a bit later in treatment, but I wanted to take advantage of Harry's crisis state. Harry asked to call his fiancée and apologize while in the session, and after a brief rehearsal, did an excellent job of taking responsibility for his actions and allowing his fiancée to express her anger without his becoming defensive. As Harry would later tell me, this session had a powerful impact on his anger control efforts.

The remainder of therapy went smoothly. Harry continued to use his cognitive and relaxation skills in session while imagining a scene that typically caused him to become angry and out of session whenever he became upset. He had no other "big blowups" and his post-CBT assessment revealed a further 50% reduction in anger since the beginning of treatment and a near absence of aggressive outbursts over the past month. Moreover, Harry had not engaged in any acts of property destruction over the last 5 weeks of therapy. His quality of life also improved. At treatment's end, Harry stated that he was much happier at work and that his relationship with his fiancée was greatly improved.

Harry returned to the clinic 6 months later. He acknowledged that his anger and aggression had increased since leaving treatment (and after stopping the fluoxetine) to about one to two heated arguments a month, including two that involved property destruction (breaking a CD and throwing his remote control against the wall). He was still far less angry and aggressive than he had been prior to treatment, and it was heartening to hear him exclaim that he wanted to learn from his "slips." Harry denied any anger-related problems at work or in his personal life, adding that he and his fiancée were in the midst of planning their wedding. Harry agreed to resume relaxation and cognitive coping skills practice and meet with us periodically to help guard against increased anger and aggression during this stressful time in his life.

The later course of Harry's IED showed a similar pattern to that of other patients in our clinic. For this reason, it might be useful to implement a more gradual "fading" of treatment of IED that includes three to six booster sessions at 2-week to 1-month intervals.

Our last contact with Harry was a phone call after he returned from his honeymoon. He informed us that he and his new wife were doing well and that, although he still had occasional flare-ups, his hothead days were behind him, to the delight of Harry, his wife, his coworkers,...and garden gnomes everywhere.

DISCUSSION

Harry's care represents a positive outcome in the treatment of IED. Individually, either CBT or selective serotonin reuptake inhibitors (SSRIs) typically reduce aggression in patients with IED. Although the degree of improvement may be quite marked in many patients, many others continue to have impulsive-aggressive symptomotology, albeit at a noticeably reduced frequency and/or intensity. No studies have yet examined the efficacy of combined SSRI and CBT treatment for IED. Our clinical work has shown that patients can often show additional improvement in remaining impulsive-aggressive symptomolotogy when the second treatment modality is added. Even in the most successful cases, total elimination of aggressive acts for an extended period may be relatively rare.

Harry initially vocalized a preference for medication over CBT. In our experience, individuals are fairly evenly split in their preference for medication or psychotherapy. Not surprisingly, those who prefer psychotherapy often point to the time investment associated with CBT as a limiting factor, whereas those stating a preference for CBT report concerns about potential medication side effects, especially sexual side effects. As there is no data suggesting one modality is superior to the other, we typically employ the treatment modality the patient prefers first and then recommend the other modality, if warranted and acceptable, to the patient.

Positive outcomes like Harry's are not unusual in our practice. However, this is not to say that all of our IED patients benefit from CBT and/or SSRIs. For some patients, mood stabilizers may be beneficial as antiaggressive agents. A direct comparison of SSRIs to a mood stabilizer has not yet been performedm, although such a study is ongoing in our research program at this time; the results of this study, however, may not be available for several years. Individuals with more limited cognitive abilities often do not respond as well to CBT. Though unknown, it is possible that other forms of psychotherapy would be more effective for these individuals. However, for the majority of IED patients CBT and SSRIs individually or in combination is an effective treatment.

REFERENCES

Coccaro EF: Intermittent explosive disorder, in Aggression: Psychiatric Assessment and Treatment. Edited by Coccaro EF. New York, Marcel Dekker, 2003, pp 149–199

Coccaro EF, Kavoussi RJ: Fluoxetine and impulsive aggressive behavior in personality disordered subjects. Arch Gen Psychiatry 54:1081–1088, 1997

Coccaro EF, Kavoussi RJ, Berman ME, et al: Intermittent explosive disorder, revised: development, reliability, and validity of research criteria. Compr Psychiatry 39:368–376, 1998

Coccaro EF, Posternak MA, Zimmerman M: Prevalence and features of intermittent explosive disorder in clinical setting. J Clin Psychiatry 66:1221-1227, 2005

Deffenbacher JL, McKay M: Overcoming Situational and General Anger: A Protocol for the Treatment of Anger Based on Relaxation, Cognitive Restructuring, and Coping Skills Training. Oakland, CA, New Harbinger, 2000

Felthous AR, Bryant G, Wingerter CB, et al: The diagnosis of intermittent explosive disorder in violent men. Bull Am Acad Psychiatry Law 19:71–79, 1991

Galovski T, Blanchard EB: The effectiveness of a brief psychological intervention on court-referred and self-referred aggressive drivers. Behav Res Ther 40:1385–1402, 2002

Mattes JA: Comparative effectiveness of carbamazepine and propranolol for rage outbursts. J Neuropsychiatry Clin Neurosci 2:159–164, 1990

McCloskey MS, Noblett KL, Gollan JK, et al: The Efficacy of Group Cognitive Behavioral Therapy in Reducing Anger Among Patients with Intermittent Explosive Disorder: A Pilot Study. Poster presented at the 2004 annual meeting of the Association for the Advancement of Behavior Therapy, New Orleans, LA, November 2004

McElroy SL, Soutullo CA, Beckman DA, et al: DSM-IV intermittent explosive disorder: a report of 27 cases. J Clin Psychiatry 59:203–210, 1998

CHAPTER 29

The Red and the Black

Integrated Treatment of Pathological Gambling

Eric Hollander, M.D.
Bernardo Dell'Osso, M.D.

Eric Hollander, M.D., is Professor of Psychiatry, Director of Clinical Psychopharmacology, Director of the Seaver and New York Autism Center of Excellence, and Director of the Compulsive, Impulsive, and Anxiety Disorders Program at the Mount Sinai School of Medicine in New York City. He has authored more than 300 scientific publications and several books in various research fields, including obsessive-compulsive spectrum disorders, autism spectrum disorders, social anxiety disorder, and impulse control disorders.

Bernardo Dell'Osso, M.D., is a Research Fellow at the Mount Sinai School of Medicine in New York City, where he is also a member of the Compulsive, Impulsive, and Anxiety Disorders Program. He is also member of the Department of Psychiatry in the Department of Clinical Sciences Luigi Sacco of the University of Milan, Italy. He is author of several scientific publications regarding the neurobiology of psychiatric disorders, including mood disorders, obsessive-compulsive spectrum disorders, autism spectrum disorders, and impulse-control disorders.

CAROLYN, A 30-YEAR-OLD bank teller, presented to our research program complaining of feeling anxious, depressed, and guilty after having been arrested for shoplifting. She denied any medical illness and acknowledged that she had experienced some mood fluctuations over the past 10 years. Carolyn struck me as being particularly anxious and depressed when she told her story, which provided important information regarding her diagnosis.

HISTORY

During her adolescence, Carolyn was a dynamic and active person, a natural leader who was involved in many activities, sports, and friendships. However, at times she experienced brief periods of depression with anxiety and rumination that lasted no more than a couple of days. Over the last 10 years, however, she had felt more affectively unstable, particularly after losing money while gambling. She had never had any prior psychiatric treatment. "When I feel nervous, anxious, or depressed, the only way to really feel better is to gamble," she said. In addition, she reported that her grandmother had lost her entire fortune at the casino after years of card playing, that her parents were occasional gamblers, and that her brother was a gambler who, after receiving treatment with a selective serotonin reuptake inhibitor for depression, never gambled again.

Carolyn's gambling began at age 18 when she would accompany her brother to the casino. She played roulette and slot machines and often won more than $100. During the next 2 years, she visited the casino once a week, generally playing roulette and video poker but also blackjack and cards. At the casino she felt satisfied and comfortable and could forget any problems in her life. When she gambled, she would smoke and drink more than usual.

Carolyn's control over her gambling was initially adequate, and she could stop gambling when she was satisfied with what she had won or when she had lost the amount of money she had foreseen for the evening. Within 2 years, however, she began gambling almost twice a week, not only at the casino but by playing bingo and numbers and betting on horses. Furthermore, she increased the amount of money she wagered to achieve the same level of excitement that she had when she first started gambling, and her degree of control over her gambling and her ability to stop gambling became less successful. During this period, her mood became less stable. She felt anxious and nervous at work, especially when she had lost money the day before; she had problems sleeping; and she sometimes became inappropriately angry with her relatives or boyfriend.

During the 3 years before I saw her, Carolyn spent $300–$1,000 per week, frequently gambled more than she intended to, and every time she lost money would return the following day to try to win it back. She could not afford this amount on her salary, and she began to borrow money from credit cards and loan sharks and finally sold personal property to obtain money for gambling. She was no longer satisfied with her work and often wandered from her office into the betting halls. Her social activities became more limited and she broke up with her boyfriend. "When I gamble, nobody can divert my attention. I am completely focused and I don't like when someone distracts me or invites me to have a drink."

Carolyn's situation had worsened in the months preceding our meeting, with gambling becoming an obsession for her. The time she was occupied by thoughts and activities related to gambling increased to more than 5 hours per day and resulted in severe interference and substantial impairment in her social and occupational performances, with frequent and unmotivated absences from her workplace and increasing disinterest toward her family. Her capacity to resist urges was completely abolished and she became more anxious and depressed. Finally, after being arrested for shoplifting that she had committed to give back money to her creditors, she had severe feelings of guilt and marked insomnia. Over the 3 weeks preceding therapy, she had experienced transient thoughts of death and suicide.

DIAGNOSIS

The diagnosis of pathological gambling (DSM-IV-TR) was not difficult to make in this case. Carolyn's symptoms met almost all the inclusion criteria for this disorder: she was preoccupied with her gambling behavior, she had made repeated unsuccessful efforts to control or stop gambling, and she felt irritable when she attempted to stop gambling. Likewise, gambling represented for her a way to relieve her anxiety and depressed mood. Moreover, she reported that any time she lost money, she returned to gamble again. She was also involved in illegal acts such as selling stolen goods to find money to gamble and, finally, she lost her romantic relationship and put her job at risk by spending considerable time gambling during office hours. These features distinguish a recreational or professional gambler from a pathological gambler, whose gambling behavior results in significant impairment in social and occupational functioning.

It is noteworthy to highlight the comorbidity with pathological gambling that might influence treatment outcome. Carolyn reported having experienced mood swings throughout her life span, which met the criteria for cyclothymic disorder (DSM-IV-TR), as well as gambling-related alcohol and nicotine abuse. Of note, she had a family history of gambling involving her grandmother and her brother.

Carolyn's baseline score on the Pathological Gambling–Yale Brown Obsessive Compulsive Scale was extremely severe (32 total: 16 on thoughts/urges and 16 on gambling behavior) and on the South Oaks Gambling Screen was extremely severe (17). The severity of her illness was rated as extreme on the Pathological Gambling-Clinical Global Impressions Scale.

TREATMENT

Carolyn approached our program at a time when we were conducting a trial to compare the effectiveness and tolerability of lithium versus placebo in patients with pathological gambling and bipolar spectrum or cyclothymic disorder. Patients, blind to their treatment condition, had a 50% chance of receiving lithium (starting at a dosage of 300 mg/day and progressing up to 1,200 mg/day) or placebo. Given Carolyn's history, I thought that she met all the inclusion criteria for such a study. Therefore, after giving informed consent, she received blinded treatment with the mood stabilizer, lithium, for 10 weeks. Lithium has been found to be helpful in the treatment of pathological gambling, especially for those with comorbid mood cycling problems (Hollander et al. 2005; Pallanti et al. 2002).

Carolyn completed the study with minimal to no side effects and with a substantial improvement in her clinical condition, resulting in a significant reduction in her thoughts and urges to gamble as well as in an increased capacity to delay or inhibit acting on impulses. Her reduction in impulsive gambling was accompanied by a reduction in affective instability and improvement in depressive symptomatology.

DISCUSSION

Carolyn's case illustrates many of the clinical features of pathological gambling. The prevalence of this disorder is 1%–3% in the U.S. adult population (Gerstein et al. 1999; Shaffer et al. 1999). It is characterized by recurrent and maladaptive patterns of gambling behavior that significantly disrupt a person's personal, familial, or vocational functioning. There has been a dramatic increase in the rates of pathological gambling over the last decade that appears to be related to the legalization and availability of new forms of gambling in most Western countries. Core psychopathological features of pathological gambling include impulsivity, a compulsive drive to gamble, addictive features such as withdrawal symptoms after abstaining from gambling, and bipolar features such as urges to gamble, pleasure-seeking behaviors, and reduced judgment capacity associated with unrealistic appraisal of one's own abilities. As in Carolyn's case, pathological gambling generally begins during adolescence, with a prevalence in adolescents (about 4%–7%) that is even larger than in adults. Within a short time, pathological gamblers usually begin to show a progressive defect in their ability to assess risk versus benefit and a failure to delay or inhibit their acting on impulses, which finally result in negative functional consequences.

Consistent with Carolyn's case, most pathological gamblers seeking treatment score significantly higher than a control population on measures of depression (Roy et al. 1988) and have high incidences of various psychiatric disorders, including depressive, bipolar, anxiety, and substance use disorders (National Research Council 1999). Gambling may, in fact, predispose vulnerable individuals to develop specific comorbid disorders, and particular psychiatric disorders may promote the development of pathological gambling in vulnerable individuals. Drinking and gambling, for example, are a common co-occurrence (Lesieur et al. 1986); moreover, several studies have linked alcohol intoxication to interference with cognitive processes involved in decision making (Baron and Dickerson 1999), risk-related judgments (Breslin et al. 1999), and attentional focus (Steele and Josephs 1988). Furthermore, some clinical features of pathological gambling resemble clinical features of bipolar disorder, and the comorbidity between pathological gambling and bipolar disorder has been estimated to be as high as 24% (Linden et al. 1986). The experience of the urge to gamble in pathological gambling seems to represent a potential overlap between pathological gambling and the spectrum of bipolar disorders. When Carolyn came for screening, she appeared to me to be more depressed than hypomanic, and her mood state gave her more insight than is normally found in pathological gamblers, especially if they are experiencing hypomanic or euphoric mood phases. It was clear that she had brief periods of mood instability, with episodes lasting from a few days to a few weeks, that were characterized by increased irritability and aggressiveness, distractibility, and decreased need for sleep. These issues, which outline the features of cyclothymic disorder, the mildest form of bipolar disorder, were the focus of our study.

I decided to offer Carolyn the possibility of enrolling in our trial because of the affective features associated with her gambling behavior. Carolyn, who was taking lithium rather than placebo, completed the study without reporting any side effects. Like most of the patients who received the active medication, she showed a substantial improvement at the end of the study in her gambling behavior and in its related scales. She shifted from a baseline time of 5 hours a day occupied by thoughts and activities related to gambling to 1 hour a day at the end point, with a better degree of control over her gambling behavior and no interference or distress associated with social and occupational performance. Moreover, during the last week of treatment, she reported no gambling episodes. Likewise, her affective instability was markedly improved; her irritability, aggressiveness, and feelings of guilt had disappeared, and she showed a stable mood with relief from anxiety, preoccupations, and sleep problems. Finally, her alcohol abuse and nicotine dependence were dramatically reduced.

In terms of pharmacotherapy, mood stabilizers (lithium, valproate, and carbamazepine) represent only one of the three classes of psychotropic medications that have been used to treat adult pathological gambling; opioid antagonists and serotonin reuptake inhibitors have also shown efficacy in treating pathological gambling and other impulse control disorders. Other single- and double-blind studies have confirmed the efficacy of mood stabilizers (lithium and valproate) in pathological gambling with or without associated bipolar features (Hollander et al. 2005; Pallanti et al. 2002). The selective serotonin reuptake inhibitors represent another valid pharmacological therapy for pathological gamblers; they have been found to be effective in some, but not all, double-blind studies. These include fluvoxamine (Luvox; mean dosage 220 mg/day; Blanco et al. 2002; Hollander et al. 1998, 2000) and paroxetine (Paxil; dosages up to 60 mg/day; Kim et al. 2002). An overlap in the phenomenology, neurobiology, and treatment response of pathological gambling and obsessive-compulsive disorder, in fact, has supported the conceptualization of pathological gambling as an obsessive-compulsive spectrum disorder (Hollander 1993). However, as our group reported in a prior single-blind study, patients like Carolyn who have bipolar comorbidity may not benefit from the use of an antidepressant because it may cause a worsening of the comorbid pathology and consequently a relapse of the impulsive condition.

Another pharmacological alternative may be treatment with opioid antagonists (e.g., naltrexone) as was demonstrated in recent studies (Kim et al. 2001). However, as Kim et al. reported, the high doses required to obtain satisfactory results with naltrexone may be associated with a risk of liver damage. Another indication for the use of naltrexone is comorbid substance abuse. Because Carolyn did not report any of these features and had bipolar comorbid features, we decided not to prescribe naltrexone.

In my experience, the choice of pharmacotherapy for a pathological gambler must include the assessment of comorbidity, with a recognition of the strong relation between impulsivity and affective instability. The observation that different types of medications for treating pathological gamblers are more or less effective depending on the patients' comorbidity suggests the existence of different pathological gambling subtypes. For example, a clinician might choose a serotonin reuptake inhibitor if obsessive-compulsive features predominate or a mood stabilizer if there is bipolar spectrum comorbidity. However, additional double-blind, placebo-controlled studies are needed to determine the long-term effectiveness of these medications.

It is noteworthy to remember that pharmacotherapies represent only one aspect in the comprehensive management of patients with this disorder. The treatment of patients like Carolyn, who have a significant family history of gambling and longitudinal and cross-sectional affective comorbidity, requires a multifactorial approach, including psychological, social, and pharmacological measures. Psychosocial approaches used to treat adult pathological gambling include Gamblers Anonymous, cognitive-behavioral therapy, and motivational enhancement therapy (MET). MET is an intervention based on motivational psychology designed to produce rapid, internally motivated change and help the patient initiate, persist in, and comply with behavioral change efforts. MET has been used in treating alcohol and other substance abuse and pathological gambling. Among adolescents, cognitive-behavioral therapy as well as eclectic therapy have been helpful in reducing problematic gambling behavior (Pietrzak et al. 2003).

Psychosocial interventions in the treatment of pathological gambling should be oriented to the modification of several factors. It is important to reduce conditioned stimuli for gambling: gambling sites or gambling images should, whenever possible, be avoided, and contact with money must be reduced by removing credit cards and access to bank accounts. There is no general agreement with regard to the need for complete abstinence from gambling; although total abstinence may be useful to prevent gambling bouts, learning new styles of gambling free of impulsive and uncontrolled decisions may be effective for some patients. Also, cognitive restructuring of a patient's unrealistic expectations of winning and belief that "chasing" is a sensible strategy to regain losses might be helpful. Several depressive attributional styles that lead patients to gamble in response to negative events should be restructured, and negative internal states must be modified. Financial needs should be addressed by counseling about job opportunities and budgeting skills. Also, the pathological dependence of the patient's self-esteem on winning at gambling should be confronted. Marital or social problems are usually associated with pathological gambling and produce increased dysphoria, which may precipitate further gambling. The role of self-help groups, such as Gamblers Anonymous, in treatment seems to be highly beneficial if long-term attendance is achieved, but most gamblers drop out after a few visits. Both clinical experience and the published literature, in fact, suggest that pathological gamblers usually show high rates of early or unauthorized departure from treatment (Nathan 2003); a marked impulsivity appears to be a significant predictor of the risk of dropping out of treatment. At the end of the trial, we suggested that Carolyn receive additional psychotherapy to maintain and consolidate the improvements she had achieved with the pharmacological treatment.

REFERENCES

Baron E, Dickerson M: Alcohol consumption and self-control of gambling behaviour. J Gambl Stud 15(1):3–15, 1999

Blanco C, Petkova E, Ibanez A, et al: A pilot placebo-controlled study of fluvoxamine for pathological gambling. Ann Clin Psychiatry 14(1):9–15, 2002

Breslin FC, Cappell H, Sobell MB, et al: The effects of alcohol, gender, and sensation seeking on the gambling choices of social drinkers. Psychol Addict Behav 13:243–252, 1999

Gerstein DR, Volberg RA, Toce MT, et al: Gambling Impact and Behavior Study: Report to the National Gambling Impact Study Commission. Chicago, IL, National Opinion Research Center at the University of Chicago, 1999

Haller R, Hinterhuber H: Treatment of pathological gambling with carbamazepine. Pharmacopsychiatry 27:129, 1994

Hollander E: Obsessive-Compulsive Related Disorders. Washington, DC, American Psychiatric Press, 1993

Hollander E, DeCaria CM, Mari E, et al: Short-term single-blind fluvoxamine treatment of pathological gambling. Am J Psychiatry 155:1781–1783, 1998

Hollander E, DeCaria CM, Finkell JM, et al: A randomized double-blind fluvoxamine/placebo crossover trial in pathological gambling. Biol Psychiatry 47:813–817, 2000

Hollander E, Pallanti S, Allen A, et al: Does sustained-release lithium reduce impulsive gambling and affective instability versus placebo in pathological gamblers with bipolar spectrum disorders? Am J Psychiatry 162:137–145, 2005

Kim SW, Grant JE, Adson DE, et al: Double-blind naltrexone and placebo comparison study in the treatment of pathological gambling. Biol Psychiatry 49(11):914–921, 2001

Kim SW, Grant JE, Adson DE, et al: A double-blind placebo-controlled study of the efficacy and safety of paroxetine in the treatment of pathological gambling. J Clin Psychiatry 63:501–507, 2002

Kim SW, Grant JE, Adson DE, et al: Disordered gambling in adolescents: epidemiology, diagnosis, and treatment. Paediatr Drugs 5(9):583–95, 2003

Lesieur HR, Blume SB, Zoppa RM: Alcoholism, drug abuse, and gambling. Alcohol Clin Exp Res 10(1):33–38, 1986

Linden RD, Pope HG, Jonas JM, et al: Pathological gambling and major affective disorder: preliminary findings. J Clin Psychiatry 47:201–203, 1986

Nathan PE: The role of natural recovery in alcoholism and pathological gambling. J Gambl Stud 19(3):279–286, 2003

National Research Council: Pathological Gambling: A Critical Review. Washington DC, National Academy Press, 1999

Pallanti S, Quercioli L, Sood E, et al: Lithium and valproate treatment of pathological gambling: a randomized single-blind study. J Clin Psychiatry 63:559–564, 2002

Roy A, Custer R, Lorenz V, et al: Depressed pathological gamblers. Acta Psychiatr Scand 77(2):163–165, 1988

Shaffer HJ, Hall MN, Vander Bilt J: Estimating the prevalence of disordered gambling behavior in the United States and Canada: a research synthesis. Am J Public Health 89:1369–1376, 1999

Steele CM, Josephs RA: Drinking your troubles away, II: An attention-allocation model of alcohol's effect on psychological stress. J Abnorm Psychol 97(2):196–205, 1988

SUGGESTED READING

DeCaria CM, Hollander E, Grossman R, et al: Diagnosis, neurobiology, and treatment of pathological gambling. J Clin Psychiatry 57:80–84, 1996

Hollander E, Buchalter AJ, DeCaria CM: Pathological gambling. Psychiatr Clin North Am 23:629–642, 2000

Lopez-Ibor JJ, Carrasco JL: Pathological gambling, in Impulsivity and Aggression. Edited by Hollander E, Stein D. New York, Wiley, 1995, pp 137–149

Sood ED, Pallanti S, Hollander E: Diagnosis and treatment of pathologic gambling. Curr Psychiatry Rep 5:9–15, 2003

PART XIV

Personality Disorders

CHAPTER 30

Volatile Vivian

STEPPS Treatment of Borderline Personality Disorder

Nancee Blum, M.S.W.
Bruce Pfohl, M.D.

Nancee Blum, M.S.W., is a Social Work Specialist in the Department of Psychiatry in the Roy J. and Lucille A. Carver College of Medicine at The University of Iowa. She is also an adjunct instructor in the College of Medicine, College of Nursing, and School of Social Work. Prior to joining the Department of Psychiatry in 1986, she spent several years as a medical writer and editor in the Department of Internal Medicine at The University of Iowa, the Department of Pediatric Neurology at Washington University in St. Louis, and the Department of Cardiology at the University of Miami. She completed the Aging Studies program at The University of Iowa, and is coauthor of *Sexual Health in Later Life*. Her current research and clinical interests are in the area of personality disorders and obsessive-compulsive disorder. She is a member of the Scientific Advisory Boards of the Obsessive-Compulsive Foundation and the Treatment and Research Advancements Association for Personality Disorder. She is one of the authors of the *Structured Interview for DSM-IV Personality (SIDP-IV)* and the STEPPS treatment program for treatment of borderline personality disorder.

Bruce Pfohl, M.D., is Professor of Psychiatry at the Roy J. and Lucille A. Carver College of Medicine at the University of Iowa. He served as a member of the DSM-III-R Advisory Committee for Personality Disorders, the DSM-IV Personality Disorders Work Group, and the DSM-IV-TR Personality Disorders Text Revision Work Group. He has published extensively in the area of personality disorders and has developed several instruments for personality disorder research including the Structure Interview for DSM Personality Disorders (SIDP-IV) and Iowa Personality Disorder Screen (IPDS). Dr. Pfohl is on the editorial board of the Journal of Personality Disorders. He is one of the authors of the STEPPS treatment program for borderline personality disorder. Dr. Pfohl received his medical degree from The University of Iowa and completed the psychiatry residency program and an National Institute of Mental Health–sponsored psychiatric epidemiology fellowship program at The University of Iowa College of Medicine. He has a master's degree in Preventive Medicine from the University of Iowa.

VIVIAN, A 53-YEAR-OLD divorced female, was referred to me (N.B.). for psychotherapy after she was discharged from the inpatient unit in which she was hospitalized for expressing suicidality during a medical evaluation in another hospital department.

HISTORY

Although this was her first hospitalization in our facility, Vivian had a long history of psychiatric treatment that included more than 25 inpatient hospitalizations, the first occurring when she was age 17. Over the years, she had received numerous diagnoses that included attention-deficit/hyperactivity disorder, bipolar I and II disorders (at different times), and alcohol dependence and abuse. Despite multiple examples of behavior patterns over a long period of time that met more than the required number of criteria for borderline personality disorder, her treatment records from outside settings and her self-report made no mention of this diagnosis except for a notation of "borderline traits" from the most recent hospitalization prior to entering our facility. By the patient's estimate, she had spent 3–4 months per year in the hospital, starting at age 17.

Vivian dated the onset of her problems to age 7 or 8 years, when she demonstrated difficulty with anger control, such as putting her foot through a wall and picking on other children. She was disruptive in the classroom, could not sit still, and had learning problems related to her vision and distinguishing sounds. At age 10, she was seen by a psychologist who gave her the diagnosis of attention-deficit/hyperactivity disorder. Her physician prescribed methylphenidate (Ritalin), and Vivian identified this as the origin of her belief that solutions to her problems would come from external sources (e.g., medication).

Vivian made the first of her estimated 30 suicide gestures at age 10 by overdosing on the Ritalin. Her dad was in the military and during her childhood, the family moved frequently. She believes the frequent moves fueled her feelings of abandonment that became a theme throughout her adult life. Many of her suicide attempts could be described as gestures, but she did make at least six serious attempts. One involved jumping from a highway overpass onto the pavement below, resulting in numerous fractures that continued to cause her chronic pain and difficulty walking many years later. Another was an overdose that left her in a coma for 3 months. For about 1 year at age 21, Vivian performed the self-harming behaviors of cutting herself to "feel if she was alive" and pushing her arms through glass windows.

Vivian described lifelong problems with anger control. During her first hospitalization at our facility, she had an anger outburst (triggered by not receiving a salad with dinner) that was expressed through her yelling, overturning tables in the dining area, throwing items off tables, and breaking glass. During a subsequent hospitalization, she was discharged to another facility after assaulting staff members. She was jailed twice for assaults outside the hospital; one incident occurred when someone cut in front of her at a gas pump.

Vivian began drinking alcohol at age 12 and drank daily by age 14. Her alcohol use continued into her 20s, when she was jailed for 3–4 days for public intoxication; after this, she joined Alcoholics Anonymous (AA) and remained abstinent from alcohol for the next 29 years. She gave a history of week-long binge eating every 2–3 months that began in high school. She engaged in periodic gambling episodes, sometimes spending as much as $400–$500 per day three to five times per month, which she could ill afford because her only income came from disability payments and student loans. Her gambling led to several incidents of illegal behavior including embezzlement, writing bad checks, and stealing money from a significant other.

Vivian described her relationships as stormy and unstable. She admitted to initially seeing a person as flawless and just as quickly becoming completely disillusioned with them. She would frequently end a relationship because she believed the other person was preparing to leave her. Significant losses included the death of her husband at a young age, a second marriage that ended in divorce, and the death of one of her sisters.

On average, Vivian was hospitalized for episodes of depression once or twice a year, during which she experienced low mood, oversleeping, decreased energy and appetite, loss of motivation, and increased risk for suicide attempts. Sometime in her 20s, she began to have periodic episodes characterized by racing thoughts, excessive energy, poor concentration, hypertalkativeness, increased irritability, and reckless driving. She was not usually hospitalized for these episodes. Outside of these specific episodes, she experienced intense mood swings and suicidal thoughts on a daily basis.

Vivian had had a very limited response to a variety of medications. She reported that antidepressants (bupropion, sertraline, paroxetine) improved her energy but also increased the risk of her acting on her suicidal thoughts. Mood stabilizers (valproate, carbamazepine, and lithium) seemed to temper her hypomanic episodes, but she still had daily mood swings.

DIAGNOSIS

Vivian's difficulties with stormy relationships, emotional dyscontrol, impulsivity, and sensitivity to abandonment easily met criteria for borderline personality disorder (BPD). She also had symptoms that might suggest additional diagnoses of major depressive disorder, bipolar II disorder, intermittent explosive disorder, alcohol dependence, pathological gambling, attention-deficit/hyperactivity disorder, and antisocial personality disorder. Even so, BPD was viewed as the primary diagnosis given that her symptoms met virtually all the criteria for BPD and that many symptoms of the other diagnoses are common in individuals with BPD.

Several studies suggest high lifetime rates among patients with BPD for a number of comorbid diagnoses including major depressive disorder (71%–83%), panic disorder (34%–49%), social phobia (20%–48%), posttraumatic stress disorder (46%–56%), alcohol abuse or dependence (52%–56%), other drug abuse or dependence (44%–53%), bulimia nervosa (12%–31%), and bipolar I (9%–12%) and II (8%–12%) disorders (McGlashan et al. 2000; Zanarini et al. 1998; Zimmerman and Mattia 1999).

In evaluating patients like Vivian, the clinician is often challenged to strike a balance between identifying all relevant comorbid diagnoses and allowing the focus of treatment to become fragmented by numerous diagnoses that may be better accounted for by another mental disorder. BPD represents a diagnosis that can account for an unusually diverse set of clinical symptoms. For example, although Vivian's behavior did meet sufficient criteria to diagnose intermittent explosive disorder, it is recommended in DSM-IV-TR that intermittent explosive disorder not be routinely diagnosed in individuals with BPD unless it has "specific clinical relevance, in which case both diagnoses should be made."

Another example of balancing diagnoses with the need to focus treatment would be Vivian's transitory difficulties with binge eating. A separate diagnosis of bulimia nervosa or eating disorder not otherwise specified would likely have distracted from the wider focus on Vivian's difficulties with impulsivity. Her symptoms of attention-deficit/hyperactivity disorder were not well defined or compelling. On the other hand, her episodes of major depression were sustained, distinct from her baseline level of transitory mood swings, and often resulted in hospitalization. Patients with BPD often endorse some symptoms of hypomania, but the episodes tend to be poorly defined or may be associated with the beginning of a new relationship. Vivian's hypomanic episodes were sufficiently detailed and distinct that a diagnosis of bipolar II disorder was probably justified. Likewise, alcohol dependence and pathological gambling may have been justified, at least as historical diagnoses.

TREATMENT

After being discharged from the inpatient unit, Vivian was initially referred for individual therapy and subsequently was enrolled in a 20-week Systems Training for Emotional Predictability and Problem Solving (STEPPS) course, a manual-guided outpatient group treatment program for BPD (Black et al. 2004; Blum et al. 2002). The STEPPS program emphasizes education about the symptoms of BPD and focuses on teaching patients emotional regulation and lifestyle behavioral skills (e.g., eating, sleeping, exercise, avoiding abusive behaviors).

The initial focus of individual therapy was to educate Vivian about the diagnosis of BPD, as this was the first time she had heard this diagnosis applied to her. Her response was, "This is the first diagnosis that really seems to fit." For the first time in her life, she no longer blamed her difficulties on someone or something else. She was seen for individual therapy approximately every 2 weeks to reinforce the material she was learning in the STEPPS group and to apply the skills to situations in her daily life. She credited the eating behavior skills section with helping her stop her binge eating episodes. She continued to attend AA meetings weekly and also attended a weekly gambling treatment group in her local community, although she intermittently experienced severe conflicts with one or more group members and had episodes of alternately overidealizing and devaluing the group facilitator.

During the first 3 months of her new treatment course, there were three or four occasions on which Vivian sent me an e-mail saying she was planning to commit suicide that day. Using the STEPPS protocol, the therapist responds to such a message either by telephone or e-mail with a series of questions: Where are you on your emotional intensity continuum (a 5-point scale)? Have you used your red STEPPS skills notebook? Which skill can you use to lower your intensity? On the occasions when Vivian could not name a skill, I reviewed the list of skills and asked her to select one or more to try for a specified period of time (e.g., 30–60 minutes). After using the skill, Vivian was instructed to phone or send another e-mail to report the observed change in intensity level. If needed, she was instructed to choose another skill and repeat the process. The process of emotion management was emphasized rather than her dwelling on the content of the perceived crisis. Almost always she would report a decrease in intensity after using the skill(s). On two occasions, it was necessary to resort to brief hospitalizations lasting 2–3 days.

Vivian periodically stopped taking her medications, sometimes because of financial difficulties but other times because she was angry at her physician or other treating professionals. As she progressed through the behavioral lessons in the STEPPS program, she became more consistently adherent to her medication regimen.

After Vivian completed the STEPPS program, she continued with a 1-year follow-up program called STAIRWAYS, a twice-monthly treatment group whose purpose is to reinforce group members' previously learned emotion management and lifestyle behavioral skills and to help members work on additional skills to help them move forward with their life. The frequency of Vivian's individual therapy sessions decreased to once monthly or less, but she would e-mail periodically between appointments to "check in" and share some of the new activities she was adding to her life (teaching a Sunday school class and volunteering at a women's shelter). She has been in a stable relationship for 7 years. She continues to attend AA meetings at least once a week or more and sponsors another person. She no longer attends the gambling support group, and her gambling behaviors are limited to buying one lottery ticket per week.

The duration of Vivian's hospitalizations decreased from 3–4 months a year to a total of 21 days in 5 years. She has not been hospitalized for the past 2 years. She continues to periodically experience suicidal thoughts, but she is much less emotionally reactive to them and has had no suicidal gestures for 7 years.

DISCUSSION

The American Psychiatric Association (2001) guidelines for the treatment of BPD include recommendations for both medication management and psychotherapy. The guidelines note that further research is essential to clearly define the role of medications in the management of BPD.

Results from available studies suggest that medications are only modestly effective, and medication without psychotherapy and psychoeducation is not recommended. Comorbid mental disorders (e.g., mood disorders, anxiety disorders, substance abuse disorders) should be considered when selecting possible medication and psychotherapy interventions. The guidelines suggest that antidepressants (especially the selective serotonin reuptake inhibitors), mood stabilizers, and antipsychotic medications may all have a role in treating this disorder, depending on the key target symptoms.

The literature on psychotherapeutic interventions for BPD is also very limited. The guidelines mention several forms of therapy that appear promising. The recommended therapies are generally well structured, if not guided by a manual, and are based on the recognition that these individuals often do poorly when faced with ambiguity in personal and professional relationships. Several controlled studies have shown the efficacy of dialectical behavioral therapy, a comprehensive, manual-guided, year-long outpatient program using group and individual therapy developed by Marsha Linehan (Linehan 1993a, 1993b). The patient's individual therapist coordinates treatment, provides weekly individual therapy, and remains available for emergency phone calls or visits as needed. The program adapts cognitive-behavioral principles to target a hierarchy of BPD symptoms, with an emphasis on controlling self-destructive behavior.

More time-limited forms of psychoanalytically oriented psychotherapy have also been tried. Bateman and Fonagy (1999) have published outcome data for their 18-month psychoanalytic therapy program that includes a partial hospital component with both individual and group therapy. The program is based on the exploration of presumed unconscious factors that interfere with the possibility of change and inconsistencies in the relationship patterns in patients with BPD. In a randomized trial, the treated group experienced improvement in depressive symptoms, and showed a decrease in suicidal and self-mutilating acts, reduced hospital days, and better social functioning. The treatment focuses on identity problems associated with BPD. Yeomans et al. (2002) have described a manual-guided approach that focuses on transference. (For further discussion of psychotherapy approaches for BPD, see Gunderson and Hoffman 2005.)

Vivian participated in STEPPS, the 20-week basic skills group, and STAIRWAYS, a follow-up group that meets twice monthly for 1 year. The program combines cognitive-behavioral techniques and skills training with a systems component. The latter teaches emotion management skills and behavior management skills not only to patients with BPD but also to those in their system—family members, significant others, and health care professionals. These members are referred to as the patient's reinforcement team.

It is not unusual for patients in STEPPS therapy to be simultaneously involved in other forms of therapy. As part of the systems model, patients learn to integrate various elements of their support system and identify what is and is not reasonable to expect from each element. The patient is encouraged to share appropriate sections from the manual with close friends and significant others as well as with his or her other mental health providers. This allows these individuals to better understand BPD, use the STEPPS terminology, and apply strategies taught in the program so that system members use a consistent manner. The systems component encourages the client to include peers, family, and others for reinforcement and reduces the tendency of patients to focus on one individual (e.g., their individual therapist) who runs the risk of being alternately overidealized and devalued. For clients receiving individual therapy, we ask the therapist to agree to support the STEPPS program by reviewing the workbook materials provided to the patient each week.

STEPPS (and the follow-up program, STAIRWAYS) and Vivian's individual therapy sessions all focused on several key principles:

- *Understanding and labeling the thoughts, feelings, and behaviors that define the syndrome of BPD*. The disorder is conceptualized as a deficit in the individual's internal ability to regulate emotional intensity; that is, the patient is periodically overwhelmed by intense emotional upheavals that drive him or her to seek relief, often in destructive ways. Patients and others in their system often view the term *personality disorder* as a sign that "I am a bad person," and the inclusion of the word "borderline" has led more than one patient to ask, "What border am I on?" We offer the term *emotional intensity disorder* (EID) as a more accurate description and one that patients find easier to understand and accept. Patients and their reinforcement team members are taught that BPD/EID is a chronic illness (similar to diabetes) that can be successfully managed through specific emotion management and behavioral skills. Reframing BPD as an illness moves patients (and those in their support system) away from viewing themselves as someone who is simply manipulative, seeking attention, or self-sabotaging; it also serves to reduce the intensity of transference and countertransference while still leaving the patient responsible for learning to manage the illness.
- *Recognizing and self-monitoring symptom severity.* This is accomplished through the use of the emotional intensity continuum, a worksheet with a 1–5 scale where 1 is feeling calm and relaxed and 5 is feeling out of control. Patients identify thoughts, feelings, maladaptive cognitive filters (schemas), physical sensations, urges to act, and behaviors that occur at each level of intensity. By using the continuum worksheet consistently, the individual becomes more adept at pre-

dicting the course of an emotional episode and anticipating stressful situations that may lead to destructive responses. In addition to the daily ratings, patients are asked to summarize the amount of time they spent at each level during the past week. Through this self-rating, patients often achieve a more balanced view and are surprised to see that they frequently have substantial periods of time when they are not at a 5.

- *Developing a series of strategies for dealing with emotional intensity.* The goal is to find ways of responding to anxiety, anger, depression, and self-destructive thoughts that can be accomplished independently or with a level of input that the support system can comfortably provide. Emotion management skills (distancing, communicating, challenging, distracting, and managing problems) are directed at the cognitive and emotional symptoms of the disorder. Patients also learn skills to manage eight behavioral areas (goal setting, eating, sleeping, exercise, leisure time, physical health, abuse avoidance, and interpersonal relationships) that have often broken down as the BPD syndrome interacts with the emotional intensity episodes and a social environment that becomes increasingly unempathic and unresponsive. Learning or relearning patterns of managing these functional areas helps the person with BPD keep these areas under control during episodes.
- *Training key members of the reinforcement team.* This is aided by a special education session and written guidelines as to how team members can respond more effectively when the patient is feeling out of control. The patient is encouraged to bring a reinforcement team member to any two group sessions. Support team members often demonstrate a remarkable capacity for change when provided with education and guidance.

Vivian described her previous experiences in psychotherapy as reinforcing her conviction that solutions would come from something external. In contrast, her STEPPS-based therapy focused on her simply accepting the reality of her symptoms and learning specific emotion management and behavioral skills for dealing with them. This allowed her to effect a cognitive shift that took her beyond the futility of trying to assign blame to herself, others, or past events.

Vivian was able to work on her anger control and impulsivity by using the emotion management skill of distancing, through which she recognized the increase in her emotional intensity and was able to "step back" by talking to a reinforcement team member or physically distancing herself by going to another room or taking a drive. She became more adept at using the skill of communicating to accurately convey her feelings and thoughts and then used the self-challenging skill to replace her distorted thoughts with more rational ones. She identified a number of activities (i.e., baking, needlework, and drawing) that were helpful to her in decreasing her emotional intensity, which then allowed her to better define the problem, consider a wider range of alternative responses, and thoughtfully evaluate the consequences of each response.

Vivian used the emotional intensity continuum to increase her awareness of her thoughts, feelings, urges, and behaviors that correlated with each level of severity. She could then apply her skills more effectively to decrease the time spent at levels 4 and 5, during which behaviors destructive to herself and her relationships were most likely to occur.

Using the goal-setting skill, Vivian agreed to take responsibility for her medication compliance as another key to controlling her emotional intensity. She made a chart and gave herself a sticker each time she took her medication. The physical health skills section helped her think more realistically about the role of her health care providers and medications. She observed, "I now realize that my medications are like my crutches. They help, but they are not the fix-it answer."

In our experience, it is not unusual for patients with BPD who have required frequent scheduled and unscheduled mental health interventions to improve over a period of years to the point that minimal, if any, services are needed. Vivian has not been in regular treatment for more than 2 years. Two or three times per year, she will e-mail or drop in to let us know how she is doing. During her last visit, she reported that she had not taken any medication for more than a year. She believes that she occasionally has symptoms of major depression and hypomania, but she feels that she is managing these episodes with the use of her emotion management and behavior skills.

REFERENCES

American Psychiatric Association: Practice guidelines for the treatment of patients with borderline personality disorder. Am J Psychiatry 158(suppl):2–52, 2001

Bateman A, Fonagy P: Effectiveness of partial hospitalization in the treatment of borderline personality disorder: a randomized controlled trial. Am J Psychiatry 156:1563–1569, 1999

Black DW, Blum N, Pfohl B, et al: The STEPPS group treatment program for outpatients with borderline personality disorder. Journal of Contemporary Psychotherapy 34:193–209, 2004

Blum N, Pfohl B, St. John D, et al: STEPPS: a cognitive-behavioral systems-based group treatment for outpatients with borderline personality disorder: a preliminary report. Compr Psychiatry 43:301–310, 2002

Gunderson JG, Hoffman PD: Psychotherapies for borderline personality disorder, in Understanding and Treating Borderline Personality Disorder: A Guide for Professionals and Families. Washington, DC, American Psychiatric Publishing, 2005, pp 21–41

Linehan MM: Cognitive-Behavioral Treatment of Borderline Personality Disorder. New York, Guilford, 1993a

Linehan MM: Skills Training Manual for Treating Borderline Personality Disorder. New York, Guilford, 1993b

McGlashan TH, Grilo CM, Skodol AE, et al: The Collaborative Longitudinal Personality Disorders Study: baseline Axis I/II and II/II diagnostic co-occurrence. Acta Psychiatr Scand 102:256–264, 2000

Yeomans FE, Clarkin JF, Kernberg OF: A Primer of Transference-Focused Psychotherapy for the Borderline Patient. Northvale, NJ, Jason Aronson, 2002

Zanarini MC, Frankenburg FR, Dubo ED, et al: Axis I comorbidity of borderline personality disorder. Am J Psychiatry 155:1733–1739, 1998

Zimmerman M, Mattia JI: Axis I diagnostic comorbidity and borderline personality disorder. Compr Psychiatry 40:245–252, 1999

CHAPTER 31

Shifts and Surprises

Psychodynamic Psychotherapy of a Mixed Personality Disorder

Daria Colombo, M.D.

Robert Michels, M.D.

Daria Colombo, M.D., is an Attending Psychiatrist at the NewYork-Presbyterian Hospital and is Assistant Professor in the Department of Psychiatry of Weill Medical College at Cornell University. She is currently a senior candidate at the New York Psychoanalytic Institute and an Editorial Associate at the *Journal of the American Psychoanalytic Association*. She is in private practice in New York City.

Robert Michels, M.D., is the Walsh McDermott University Professor of Medicine and Psychiatry at Weill Medical College of Cornell University and a Training and Supervising Analyst at the Center for Psychoanalytic Training and Research, Columbia University College of Physicians and Surgeons. Dr. Michels is the former Dean and Provost of Cornell University Medical College, where he served as Chairman of the Department of Psychiatry. He has published more than 250 scientific articles, is or has been on the editorial boards of the *Journal of the American Psychoanalytic Association,* the *International Journal of Psychoanalysis,* the *Psychoanalytic Quarterly,* and the *New England Journal of Medicine*. He is Deputy Editor of the *American Journal of Psychiatry*.

GLORIA, A 21-YEAR-OLD single woman, was referred to me (D.C.) by a psychiatrist who had been treating her for 2 years but had since moved from the city. She had been seeing the original psychiatrist for weekly supportive psychotherapy as well as for pharmacotherapy.

The referring psychiatrist described Gloria as having only a limited response to treatment for a moderate depression and noted that she was difficult to treat. Although she appeared to have made some improvement with psychotherapy and medication (fluoxetine, an antidepressant), it was a modest one; her mood was now bland as opposed to sad and her neurovegetative symptoms (insomnia, loss of appetite) were resolved, but she did not have any greater engagement with the outside world. Gloria spent most of her time alone, surfing the Internet, reading music magazines, playing with her dog, and occasionally seeing one of the few friends she had kept from school. She had dropped out of high school in the middle of her senior year and had no plan to return to school, no desire to work, and no financial need to do so. The referring psychiatrist had considered whether Gloria might have prodromal schizophrenia, given the paucity of her current relationships, her poor functioning, her consistently withdrawn and distant manner during sessions, and her often vague, tangential thinking. I started treatment with the impression that she would need supportive psychotherapy and ongoing pharmacotherapy and that my goals for this young woman might be circumscribed ones.

HISTORY

Gloria's history was marked by an early refusal to attend school, beginning in the third grade. Shortly before that, when Gloria was age 8, her mother died after an operation related to metastatic breast cancer and a postoperative course complicated by a medical error. Initially Gloria recalled little of this time and had few memories of her mother. She did remember having increasing difficulty at school and being bullied by other girls. After attending a public school in a gifted academic track, she transferred to a small private school for junior high school. She noted that she had never been part of a crowd but always had one or two close friends. She mentioned that she would slowly make friends and become attached to them, but that they would then switch schools or move out of the city. She was in touch with only one of these friends now.

Gloria's first contact with a therapist was when she was in eighth grade. Along with a continuing intermittent refusal to attend school, she had developed a phobia about riding on buses and subways by herself and needed to be accompanied by her father. She saw a behavioral therapist for her phobia, which she said subsequently resolved. She also was evaluated for attention-deficit/hyperactivity disorder because there was a feeling that her school performance did not match her level of intelligence, but she said that no specific diagnosis was made. She recalled being very messy as a child and avoided cleaning up because she would be too obsessive to get much done; for example, she would repack her pencil case and book bag repeatedly while ignoring larger projects. Although she did not recall ever feeling happy, she believed that she first became depressed at around age 16. She remembered feeling sad and withdrawn, taking no pleasure or interest in anything, and having trouble sleeping, poor appetite, fatigue, and ruminative, self-denigrating thoughts. She was never suicidal but recalled feeling hopeless. She had trouble with concentration and fell increasingly behind in school. She gradually stopped attending most of her classes during her senior year in high school and did not take part in any activities related to applying to colleges. She was brought to a child psychiatrist for a consultation but at that time refused treatment; her father apparently did not insist that she pursue treatment. She spent the next 2 years being isolated and inactive, filling her time with television, reading, and music and with few social contacts beyond her immediate family. Only at age 19 did she agree to try treatment, and she saw her previous psychiatrist from that age until coming to me.

Gloria denied any psychotic symptoms or manic or hypomanic episodes. She denied any drug or alcohol use, apart from having tried marijuana twice while in high school. She had never had a romantic relationship or sexual contact. She had no plans for further education and had never worked. She was supported by a large settlement the family received after her mother's death.

DIAGNOSIS

My working diagnosis for Gloria was as follows:

Axis I: Major depressive disorder, in partial remission, versus major depressive disorder and dysthymia (double depression)

Axis II: Features of obsessive-compulsive personality disorder and avoidant personality disorder; possible schizoid personality disorder

Axis III: No medical problems

Axis IV: Poor social and occupational functioning, but no evidence of an inability to care for her basic needs, no suicidality, and intact reality testing

Axis V: 60

TREATMENT

My treatment prescription when I first started with Gloria was that we would meet once a week and that I would continue her medication while I made a fuller assessment of her pathology and what the appropriate psychotherapeutic and pharmacological interventions might be. She agreed rather passively and gave me the impression that she was being transferred, like a child, from one set of arms into another.

At our first meeting, Gloria in fact looked several years younger than her age. She was pale and soft spoken and, although she was childishly chubby, seemed insubstantial, an effect heightened rather than counteracted by her harshly dyed black hair, her dark eyeliner, and her button-studded army fatigue jacket. She initially spoke little and had a disturbingly blank facial expression and poor eye contact. The first few sessions left me foraging among her "okays" and "fines," her shrugs and sighs, for nuggets of psychological information.

Her thinking initially appeared tangential, but by piecing together her rare comments and observations, I began to realize that she was presenting a central narrative about herself, one that would dominate her first few months in treatment. She saw herself as a detached critic of a hypocritical, hollow world. She was a connoisseur of society's foibles, and the sparse content she brought to her sessions consisted largely of trivial details of social life that she tediously and humorlessly attacked as meaningless and absurd. She felt people ignored the true worth of things while focusing on superficialities, such as degrees, looks, and charm. Her rejection of society was clearly defensive and preemptive, but it was difficult to imagine how she could gain any insight into this, given what appeared to be the rigidity of her defenses. There was a striking contrast between her stance as a conscientious objector and her fragile position as a profoundly dependent and powerless young girl within her family. It was also unclear to what extent her father had abdicated some responsibility toward her in not insisting on earlier and more intensive treatment and in allowing her to drop out of school and to what extent she had refused to let him help her.

In the first few months of treatment, Gloria's rigid defenses, highly intellectualized discussion of minutiae interspersed with long silences, and absent affect, rendered the sessions excruciatingly boring. I was fairly active in this phase of treatment, trying to foster some sort of therapeutic alliance, learn more about her inner world, and clarify her diagnosis. It seemed that she did not have a major depressive disorder, which she appeared to have had in the past, but did currently have dysthymia. I decided to continue the fluoxetine, which Gloria had been tolerating well with no side effects. This medication, at the same dosage of 60 mg/day, continued throughout the treatment course.

I began to reconceptualize Gloria's blandness and negativity as a dynamic strategy unconsciously chosen to manage her severe loss and disappointment and thought of her as having a predominantly obsessional character, relying on isolation of affect and reaction formation—in the form of her extreme passivity—to control her rage. This hypothesis was bolstered by her unexpected responsiveness to some simple trial interpretations. Initially she was frequently late to sessions and occasionally missed them. I pointed out how little emotion she showed and asked her if she thought part of her wanted to avoid coming to sessions to avoid speaking about her feelings. She responded with associations about school, being compelled to do things she did not want to do, how avoidance felt like the only power she had. She also described her extreme anxiety about leaving her home and how she was often late for appointments because of her obsessive ordering. After this exchange, she began to come to our sessions more consistently. She reacted to some tentative interpretations about loss with associations and new information. It turned out she had finally agreed to treatment when her best friend became involved with a boyfriend, which had been a huge blow. Without being asked, she began to bring in dreams. Her thinking appeared less tangential and, most notably, she began to be curious about her own psychological functioning.

After Gloria reported one dream in which she had visited her now abandoned childhood playground, I asked her about memories of her mother. She said she never thought about her childhood. She then had a severe coughing fit, which troubled her for the rest of the session and impeded her from saying much. In the next session, she spontaneously associated her coughing to the asthma which she had had as a child and wondered if she had experienced this in the previous session to "choke my words off." She began to relate fragments from her childhood of which she had only recently become aware—a red mitten knit by her mother lost in a park, a game they had played—in a vivid, impressionistic manner. Although her face remained largely unexpressive, her words became more lively and her tone less monotonous. In response to my comments about how she had sustained important losses, she said she had never thought of it that way and that "for some reason" she had largely avoided thinking about her mother and her death. She began to acknowledge feeling sad at times, and her negativity became increasingly connected to an awareness of feeling angry. She thought adulthood was "full of dumb rules." She felt empty, as she had trouble identifying anything she wanted for herself and resented her family's expectations for her—that she should attend college, be more productive or, in her words, "whatever." I began to see her as having become a ghost in an identification with her dead mother and perhaps as an expiation of her guilt about her mother's death. Gloria was refusing to participate in the world and rejected the internal and external tasks of growing up, as well as, of course, the potential rewards.

As our work continued, I noticed that Gloria spent her sessions denigrating the establishment while glancing at my degrees; presenting theories about why words were useless while continuing, if haltingly, to talk to me; and discussing her rejection of everyone while being interested in and deferential toward me. I wondered to myself about the difference from her reaction to her previous therapist. I learned that it was actually not so different; she had felt extremely connected with the therapist, but the treatment framework had been different. Her previous psychiatrist, who worked in an inpatient setting, would schedule her from week to week and often had patient emergencies that would lead to cancelled sessions. Gloria was responding, in part, to my consistency and presence.

I gradually became aware of a growing transference-countertransference enactment. Despite the sessions that she would still fill with minutiae and intellectual detours, I felt less bored and instead increasingly protective of her, as if she were a stubborn girl turning her back to the world while her chin quivered with tears. Finally, she had found an adult whom she experienced as unlike those others, one who could understand and help her. I understood that my continuing in a supportive mode would be a transference-countertransference enactment in which her masked dependency and vulnerability would be gratified rather than explored and understood. It would mean enacting a scenario to allow Gloria to feel that she had finally found a good object. Although it might have been satisfying for both of us, it would have limited what I increasingly saw as her potential. It would also mean not addressing the destructive, angry fantasies that I suspected lurked beneath her passive exterior. An external event facilitated this exploration.

After 4 months of treatment, I informed Gloria that in 3 months I would be going on maternity leave. She was shocked and disorganized, said her thoughts were jumbled, and retreated to very sparse communication for a few sessions. She then spoke more about her mother's death. She recalled not being sad when her mother died, being impatient to get out and play during the funeral, and feeling very guilty about that. I pointed out that mothers were not supposed to die and asked whether she thought this was part of her protest against society and convention?

She said this was possible. She described fantasies about avenging, murderous women and was curious about how these thoughts coexisted with what she saw as her extreme passivity. She also described how her teachers had all let her down and wondered if she did not want to learn things without her mother being the one to teach her.

As these issues were coming up before my leave, Gloria came in one day and said that she felt that for a long time there had been a "crust" over her feelings of sadness and anger and that she was worried this containment was in danger. She was able to say that she was anxious and angry about my leaving, that I had agreed to see her knowing I was pregnant, and that she saw this as another betrayal and another loss. She also shared the fantasy that when I returned she "would have fixed everything." She said, "I would have a boyfriend and a job....I would do it all by myself." Gloria was able to acknowledge longings and wants. I was struck by how strong an attachment she had formed to me and by her responsiveness to an increasingly exploratory approach. The interruption forced by my maternity leave actually laid bare the intensity of her attachment to me and forced me to address a countertransference in which I saw myself as protecting and caring for her. Instead of replacing and resurrecting her dead mother, I reiterated her experience of abandonment. The resonance of my leave led to exploration and insight rather than only a soothing repair and was more fruitful for the treatment than an uninterrupted course would have been.

Soon after my return, I proposed to Gloria that we increase the frequency of our meetings to regularly scheduled sessions twice a week and at a fixed time. When we had been meeting once a week, she had wanted to set the time for the next meeting at each session. She was increasingly open to thinking about the meanings behind this, primarily that I would always be available to her and have no other patients. Shortly after my return, she agreed to twice-weekly meetings at a set time. She was eager to meet more often and noted herself that "we could get deeper into things" and that often, after a session, she felt that many thoughts had been stirred up. Even as she started to see me more often, she described a fantasy of being self-sufficient, "a hermit." She accepted that this was in reaction to feeling increasingly tied to me. She became more vivid in sessions, humorous at times, angry and tearful at others. She noticed that she was "less numb" but was worried about how sad she would become.

Gloria also began for the first time to present material about her sexual life. She described being in love with a boy all throughout high school and remembered how humiliating it had felt to see him pick girls "who weren't as good as I am." She spoke about her insecurity about her own body and whether it was feminine enough. This led to associations about her father. She was very close to him growing up and accused him of making her "too masculine." She was furious when, in her mid-teens, her father remarried "a skinny woman who stinks of perfume and wears all this makeup." She added, "If that's the kind of woman he wanted, he shouldn't have made me such a boy." She also felt he had betrayed her mother by picking for his second wife a woman she felt was so different from the earthy, practical, plumpish mother with whom Gloria identified. She said her father alternated between being gruff and supportive ("Oh, I just know you'll get on the right track, kid") and losing his temper and yelling at her about ruining her life. Gloria's blandness was in part a reaction to her father's temper.

Gloria described strong feelings about my returning to work after having a baby; she was worried I would not be able to take care of her and the baby at the same time, that the baby would be neglected, and that women did not take their maternal role seriously enough. She noted how different it was to come to twice-weekly sessions and was aware of feeling more dependent on me. She began to develop a classic transference neurosis, in which her increasing acute awareness of her dependence on me led her to reexperiencing feelings from childhood, longings and rages she had long suppressed. She became increasingly aware of thoughts about sessions after leaving and in between sessions and often arrived discussing something that had come up at our last meeting. She had a fantasy that my office was filled with music and that I would turn the concert off before she came in, shutting her out of my own vibrant life. Her own life became less restricted as she shifted from total passive withdrawal to more active engagement; she took a part-time job, reconnected with old friends, and began to consider obtaining a General Education Developement (GED) degree and going to college. She was increasingly psychologically minded and was aware of her strong reactions to interruptions and absences.

DISCUSSION

Ultimately, this patient who had begun in a supportive treatment with the specter of prodromal schizophrenia hanging over her, did well in dynamic , exploratory treatment. Her case illustrates the importance of shifting treatment paradigms in light of growing clinical information about diagnosis, character structure, and patient response to various therapeutic modes. I could not have anticipated the sort of treatment that would have most benefited Gloria when we first met nor the ways in which she would be able to engage in an intensive, dynamic therapy. One of the joys of our profession is how wonderfully wrong we can sometimes be about our initial impressions and how the treatment course is in itself a diagnostic instrument. I often wonder whether, if I had seen Gloria in a more extended consultation, what I might have concluded and whether every consultation should better be thought of as a speculation in which, when there is any doubt, multiple roads—diagnostically, dynamically, and therapeutically—should be kept open.

SUGGESTED READING

Colombo D, Abend S: Psychoanalysis: the early years, in The American Psychiatric Publishing Textbook of Psychoanalysis. Edited by Person ES, Cooper AM, Gabbard GO. Washington, DC, American Psychiatric Publishing, 2005, pp 375–385

Michels R: Psychodynamic psychotherapy in modern psychiatry. Journal of Practical Psychiatry and Behavioral Health 3:95–98, 1997

Michels R: Psychotherapeutic approaches to the treatment of anxiety and depressive disorders. J Clin Psychiatry 58 (suppl 13):30–32, 1997

Michels R: Psychoanalysts' theories, in Psychoanalysis on the Move: The Work of Joseph Sandler. Edited by Fonagy P, Cooper AM, Wallerstein R. New York, Routledge, 1999, pp 187–200

Michels R: Psychoanalysis in practice, in Contemporary Psychiatry, Vol 1: Foundations of Psychiatry. Edited by Henn F, Sartorius N, Helmchen H, et al. Berlin, Springer-Verlag, 2000, pp 371–381

Michels R, Abensour L, Eizirik C, et al. (eds): Key Papers on Countertransference. London, Karnac, 2002

CHAPTER 32

The Serial Killer Who Ticked

A Diagnostic Debate in Criminal Court

Park Dietz, M.D., M.P.H., Ph.D.

Park Dietz, M.D., M.P.H., Ph.D., is Clinical Professor of Psychiatry and Biobehavioral Sciences at the David Geffen School of Medicine at the University of California, Los Angeles. He is also President of Park Dietz and Associates, Inc., and the Threat Assessment Group, Inc., in Newport Beach, California. He received his undergraduate education at Cornell University and received his M.D., M.P.H., and Ph.D. in sociology from Johns Hopkins University. He completed his residency in psychiatry at Johns Hopkins Hospital and the Hospital of the University of Pennsylvania, where he also completed a fellowship in forensic psychiatry. He specializes in forensic psychiatry, workplace violence prevention, and the protection of public figures and their families. He has consulted or testified in criminal and civil litigation in all 50 states, working on such notable cases as those involving John Hinckley, Jeffrey Dahmer, the Menendez brothers, Theodore Kaczynski, the D.C. snipers, and hundreds of civil suits alleging sexual abuse by clergy. His primary research interests are sexual sadism, threats, stalking, and kidnapping. Dr. Dietz is a consultant to the FBI, the U.S. Department of Justice, and over 100 Fortune 1,000 companies. He is a Past President of the American Academy of Psychiatry and the Law, a Distinguished Fellow of the American Psychiatric Association, and a Fellow of the American Academy of Forensic Sciences.

LUIS, A 40-YEAR-OLD, Hispanic male who confessed to eight homicides committed over a 10-year span, sparked a diagnostic controversy. A therapist who had seen him for more than 100 sessions before his arrest—primarily for his dissatisfaction with his career as a security guard, social isolation, and risky practice of unprotected sex with prostitutes—had diagnosed him with dysthymia and avoidant personality disorder. Luis was charged in multiple jurisdictions for each of the eight homicides, and the first to come to trial was his seventh known homicide. In preparing for that trial, Luis's lawyers pursued a defense of not guilty by reason of insanity. Psychiatrists and psychologists retained by the defense diagnosed him as having paranoid schizophrenia, bipolar disorder, left hemisphere brain damage, and posttraumatic stress disorder. They claimed that at the time of the homicide, Luis was psychotic, had a mental disease, and could not appreciate the criminality of his conduct.

As a forensic psychiatrist working for the prosecution, I examined Luis to evaluate his criminal responsibility at the time of the crime. The forensic psychiatric evaluation of criminal responsibility is not focused on specific diagnoses but on the presence or absence of such legal constructs as "mental disease or defect" or "severe mental illness" and on particular functional impairments such as "not knowing the wrongfulness of his conduct" or "lacking substantial capacity to appreciate the criminality of his conduct" at the time of an offense. Even though a precise diagnosis is not always necessary in this context, it often helps inform the legally relevant determinations. The most important diagnostic issue to consider is usually whether a defendant was psychotic at the time of the charged offense, as psychosis is the medical concept that most closely approximates what the law calls "mental disease" or "severe mental illness." Often these terms are undefined by the law, leading to disagreements among experts in those cases that come to trial claiming a defense of insanity.

The functional assessment of a person's knowledge of wrongfulness or capacity to appreciate criminality is based on all sources of information; in this case, the evidence included statements by Luis and witnesses as well as autopsy and physical evidence that showed what Luis thought and did before, during, and after the offense. Defendants who are determined to have been psychotic at the time of the offense and thereby meet the threshold test of mental disease or severe mental illness may or may not have known their conduct was wrong or appreciated its criminality. These elements are evaluated by analyzing whether the defendant took steps to act secretly, avoid detection or identification, and conceal evidence and by examining the defendant's statements to determine whether he or she believed what he or she was doing was illegal or legal, immoral or moral, and blameworthy or praiseworthy.

HISTORY

Luis carried a heavy burden of resentment stemming from his parents' focus on his brother, molestation by his sister, being teased and bullied by peers, being disappointed with his military service, acquiring venereal diseases from prostitutes, being fired by a woman, and financial floundering that left him living with his parents. When asked questions designed to elicit whether he had more negative sentiments toward women than men, he was able to identify people of both sexes toward whom he felt negatively but no woman toward whom he felt particularly positively. These life experiences probably contributed to the shaping of his personality and to his level of anger.

Often, persons charged with heinous offenses have had horrible childhoods that elicit the empathy of the examiner, just as the suffering of the victims elicits empathy for their plight. In the role of forensic examiner, however, the evaluator must recognize and put aside these feelings in an effort to remain as objective as possible. This is one of the challenges of forensic psychiatry. The evaluator's empathy for victims or offenders is often a useful tool in asking the right questions and eliciting information but must not be allowed to influence his or her opinion on the legally relevant questions, which should be based solely on the objective evidence.

DIAGNOSIS

During my examination of Luis, which covered all of the homicides to which he had confessed, he used the passive voice to describe his crimes, claimed to be "hazy" or not remember parts of crimes, and sought to portray some of his victims as the aggressors. Such statements all seemed designed to reduce his apparent blameworthiness for the brutal rapes and homicides of which he was accused. Although he was willing to confess to murder and sex with prostitutes, Luis was understandably reluctant to reveal perverse activities or the true reasons for the murders.

Luis made references to hearing voices or noises, being guided by some force, and experiencing out-of-body experiences, memory lapses, and other seemingly strange and unusual events, but these claims were made inconsistently and did not fit known patterns of psychotic illness. When questioned in any detail about his possible psychotic symptoms, Luis described subjective experiences within the normal range and gave no plausible example of a true psychotic symptom.

Luis frequently used the plural pronoun ("we") or the third person pronoun ("he") when describing his criminal actions. His references to other parties was interpreted by defense experts as evidence of dissociation at the time, but I thought they could reflect a problem in language processing or an effort to feign insanity. This issue was clarified I asked Luis why he used pronouns this way and he explained that changing pronouns made it easier for him to talk about what he had done.

Luis was of normal intelligence despite having academic weaknesses consistent with learning disability. Claims of brain damage were without objective support. There was no documented history of head trauma sufficiently severe to suggest a likelihood of relevant functional impairment, and the objective tests (magnetic resonance imaging, electroencephalogram, single-photon emission computed tomography [SPECT], and neuropsychological testing) were within normal limits.

The claim of posttraumatic stress disorder could not be corroborated, as he had only nonspecific symptoms such as difficulty sleeping and outbursts of anger. Objective psychological testing (MMPI-II) indicated malingering, exaggeration, and personality disorder—all of which were consistent with my findings. Based on my evaluation and the psychological testing, I concluded that at the time of the charged homicide Luis did not have any mental disease or defect, although he did give evidence of several other less severe mental disorders.

Tourette's Disorder

The most striking feature of the mental status examination was Luis's frequent tics. He had a history beginning in childhood of simple motor tics (including blinking, grimacing, and other facial tics) and verbal tics (most noticeably sniffing). He had experienced a compulsion for symmetrical movements and a checking compulsion, but these were not sufficiently severe to warrant an additional diagnosis of obsessive-compulsive disorder. He also had a history of hyperactivity (fidgeting, squirming, and talking excessively), distractibility, and impulsivity, but without a well-documented history of attention-deficit/hyperactivity disorder. His tics had played a part in socially isolating him, as he had been the target of mean-spirited teasing by peers as a boy and had often been rejected by women.

Personality Disorder

Lacking reliable information about whether he had the onset of a conduct disorder in childhood, I made a preliminary diagnosis of personality disorder not otherwise specified with antisocial and schizotypal traits, including

- Failure to conform to social norms with respect to lawful behaviors
- Deceitfulness
- Impulsivity
- Irritability and aggressiveness
- Reckless disregard for safety of self and others
- Lack of remorse
- Unusual perceptual experiences
- Odd thinking and speech
- Lack of close friends or confidants
- Excessive social anxiety

Sexual Sadism

Although Luis sought to minimize his sexual deviance and refused to discuss his sexual fantasies, he had carried handcuffs, binding materials, guns, and knives at the time of several of his crimes, and many of his homicide victims showed excessive wounding suggestive of a sadistic motive. Most telling, two of the crimes he committed against surviving victims provided evidence of sexual sadism.

In the kidnapping and rape of his first victim, who survived, Luis had called her "bitch"; held a knife to her throat; pushed her head into the dashboard; bound her hands behind her back; pulled her by the hair to force fellatio; cut off her shorts, underwear, and bra; gagged her with her underwear and bra; called her "a bitch, a whore, a slut" as he raped her vaginally; scripted her language (telling her to say she loved him); hit her; strangled her to the point of unconsciousness; and bit her neck, drawing blood.

In a sexual encounter with a prostitute five years later, he requested that she accompany him to an isolated area (where he had killed several of his victims) and allow him to handcuff her, secure her with duct tape, tie her up, and have sex with her in the back of his truck.

DISCUSSION

The physical evidence and autopsy proved that the victim of the homicide for which Luis was first brought to trial was badly beaten (with three broken teeth and hundreds of abrasions and contusions to the face, chin, shoulders, neck, chest, arms, legs, and hands), strangled (with fracture of the hyoid bone and hemorrhage around the larynx), bound and kidnapped, stripped naked, shot in the head, stabbed seven times, and dumped at a location remote from the point of abduction. These elements of the crime were entirely consistent with the defendant's personality disorder and sexual sadism.

The test of insanity that was applicable for this trail was that "[a] person is not criminally responsible for conduct if at the time of such conduct, as a result of mental disease or mental defect, he lacks substantial capacity to appreciate the criminality of his conduct." However, Luis had engaged in behaviors that demonstrated a capacity to appreciate the criminality of his conduct: binding and gagging his victim, transporting her to a remote location, killing her after a substantial opportunity to reflect upon his prior assault and kidnapping, disposing of physical evidence, and remaining silent about these crimes until confronted with ballistic evidence.

Luis was convicted and faces trial for murders in other jurisdictions.

CHAPTER 33

Abused Survivor

Psychodynamic Psychotherapy With a Borderline Personality Disorder Patient

Michael H. Stone, M.D.

Michael H. Stone, Ph.D., is Professor of Clinical Psychiatry at the Columbia University College of Physicians and Surgeons and Attending Psychiatrist in Forensics at MidHudson Psychiatric Center. He also serves as a consultant to the Personality Disorder Institute at New York Hospital/Westchester, directed by Dr. Otto Kernberg. He completed his psychoanalytic training at the Columbia Psychoanalytic Institute.

Dr. Stone has been involved in the study of personality disorders, particularly borderline personality disorder, for the past 40 years. In recent years he has also worked in forensic psychiatric hospitals. He has done long-term follow-up research on borderline and related disorders in patients who were admitted to the New York State Psychiatric Institute in the 1960s and 1970s and on forensic patients who were at the MidHudson Forensic Hospital in the 1980s. His 10 books and 200 articles have focused on borderline and other personality disorders, although some of his writing is devoted to the history of psychiatry, aided by his large collection of antiquarian books in psychology and psychiatry. He has lectured widely on the diagnosis, treatment, and outcome of borderline patients and in recent years has also lectured on forensic topics such as serial sexual homicide, sadistic personality, psychopathy, and infanticide. Currently he is involved in a long-term follow-up project in which he is contacting former patients of the New York State Psychiatric Institute from 40 years ago.

WENDY, A 20-YEAR-OLD college student, was referred to me by a colleague because of an eating disorder that was not responding to the treatment program offered her at the clinic she had been attending. What impressed me the most during the initial consultation was that the eating disorder, bulimia nervosa, appeared to be merely the tip of a very deep iceberg of disabling symptoms and behaviors.

Wendy's overall condition met most of the criteria for borderline personality disorder (BPD) as defined in DSM-IV-TR. She was in a close relationship with a boyfriend at the time but was desperate over the prospect that he might leave her, as she had almost no other friends and was dependent on him financially as well as emotionally. Their relationship was stormy, characterized by frequent arguments and "scenes" (in which she would break pottery or hurl food to the floor). After Wendy would binge eat, an almost daily occurrence, she would induce regurgitation to preserve what she perceived as a normal weight. This binge eating/regurgitating pattern was a habit that had begun shortly after her menarche at age 13 years. Occasionally she would take appetite suppressants, hoping to reduce the urge to binge, but they had no benefit. Wendy had struggled for several years with bouts of depression, capped at times with suicidal feelings, and had cut her wrists (albeit not deeply) two or three times in the preceding year. She had begun engaging in self-mutilative acts by age 10 when she was living in Hong Kong: she would scratch herself with pieces of glass or else cut her arms as a means to relieve unbearable tension or curb rage that threatened to get out of control. She did not, however, abuse substances or engage in promiscuity. Once I began treating her in earnest, other facets of BPD became apparent, such as her marked lability of mood; she would shift rapidly from one strong emotion to another, becoming tearful or cheerful, rageful or sweet, by turns. She was at times consumed by her anger, particularly whenever she would recount painful episodes from the past. Her habit of tuning out and staring into space sometimes became activated at such moments. These dissociative reactions were usually of short duration.

So many patients with borderline pathology have experienced trauma of one sort or another in their early years that some clinicians regard BPD as a mere variant of posttraumatic stress disorder, an approach that, in my opinion, is mistaken. Still, the traumas experienced by this young woman were of a severity and chronicity that surpassed the levels I had encountered in the dozens patients with BPD that I have worked with over the past four decades. As a seasoned clinician who has recently practiced forensic psychiatry in addition to my ordinary practice, I have become inured to horror stories about what certain patients have suffered or about the suffering they have caused others. But the story of this woman is the only one where I myself become tearful at the recounting of it.

HISTORY

Both of Wendy's parents, originally from Hong Kong, were physicians who worked in America when Wendy and her older sister were quite young. When the family returned to Hong Kong, where promising work opportunities had become available for the parents, a freak electrical accident led to their house burning down. Wendy, age 5 at the time, and her sister, age 12, survived, but both parents died. The girls were then placed in the hands of a paternal uncle and aunt who had adolescent children of their own. For the next 6 years, Wendy was sexually abused by her uncle and male cousin. Both girls were effectively enslaved by the uncle and forced to do all the chores, launder the clothes, and cook the food; they were allowed but one meal a day and at that a very meager one. If Wendy snuck into the refrigerator at 2:00 A.M. in an effort to snitch a few forkfuls of rice, this "theft" would be invariably detected the next morning. For her punishment, the uncle would lead her into the backyard and command that she choose a stick with which he would then beat her. She quickly learned to pick a stick of intermediate thickness, knowing that a bigger stick would lead to serious injuries. If she chose a smaller one in the hopes of "getting off easy," the uncle, intolerant of such a ruse, would toss the little stick and himself choose a thick one.

The women in the house were no better. Wendy's aunt and female cousin took great delight in taunting Wendy with the promise of extra food, only at the last second to shove the fork into the back of her throat and then quickly remove it (with the morsel of food still on it), leading at times to Wendy's sustaining a bleeding wound in the pharynx. This sadistic treatment was meted out more to Wendy than to her sister, as the latter was older and less easily targeted. Worse still, Wendy, the prettier of the two sisters, was from the beginning an object of illicit desire by the male members of the family, an object of envy by the female members, and an object of exploitation by all the members of the adoptive family. Economic exploitation was later added, when the uncle seized an opportunity to send Wendy (who was now age 11) and her sister back to America to live with some distant relatives. As a "favor" for being allowed to return to the United States, the uncle had the girls sign over to him their inheritance from the dead parents. This they did, little understanding that in so doing they were forfeiting a very large sum of money. The family they then lived with in rural Pennsylvania did not treat them harshly but did expect a great deal of work from them around the house and in their store.

Wendy met with a series of stressful situations at ages 12 and 13, especially at school. She became the victim of prejudice as the only Chinese student in her class; she was also envied as the brightest student. In addition, she was stalked by several of her male classmates both because of her attractiveness and because she refused to date any of them. Because the new family did not limit her food intake, she began to gorge herself, as if to make up for the food she was denied while living with her uncle's family in Hong Kong. This was the beginning of the bulimia symptoms.

Thanks to her high grades, Wendy was able to obtain a scholarship to a university in the Bronx. In one of her classes she met her boyfriend. The relationship that evolved became turbulent from the beginning. She grew dependent on him but at the same time was mistrustful and prone to angry outbursts, triggered by any sign of inattention or forgetfulness on his part. In this context she became depressed and agoraphobic. She was also subject to panic attacks, but these could occur within as well as outside her apartment. The agoraphobia itself was related primarily to a dread of being out in the world among people, whom she viewed as poised to regard her with hostility as some sort of outcast (as she had come to see herself when living with her uncle). As a result, she withdrew from some classes and took a lighter load of courses for the next semester. It was after she engaged in several self-mutilative acts, consisting of cutting herself in several parts of her body (arms, legs, abdomen), that she was referred to me for treatment by a psychiatrist at the emergency department of a hospital near her university.

TREATMENT

Psychotherapy in the beginning consisted of three sessions a week. My initial goals were to alleviate Wendy's symptoms as much as possible: her depression, eating disorder, agoraphobia, panic attacks, and self-cutting, all of which combined to interfere significantly with her academic pursuits and also with the preservation of the relationship with her boyfriend, on whom she was realistically (and in the absence of any family support) so dependent. I also sought to establish a positive relationship of a sort that would help her overcome, or at least minimize, her profound distrust of others. Helping her to contain her rage was another goal—teaching her not to bottle it up but rather to channel it within our sessions by talking about the true sources of her anger so that she would be less disposed to take it out on her boyfriend for the minor lapses and faults to which she overreacted. At the same time, I avoided plunging her too quickly into sharing with me all the details of the early abuse, as I believed this would prove overwhelming for her. Instead, I let Wendy know that by working together, she and I could handle the memories of her past abuse, but that it was important for her to go at her own pace.

The thrice-weekly frequency of our sessions was chosen based on the depth of Wendy's depression and the precariousness of her day-to-day situation. I also felt it was important to add medication to her treatment and prescribed fluoxetine (an antidepressant) 40 mg/day. To help stabilize Wendy's moods and perhaps decrease the intensity of her anger, I also added valproic acid (a mood stabilizer) 500 mg/day. Nothing seemed to control her anxiety except for clonazepam (an antianxiety medication similar in action to valium), which she used on an as-needed basis, taking 1–4 mg/day.

This regimen was maintained for the first 2½ years, at which point these medications were tapered and discontinued. The clonazepam had the most clear-cut effect in minimizing Wendy's tendency to panic. The fluoxetine correlated with, and probably contributed to, the gradual alleviation of her depression. Lamotrigine (another mood stabilizer)—the only medication she is currently taking—was substituted for the valproic acid because the latter made her feel drowsy. Wendy's bingeing episodes are now infrequent, but in the early stages of therapy, she found she could sometimes abort an episode with clonazepam. Without the pharmacotherapy, it would not have been possible to control the complex array of symptoms that dominated the initial stages of her treatment.

My approach in treating Wendy was primarily supportive throughout most of the treatment. I felt this was appropriate because for a long time her life was a string of crises that called for either her containment of overpowering affects or else intervention by college authorities who were at times dubious about letting her continue her studies. She was not at first able to take more than a few courses at a time. Although she would earn A's in the courses she was able to complete, there were others from which she had to withdraw because of multiple absences (the result of her agoraphobia). I spoke, and at various times, wrote to her professors and deans, urging them to let her continue. This proved helpful; eventually (3½ years later), as Wendy became able to work more consistently and continued to maintain an A average, she was given an additional scholarship.

I consider the therapy to have been largely supportive because I relied on such interventions as giving advice, exhorting and encouraging Wendy, offering her sympathy and the opportunity to ventilate (through which she would express her intense feelings and painful memories), interceding on her behalf with school authorities, and arranging joint meetings with her and her boyfriend. The latter allowed me to make my own assessment of the boyfriend's personality and his overall attitude toward Wendy. He was a decent person who cared for her deeply. Guided by this impression, I could then convince her to adopt a more accepting and forgiving attitude toward him, which then strengthened this important relationship.

As Wendy's symptoms gradually grew less intense, I was able to shift into an approach where insight and support were combined, in what is sometimes called an analytically informed supportive therapy (as described by Rockland [1989] and Winston et al. [2004]). My main objective at this point (now the second year of treatment) was to enable Wendy to distinguish between those individuals who were apt to be hurtful or at best exploitative (pretty much the whole human race, from which she felt so alienated in the beginning) and those who were trustworthy and genuinely caring. The work we had done in the first year, including the joint meetings with her boyfriend, solidified her relationship with her boyfriend, and through his continuing emotional and economic help she was able to get through this difficult period, even though she could barely attend classes. She was eventually given additional scholarship funds, which made her feel more secure.

In the early months of therapy, there were many sessions in which Wendy exploded with rage as she recounted her memories of the years she had spent in Hong Kong. Here was a young woman—extremely respectful, humble, and polite toward me—who was so consumed with murderous impulses toward the adoptive family that I felt she might have acted on them had there not been 10,000 miles between them. As it happened, these outbursts served as *abreactions*—the psychic equivalents of lancing a boil—after which she grew calmer. I found myself unable to say much about her murderous feelings at first, because her feelings as a victim of sustained torture (there is no other word for it) were understandable and even expected. Once she became calmer (partly through the medications mentioned above), however, I shared with her my own sentiments, namely that although murderous rage was part of the "normal" reaction to what she had suffered, exacting revenge in the form of murder would afford her several days of joyful relief, but her grim view of the world would not be ameliorated. I emphasized that she would continue to see the world as a totally dangerous place, anticipate malice and maltreatment from everyone, and remain blind to the goodness of at least some people who might genuinely love her and want to take care of her.

As she began to grasp this point, I felt she was ready to hear some interpretive remarks I had to offer relating to her boyfriend. By now I had already met with the two of them together on several occasions. What made her particularly angry toward him was his unemotional demeanor and lack of demonstrativeness. This may have reflected a cultural factor, as he was of Japanese descent and was not used to open expression of feelings. I initially explained that because of all she had been through, Wendy held him to impossibly high standards of perfection as a friend and a lover; the reason for this was that because she was so used to being taken advantage of or neglected, she was hypersensitive to the tiniest signs of negativity. This led her to misinterpret others' actions and overreact in many quite ordinary situations. Second, it seemed to me that a more emotionally responsive and reactive man who was exposed to her roller-coaster of extreme moods would have tired of the relationship early on and left her. Thus her boyfriend's "faults" were what allowed the bond between them to remain unbroken. Of course it would not have been appropriate for me to address Wendy's contributions to the shortcomings of their relationship until she was comfortable enough and trusting enough with me to understand that I was saying these things to benefit her and not to scold her.

About 6 months into my work with her, there was a time when two stressful situations coincided: a more bitter than usual fight with her boyfriend and my preparing to travel to Europe for a week. The day before I left, she cut her arms fairly deeply with a razor and showed up at my office with blood on her dress. I put sterile dressings on the wounds and called her boyfriend to come and take her to a local emergency department. The doctors there insisted on hospitalizing her for a few days' observation. She was opposed to the idea; however, after I had a chance to speak with the psychiatrist on call, I urged her to stay as they had recommended. I gave her my phone numbers in Europe, as I always do for patients about whom I have worries, and we spoke each of the 4 days she remained at the hospital.

Between the first and second years of therapy, there were improvements on some fronts, worsening on others. She and her boyfriend had a falling out, after which they lived separately, although they remained in touch with one another. Now more alone than ever, Wendy became intensely agoraphobic and had to take a leave of absence from college. She still received financial help from her former boyfriend and the university. Her one consolation was a kitten someone had given her. She lavished considerable affection on the kitten and felt comforted by the unambivalent love she received in return, something she little expected to receive in her relationships with people. Toward the end of that year, she was able to do part-time work, using her artistic skills to do graphic design. We met less often, sometimes for two sessions a week and sometimes for only one. There were moments when Wendy felt discouraged about ever being able to graduate from college because of the unpredictable recrudescence of her symptoms. I emphasized the absolute importance, nonetheless, of her soldiering on and finishing her courses, because the diploma would greatly facilitate her obtaining a job that would allow her to support herself. This would end her dependency on the kindness of strangers, given that she was alone in the world with no family to support her. Her symptoms were beginning to subside. She never again cut herself. Whereas in the past she would feel quite desperate when alone, she was able now to read while alone without becoming unduly anxious.

In the third year of her therapy, Wendy returned to college and was again able to maintain an A average despite missing a fair number of classes because of occasional bouts of agoraphobia or depression. The relationship with her former boyfriend had changed into a simple, but solid, friendship—free of the tempestuousness that had characterized their romantic relationship.

Through the Internet, during the fourth year of treatment, Wendy was able to locate an elderly neighbor in Hong Kong who knew her parents before they had moved to America. This woman imparted some facts and recollections about the kind of people they were. Wendy herself had almost no memory of them at all, but learned that her father was a highly respected man who could be quite stern, although he also enjoyed playing with his two girls. Her mother was described as an affectionate and devoted woman, indulgent toward her daughters, for whom she always found plenty of time despite her duties as a physician. I speculated with Wendy that perhaps her parents—although they were no more than ghostlike figures, not even recognizable images, in her life—may have given her the genes and also the warm attention that allowed Wendy to develop the high moral character and goal orientedness that ultimately persisted despite her traumatic loss of her parents and the suffering to which she was subjected in the years that followed.

In the fourth year of treatment, we met only once weekly, with the psychotherapy continuing mostly along supportive lines. There were occasional allusions to the transference—or perhaps more accurately, to myself as a real person in her life. When she referred to me as a "fatherly person" or as someone who was "like a father" to her, these impressions did not hearken back to actual memories of her father because she had none. In this regard, the transference was always positive. For example, she never saw me, even briefly, in the guise of her exploitative uncle. In this respect, our relationship differed from what is considered typical in the treatment of a BPD patient. Many of these patients, for example, in the beginning of therapy, oscillate between periods of intense positive and negative feelings, with admiration and trust alternating with anger (or even hatred) and mistrust. Still others manifest a paradoxical reaction, the "negative therapeutic reaction," where helpful interventions on the part of the therapist elicit guilt and discomfort rather than relief. But these patterns are by no means universal in work with BPD patients and did not emerge in my work with Wendy.

I became, and remained, Wendy's ally and indeed at times was her only ally in a world she viewed as hostile. One might ask how, given her past, she could develop trust in anyone and how she could avoid the fate of many abused BPD patients, which is an engulfment in bitterness. My guess is that her exposure to a "good-enough" mother (in Winnicott's terms [Winnicott 1965]) and adequate parenting in general before the death of her parents formed the template allowing for the possibility of trust, even though her parents' deaths occurred before she could develop conscious memories of her (presumably) positive experiences with them. Another positive factor might have been her fairly calm innate temperament; in many BPD patients, a genetic predisposition to affective illness contributes to (and intensifies) their extreme lability of mood and tendency to depression. Once Wendy's anger and depression were dealt with in the therapy, they almost disappeared (the overt anger at her uncle was gone after 2 years; the depression, after 3 years) rather than being kept alive by genetic vulnerability, even when her life circumstances improved. Also, Wendy's attractiveness and high intelligence should not be discounted as these constitutional advantages can help pave the way to positive experiences both in work and in one's intimate life, thereby ultimately canceling the ill effects of a wretched past.

In the latter half of her therapy, Wendy was able to expand her world of allies from the miniature domain of myself and (at times) her boyfriend to include others: teachers, friends of either sex, employers, and even her sister, from whom she had been estranged for many years. Shortly before she graduated, she was able to obtain part-time work in graphic design with a publishing company. This gave her a measure of financial independence and enhanced her self-confidence and stability. She became more forgiving toward her sister (who had used some of the monies that belonged to Wendy) and was able to effect a rapprochement with her. Neither, of course, could ever forgive their uncle and his family. Wendy's relationship with her boyfriend, although cooler than it once was, is now one of a close friendship with "possibilities for a future." Wendy continues in treatment with me, although currently on a less frequent (once every few weeks) schedule; our sessions focus on sorting out Wendy's feelings about her former boyfriend and about marriage as a goal, given that she has conflicting attitudes about both.

DISCUSSION

My treatment of Wendy was similar to the way in which I treat other patients with BPD in which extreme abuse has dominated their early lives. These patients usually present with such a panoply of severe symptoms and string of life crises that a prolonged period of supportive-dynamic therapy is needed to strengthen them to the level where a more transference-focused therapy becomes possible and desirable. For some of these patients, depending on their cognitive style and life circumstances, the supportive approach will prove successful by itself, as it did with Wendy. I never had the slightest doubt as to the veracity of Wendy's story of abuse; the unique features of her story coupled with the profound affects (and at times, dissociation) that accompanied their recounting was altogether convincing. Wendy did better than most of the severely traumatized BPD patients with whom I have worked. Some have been permanently crushed by their experiences. Wendy's resilience is remarkable, but the reasons for it are mysterious. I mentioned above the probability that she had 4 years of a "good-enough" mother. There must also have been favorable innate factors—not just her intelligence and attractiveness, but whatever brain-wiring it is that lets some people withstand traumas and develop serenity in the face of cruelty and loss. Psychiatry understands mental illness better at present than it does mental health—hence the difficulty in pinpointing what allowed this woman to flourish after not too many years of therapy, whereas others struggle with their BPD with less success even after a longer time in treatment.

REFERENCES

Rockland L: Supportive Therapy: A Psychodynamic Approach. New York, Basic Books, 1989

Winnicott DW: The Maturational Process and the Facilitating Environment. New York, International University Press, 1965

Winston A, Rosenthal RN, Pinsker H: Introduction to Supportive Psychotherapy. Washington, DC, American Psychiatric Publishing, 2004

SUGGESTED READING

Bateman A, Fonagy P: Psychotherapy for Borderline Personality Disorder. Oxford, Oxford University Press, 2004
Clarkin JF, Yeomans FE, Kernberg OF: Psychotherapy for Borderline Personality. New York, Wiley, 1999
Gunderson JG: Borderline Personality Disorder: A Clinical Guide. Washington, DC, American Psychiatric Publishing, 2001
Judd PH, McGlashan TH: A Developmental Model of Borderline Personality Disorder. Washington, DC, American Psychiatric Publishing, 2003
Koenigsberg HW, Kernberg OF, Stone MH, et al: Borderline Patients: Extending the Limits of Treatability. New York, Basic Books, 2000
Stone MH: The Fate of Borderline Patients. New York, Guilford, 1990
Stone MH: Treatment of borderline patients: a pragmatic approach to psychotherapy and psychopharmacology. Psychiatr Clin North Am 13:265–285, 1990
Stone MH: Abnormalities of Personality: Within and Beyond the Realm of Treatment. New York, WW Norton, 1993
Stone MH: Determining amenability to psychotherapy in patients with borderline disorders. Psychiatr Ann 34:437–445, 2004

Index